ISCHEMIC STROKE - UPDATES

Edited by **Bernhard Schaller**

Ischemic Stroke - Updates
http://dx.doi.org/10.5772/59738
Edited by Bernhard Schaller

Contributors

Kazuo Yamagata, David Mazensky, Slavka Flesarova, Ján Lehotský, Maria Kovalska, Barbara Tothova, Anna Benova, Peter Kaplan, Bernhard Schaller, Erion Musabelliu, Ramon Rama, Julio Cesar García, Rubens Gagliardi, Vivian Gagliardi, Wen-Long Hu, Po-Yu Huang, Yu-Chiang Hung, Antonio Ibarra, Yolanda Cruz, Karla Cantu-Saldaña, John Cole, Christopher Stack, Robert Rennert, Christine Carico, J. Scott Pannell, Alexander Khalessi, Arvin Wali

Published by InTech

Janeza Trdine 9, 51000 Rijeka, Croatia

Publishing Process Manager Iva Lipovic

Technical Editor SPi Global

Cover InTech Design team

First published October, 2016

Printed in Croatia

Additional hard copies can be obtained from orders@intechopen.com

Ischemic Stroke - Updates , Edited by Bernhard Schaller

p. cm.

Print ISBN 978-953-51-2712-3
Online ISBN 978-953-51-2713-0

For EU product safety concerns:
IN TECH d.o.o., Prolaz Marije Krucifikse Kozulić 3, 51000 Rijeka, Croatia,
info@intechopen.com or visit our website at intechopen.com.

Contents

Preface VII

Section 1 Introduction 1

Chapter 1 **Ischemic Postconditioning after Stroke: Another Concept for the Trigeminocardiac Reflex? 3**
Nora Sandu and Bernhard Schaller

Section 2 Basic Science 15

Chapter 2 **Excitotoxicity and Oxidative Stress in Acute Stroke 17**
Ramon Rama and Julio César García

Chapter 3 **Cerebral Ischemia Induces Neuronal Vulnerability and Astrocytic Dysfunction in Stroke-Prone Spontaneously Hypertensive Rats 43**
Kazuo Yamagata

Chapter 4 **Importance of the Arterial Blood Supply to the Rabbit and Guinea Pig Spinal Cord in Experimental Ischemia 59**
David Mazensky and Slavka Flesarova

Section 3 Translational Science 87

Chapter 5 **Forebrain Ischemic Stroke and the Phenomenon of Ischemic Tolerance: Is Homocysteine Foe or Friend? 89**
Ján Lehotský, Maria Kovalská, Barbara Tothová, Anna Beňová, Dagmar Kalenská and Peter Kaplán

Chapter 6 **Immune System Involvement in the Degeneration, Neuroprotection, and Restoration after Stroke 107**
Yolanda Cruz, Karla A Cantú-Saldaña and Antonio Ibarra

Section 4 Clinical Science 135

Chapter 7 **Cerebrovascular Anatomy, Neuropathology, Clinics of Stroke: Endovascular Treatment, Decompressive Craniectomy 137**
Erion Musabelliu, Masahiro Oomura and Yoko Kato

Chapter 8 **Cryptogenic Stroke 181**
Rubens J. Gagliardi and Vivian D.B. Gagliardi

Chapter 9 **Updates in Mechanical Thrombectomy 189**
Robert C. Rennert, Arvin R. Wali, Christine Carico, Jeffrey Scott Pannell and Alexander A. Khalessi

Chapter 10 **Large Artery Occlusive Disease 203**
John W. Cole and Christopher A. Stack

Chapter 11 **Complementary Therapy with Traditional Chinese Medicine for Ischemic Stroke 241**
Po-Yu Huang, Yu-Chiang Hung and Wen-Long Hu

Preface

The current book gives an overview of basic science to translational and clinical sciences and shows the broad spectrum of current stroke research. In its diversity, the book also indicates that only a combination of existing concepts can push stroke research to great results.

We are in times where only the combination of different models helps us to overcome the complexity of matter; ischemic stroke research is a good example for this. However, we must first have these models and the proof of them showing how demanding and knowledge-based today's research has become. Applied or better translational research is needed today: that means that basic researchers must understand the clinics of the stroke and clinicians must understand the cellular and molecular actions.

In such a context, the current book also shows how vibrant and exciting the current concepts in ischemic stroke research are. It is a bouquet covering the major aspects of current stroke research, giving an overview for the beginners in the field, but also streaks newer concepts, so that everybody interested in ischemic stroke research finds interesting parts in this book!

Enjoy this multi-author book! We hope to read perhaps your chapter in the future.

Bernhard Schaller
University of Southampton, UK

Section 1

Introduction

Chapter 1

Ischemic Postconditioning after Stroke: Another Concept for the Trigeminocardiac Reflex?

Nora Sandu and Bernhard Schaller

Additional information is available at the end of the chapter

http://dx.doi.org/10.5772/65201

Abstract

Ischemic postconditioning is a concept for preventing ischemia/reperfusion injury in cerebral infarction. It has been evolved into experimental research by a broad range of stimuli/triggers and has not yet found its place in translational research. This review, therefore, first examines a potential clinical application of this concept and also provides insight into the phenomenon of trigeminocardiac reflex (TCR) and its oxygen-conserving component as a pillar of the ischemic postconditioning concept in humans. This concept serves as an example that only innovative therapeutic approach will substantially improve the current stroke research.

Keywords: ischemic tolerance, stroke, treatment

1. Introduction

Extensive experimental studies have shown that the mechanisms of cerebral ischemia include glutamate excitotoxicity, calcium toxicity, free radicals, nitric oxide, and inflammatory reactions, as well as dysfunctions of endoplasmic reticulum and mitochondrion, and it is an evolving topic from basic research to clinical applications during the past two to three decades [1–5]. These injury cascades are interconnected in complex ways, suggesting that only a few neuroprotective substances can offer therapeutic effects [6–10]. Thus, it is necessary to compare the novel and innovative therapeutic approaches in ischemia models. All these tremendous works have led to some substantial research in cellular and molecular pathways that have spurred the studies in potential neuroprotection, mainly in pharmacological fields, such as anti-excitotoxic treatment, calcium channel antagonist, approaches for inhibition of oxidation, inflammation, and apoptosis. However, several decades of research have not led to a new breakthrough concept of stroke treatment [11–21]. Nevertheless, there are still the same topics that we are dealing with our work. This chapter, therefore, shows the wide range of today's stroke research and also opens the door to the need for some innovative areas of studies in this topic, such as ischemic postconditioning, a strategy that has emerged during the past years.

Here, we present an innovative therapeutic approach covering several of the already known concepts of ischemic stroke treatment, leading to an easy clinical application.

2. Trigeminocardiac reflex

The trigeminocardiac reflex (TCR) is defined as the sudden onset of parasympathetic dysrhythmia, sympathetic hypotension, apnea, and/or gastric hypermotility during mechanical/thermic stimulation of any of the sensory branches of the trigeminal nerve [22–65]. The sensory nerve endings of the trigeminal nerve send neuronal signals through the Gasserian ganglion to the sensory nucleus of the trigeminal nerve, forming the afferent pathway of the reflex arc (see **Figure 1**) [45, 48, 49]. This afferent reflex pathway continues along the short internuncial nerve fibers in the reticular formation to connect with the efferent reflex pathway to the motor nucleus of the vagus nerve [45, 49, 65]. Clinically, the TCR has been reported to occur during nearly all skull base surgeries [22, 28, 53, 61]. Apart from these clinical reports, the physiological function of this brainstem reflex has not yet been fully explored, but different connections to the oxygen-conserving reflex are found [34–38, 55, 56, 63, 64].

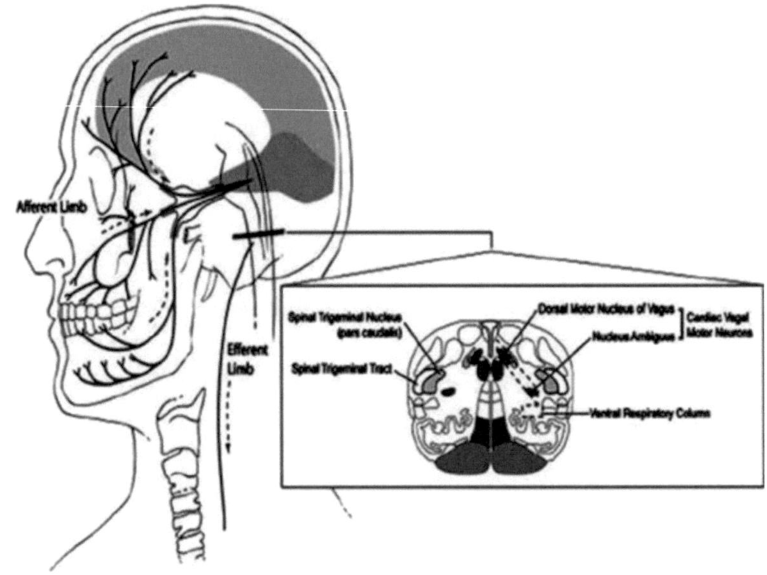

Figure 1. Summary of the trigeminocardiac reflex.

3. Oxygen-conserving reflex

From experimental findings, it may be suggested that the TCR represents an expression of a central neurogenic reflex, leading to rapid cerebrovascular vasodilatation generated from excitation of oxygen-sensitive neurons in the rostral ventrolateral medulla oblongata [39, 55, 56]. By this physiological response, the adjustments of the systemic and cerebral circulations are initiated to divert blood to the brain or to increase blood flow to it (see **Figure 2**) [25, 39]. As it is accepted that the diving reflex and ischemic tolerance appear to involve at least partially similar physiological mechanisms, the existence of such endogenous neuroprotective strategies may extend the known clinical appearance of the TCR and include the prevention of other potential brain injury states as well [25]. This existence of an oxygen-conserving reflex may be in line with the suggestion that the TCR is physiological, but not a pathophysiological entity.

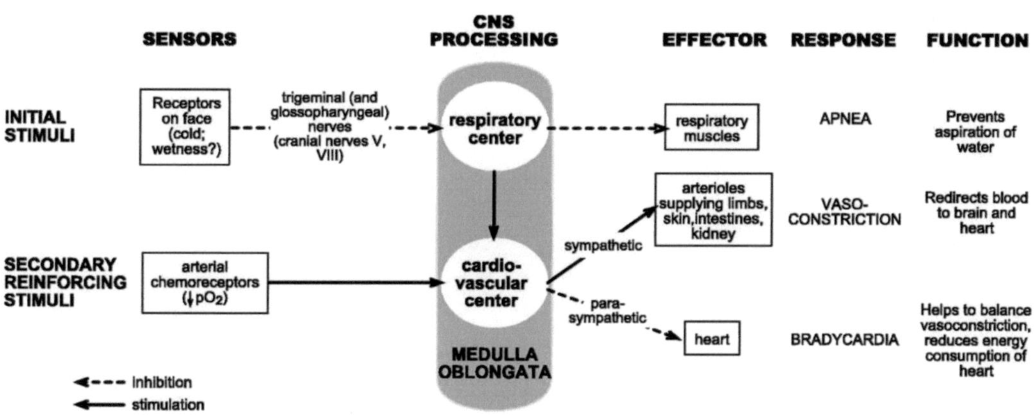

Figure 2. Oxygen-conserving reflex (adapted with permission from Hiebert and Burch [66]).

4. Postconditioning

Brief interruption (10–60 s, depending on the model) of the blood flow, applied immediately after the onset of reperfusion following an ischemic event, is observed to provide protection [19–21]. In the initial study in an anesthetized canine model of coronary artery occlusion-reperfusion, three cycles of coronary artery reperfusion alternating with 30 s of reocclusion were associated with a significant reduction in both the infarct size and the endothelial dysfunction [14–18]. Similar findings are now also demonstrated in the rat's brain. This "postconditioning" is so named because the stimulus is applied after the ischemia and is now also conferred by other species.

The protective effect of postconditioning can be achieved by occluding the ipsilateral common carotid artery (CCA), which is clinically relevant, for the ipsilateral CCA is accessible. Also, postconditioning can also be induced through volatile anesthetics. Isoflurane, for example, reduces the infarct size by 50%, if administered early during reperfusion. Likely, this effect is mediated through the PI3K pathway. Other pharmacological agents administered at the start of reperfusion have been shown to be cardioprotective (see **Figure 3**). This includes the following:

1. Adenosine
2. Nitric oxide
3. Cytokines
4. Complement inhibitors

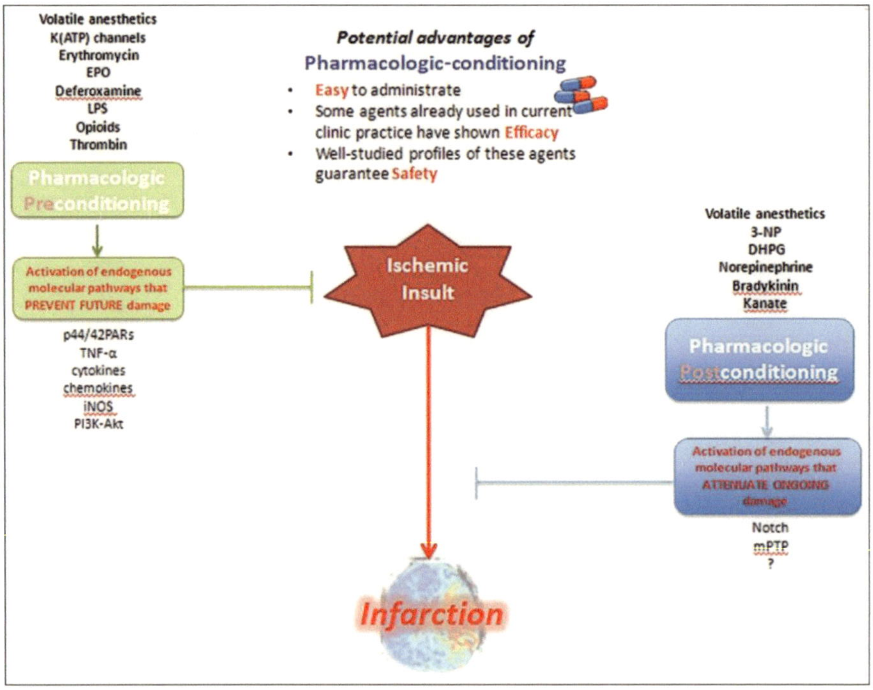

Figure 3. Postconditioning (adapted with permission from Esposito et al. [67]).

However, whether this approach should be described as "pharmacological postconditioning" or as a "postreperfusion treatment" has been debated [20]. Since the mechanisms of postconditioning have not been fully elucidated and the importance of the alternating cycles of ischemia-reperfusion has not been appreciated nor determined to be critical to protection, direct association to 'postconditioning' (whatever 'conditioning' means at reperfusion) should be debated.

Experimental studies support the neuroprotective potency of postconditioning to reduce the infarct size, endothelial dysfunction, and neutrophil accumulation in the jeopardized area [21].

http://dx.doi.org/10.5772/65201

These experimental results suggest that within the first minutes of reperfusion, endogenous processes are initiated, which help to reduce reperfusion injury after a limited duration of ischemia. The multiplicity of cell types that are affected by postconditioning (i.e., vascular endothelial cells and inflammatory cells) reflects the complexity of reperfusion injury and suggests a broad network of effects within this complex interactive web of responses. Also, delayed postconditioning, which is clinically more relevant, also improved glucose uptake, inhibited edema, and mitigated blood-brain barrier leakage in the penumbra, and finally, attenuated the exacerbating effect of tissue plasminogen activator (t-PA).

5. Trigeminocardiac reflex and postconditioning in stroke

Some studies have shown that postconditioning reduces infarction in the period immediate after a stroke [20]. However, more studies are needed to better understand this phenomenon and to translate it into the clinic. Postconditioning seems to reduce the cerebral ischemic injury by blocking the overproduction of ROS and lipid peroxidation, and by inhibiting apoptosis. The initial inhibiting effect on ROS may lead to an improved activity of the Akt and K_{ATP} channels, which contributes to the protection of postconditioning. Also, the changes in the MAPK pathways and the δPKC and εPKC activities are also associated with the protection of postconditioning.

However, what is the connection with the TCR? The TCR is, in our opinion, a specific example of a group of related responses generically defined by Wolf as oxygen-conserving reflexes. Within seconds after this TCR initiation, there is a vast and differentiated activation of sympathetic nerves. The suggested effect of the TCR in the brain is a constant elevation in cerebral blood flow (CBF) that is not associated with changes in the cerebral metabolic rate of oxygen (CMRO2) or cerebral glucose metabolic rate (CMRglc) and hence represents a primary cerebrovascular vasodilatation. The brain can protect itself from ischemia by distinct (endogenous) physiological mechanisms, which probably involve two separate systems of neurons in the CNS. The one who mediates a reflexive neurogenic neuroprotection emanates from oxygen-sensitive sympathoexcitatory reticulospinal neurons of the rostral ventrolateral medulla (RVLM). These cells, excited within seconds by a reduction in CBF or CMRO2, initiate the systemic vascular components of the oxygen-conserving diving reflex. They profoundly increase CBF without changing CMRO2 and CMRglc and, hence, rapidly and efficiently provide the brain with oxygen [39]. Upon cessation of the stimulus, the systemic and cerebrovascular adjustments return to normal. The system mediating reflex protection projects through as-yet-undefined projections from the RVLM to the upper brainstem and/or thalamus to engage a small population of neurons in the cortex, which appear to be dedicated to transducing a neuronal signal into vasodilation [39]. Two lines of evidence indicate that the RVLM neurons are essential for the expression of the cerebrovascular vasodilation elicited by hypoxia [55]. First, electrical stimulation of RVLM in intact or spinalized rats site-specifically and dose-dependently elevates rCBF, but not CMRO2 or CMRglc [39]. In this manner, these data replicate hypoxic vasodilatation. The response can only be attributed to stimulation of the reticulospinal sympathoexcitatory neurons since these are the only neurons in the region excited by over 50% elevation of CBF produced by hypoxemia [39]. The fact that such lesions do not affect the vasodilatation elicited by hypercarbia indicates that the response is stimulus selective. Thus, much of the cerebrovascular vasodilatation elicited in the cerebral cortex by hypoxemia is a reflex that results from excitation of oxygen-sensitive brainstem neurons, and not by a direct effect of hypoxia on blood vessels nor by stimulation of arterial chemoreceptors whose activity, while regulating blood flow to most vascular beds, is without force in the cerebral circulation [55, 56]. It also appears to relay the central neurogenic vasodilatation elicited from other brain regions, including excitation of axons innervating the fastigial nucleus. This mode of protection would be initiated under conditions of global ischemia and/or hypoxemia because the signal is detected by medullary neurons. The concept that the brain may have neuronal systems dedicated to protecting itself from (ischemic) damage, at first appearing to be a novel concept, is, upon reflection, not surprising since the brain is not injured in naturalistic behaviors characterized by very low levels of rCBF, such as diving or hibernation.

Such neuroprotective adaptations may also underlie preconditioning strategies. The diving reflex, hibernation, and ischemic tolerance appear to involve at least partially similar physiological mechanisms because most of the signals, transducers, and effectors that are well established in ischemic tolerance have also been demonstrated in hypoxia-tolerant or hibernating animals. A better and more detailed understanding of the pathways, transmitters, and molecules engaged in such protection may provide new insights into novel therapies for a range of disorders characterized by neuronal death. Recent clinical studies suggest such an endogenous neuroprotective effect in the human brain.

6. Conclusions and take-home message

The TCR is certainly the most influential and most innovative concept in skull base surgery of the past 20 years. In addition, the TCR steps out of this shadow and opens the door to significant therapeutical options in neurological disorders.

The here presented concept is also exemplary for this book: to think out of the box is needed to make further substantial improvements in today's stroke research and its clinical application. The time that simple systematic reviews with its not negligible bias lead to improved therapeutic approaches is over. Now the time of concepts integrating knowledge from different sources has begun: the ischemic preconditioning by the TCR is one such approach, the use of 3-D-printing in neuroradiology aneurysm treatment another. However, this book also shows that we have to prove these concepts in different ways.

"Tempora mutantur, et nos mutamur in illis" shows that stroke research has to make the next step to overcome the standstill of the last years. This book is—if any—a subtle step in this direction, but it shows that we need newer models to cover and explain all important aspect of stroke and its treatment.

http://dx.doi.org/10.5772/65201

Author details

Nora Sandu and Bernhard Schaller*

*Address all correspondence to: bernhardjschaller@gmail.com

Departement of Research, University of Southampton, Southampton, UK

References

[1] Schaller B, Graf R (2002) Cerebral ischemia tolerance. Praxis (Bern 1994);91(40): 1639-1644.

[2] Schaller B, Graf R (2002) Cerebral ischemic preconditioning. An experimental phenomenon or a clinical important entity of stroke prevention? J Neurol;249(11): 1503-1511.

[3] Schaller B, Graf R, Sanada Y, Rosner G, Wienhard K, Heiss WD (2003) Hemodynamic and metabolic effects of decompressive hemicraniectomy in normal brain. An experimental PET-study in cats. Brain Res;982(1):31-37.

[4] Schaller B, Graf R, Sanada Y, Tolnay M, Rosner G, Wienhard K, Heiss WD (2003) Hemodynamic changes after occlusion of the posterior superior sagittal sinus: an experimental PET study in cats. AJNR Am J Neuroradiol;24(9):1876-1880.

[5] Schaller B, Graf R, Wienhard K, Heiss WD (2003) A new animal model of cerebral venous infarction: ligation of the posterior part of the superior sagittal sinus in the cat. Swiss Med Wkly;133(29-30):412-418.

[6] Schaller B, Graf R (2003) Hypothermia and stroke: the pathophysiological background. Pathophysiology;10(1):7-35.

[7] Schaller B (2003) Educational attainment and risk of stroke and myocardial infarction. Med Sci Monit;9(12): LE27.

[8] Schaller B, Graf R (2004) Cerebral ischemia, and reperfusion: the pathophysiologic concept as a basis for clinical therapy. J Cereb Blood Flow Metab;24(4):351-371.

[9] Schaller B, Graf R (2004) Cerebral venous infarction: the pathophysiological concept. Cerebrovasc Dis;18(3):179-188.

[10] Schaller B, Jacobs AH, Graf R (2004) Hemispheric dominance for the cortical control of swallowing in humans: a contribution to better understand cortical organization? Eur J Radiol;51(3):290-291.

[11] Schaller B (2005) Ischemic preconditioning as induction of ischemic tolerance after transient ischemic attacks in human brain: its clinical relevance. Neurosci Lett;377(3): 206-211.

[12] Schaller BJ (2007) Influence of age on stroke and preconditioning-induced ischemic tolerance in the brain. Exp Neurol;205(1):9-19.

[13] Schaller BJ, Graf R, Jacobs AH (2006) Pathophysiological changes of the gastrointestinal tract in ischemic stroke. Am J Gastroenterol;101(7):1655-1665.

[14] Schaller B (2007) Extracranial-intracranial bypass surgery to reduce the risk of hemodynamic stroke in cerebroocclusive atherosclerotic disease of the anterior cerebral circulation—a systematic review. Neurol Neurochir Pol;41(5):457-471.

[15] Schaller B, Cornelius JF, Sandu N (2008) Molecular medicine successes in neuroscience. Mol Med;14(7-8):361-364.

[16] Schaller B (2008) Extracranial-intracranial bypass to reduce the risk of ischemic stroke in intracranial aneurysms of the anterior cerebral circulation: a systematic review. J Stroke Cerebrovasc Dis;17(5):287-298.

[17] Schaller BJ (2008) Strategies for molecular imaging dementia and neurodegenerative diseases. Neuropsychiatr Dis Treat;4(3):585-612.

[18] Cornelius JF, Sandu N, Perez-Pinzon MA, Schaller B (2009) Treatment of acute ischemic stroke: Role of ischemic tolerance in intravenous and endovascular therapies. Expert Rev Cardiovasc Ther;7(4):331-332.

[19] Sandu N, Cornelius J, Filis A, Arasho B, Perez-Pinzon M, Schaller B (2009) Ischemic tolerance in stroke treatment. Expert Rev Cardiovasc Ther;7(10):1255-1261.

[20] Sandu N, Schaller B (2010) Postconditioning: a new or old option after ischemic stroke? Expert Rev Cardiovasc Ther;8(4):479-482.

[21] Schaller B, Graf R, Jacobs AH (2003) Ischaemic tolerance: a window to endogenous neuroprotection? Lancet 2003: 362:1007-1008.

[22] Sandu N, Chowdhury T, Schaller BJ (2016) How to apply case reports in clinical practice using surrogate models via example of the trigeminocardiac reflex. J Med Case Rep.; 10:84.

[23] Chowdhury T, Ahuja N, Schaller B (2015) Severe bradycardia during neurosurgical procedure: depth of anesthesia matters and leads to a new surrogate model of the trigeminocardiac reflex: a case report. Medicine (Baltimore);94(49):e2118.

[24] Chowdhury T, Nöthen C, Filis A, Sandu N, Buchfelder M, Schaller B (2015) Functional outcome changes in surgery for pituitary adenomas after intraoperative occurrence of the trigeminocardiac reflex: first description in a retrospective observational study. Medicine (Baltimore);94(37):e1463.

[25] Lemaitre F, Chowdhury T, Schaller B (2015) The trigeminocardiac reflex—a comparison with the diving reflex in humans. Arch Med Sci.;11(2):419-426.

[26] Meuwly C, Chowdhury T, Sandu N, Reck M, Erne P, Schaller B (2015) Anesthetic influence on occurrence and treatment of the trigemino-cardiac reflex: a systematic literature review. Medicine (Baltimore);94(18):e807.

[27] Meuwly C, Golanov E, Chowdhury T, Erne P, Schaller B (2015) Trigeminal cardiac reflex: new thinking model about the definition based on a literature review. Medicine (Baltimore);94(5):e484.

[28] Chowdhury T, Mendelowith D, Golanov E, Spiriev T, Arasho B, Sandu N, Sadr-Eshkevari P, Meuwly C, Schaller B (2015) Trigeminocardiac reflex: the current clinical and physiological knowledge. J Neurosurg Anesthesiol;27(2): 136-147.

[29] Sadr-Eshkevari P, Schaller BJ, Bohluli B (2014) Trigeminocardiac reflex: Some thought to the definition. Surg Neurol Int;5:43.

[30] Chowdhury T, Meuwly C, Sandu N, Cappellani RB, Schaller B (2014) Coronary spasm in neurosurgical patients and role of trigeminocardiac reflex. Neurol Res Int; 2014:974930.

[31] Chowdhury T, Sandu N, Sadr-Eshkevari P, Meuwly C, Schaller B (2014) Trigeminocardiac reflex: current trends. Expert Rev Cardiovasc Ther;12(1):9-11.

[32] Chowdhury T, Cappellani RB, Schaller B (2014) Chronic trigemino-cardiac reflex in patient with orbital floor fracture: role of surgery and first description. J Neurosurg Anesthesiol.;26(1):91-92.

[33] Meuwly C, Chowdhury T, Schaller B (2013) Topical lidocaine to suppress trigeminocardiac reflex. Br J Anaesth;111(2):302.

[34] Chowdhury T, Cappellani RB, Schaller B (2014) Retrogasserian glycerol rhizolysis: first description of occurrence trigeminocardiac reflex. J Neurosurg Anesthesiol.;26(1): 86-87.

[35] Spiriev T, Tzekov C, Laleva L, Kostadinova C, Kondoff S, Sandu N, Schaller B (2012) Central trigeminocardiac reflex in pediatric neurosurgery: a case report and review of the literature. J Med Case Rep.;6:372.

[36] Spiriev T, Prabhakar H, Sandu N, Tzekov C, Kondoff S, Laleva L, Schaller B (2012) Use of hydrogen peroxide in neurosurgery: case series of cardiovascular complications. JRSM Short Rep;3(1):6.

[37] Spiriev T, Kondoff S, Schaller B (2011) Cardiovascular changes after subarachnoid hemorrhage initiated by the trigeminocardiac reflex-first description of a case series. J Neurosurg Anesthesiol.;23(4):379-380.

[38] Spiriev T, Kondoff S, Schaller B (2011) Trigeminocardiac reflex during temporary clipping in aneurismal surgery: first description. J Neurosurg Anesthesiol.;23(3): 271-272.

[39] Sandu N, Cornelius J, Filis A, Nöthen C, Rasper J, Kulinsky VI, Schaller BJ (2010) Cerebral hemodynamic changes during the trigeminocardiac reflex: description of a new animal model protocol. ScientificWorldJournal;10:1416-1423.

[40] Arasho B, Sandu N, Spiriev T, Prabhakar H, Schaller B (2009) Management of the trigeminocardiac reflex: facts and own experience. Neurol India. 2009;57(4):375-380.

[41] Schaller B, Sandu N, Filis A, Buchfelder M (2008) Cardiovascular responses during percutaneous radiofrequency thermocoagulation therapy in primary trigeminal neuralgia: an explanation of the trigeminocardiac reflex? J Neurosurg Anesthesiol; 20(4):270.

[42] Schaller B, Sandu N, Ottoviani G, Filis A, Noethen C, Buchfelder M (2009) Transient asystole during endoscopic transsphenoidal surgery: an example of trigeminocardiac reflex. Pituitary;12(3):271-272.

[43] Schaller B, Filis A, Buchfelder M (2008) Trigeminocardiac reflex in embolization of intracranial dural arteriovenous fistula. AJNR Am J Neuroradiol;29(7): E55.

[44] Filis A, Schaller B, Buchfelder M (2008) Trigeminocardiac reflex in pituitary surgery. A prospective pilot study. Nervenarzt;79(6):669-675.

[45] Schaller BJ (2007) Trigeminocardiac reflex. J Neurosurg;107(1): 243.

[46] Schaller BJ, Filis A, Buchfelder M (2007) Detection and prevention of the trigeminocardiac reflex during skull base surgery. Acta Neurochir (Wien);149(3):331.

[47] Schaller BJ, Buchfelder M (2006) Delayed trigeminocardiac reflex induced by an intraorbital foreign body. Ophthalmologica;220(5):348.

[48] Schaller B (2004) Trigeminocardiac reflex. A clinical phenomenon or a new physiological entity? J Neurol.;251(6):658-665.

[49] Schaller B, Probst R, Strebel S, Gratzl O (1999) Trigeminocardiac reflex during surgery in the cerebellopontine angle. J Neurosurg;90(2):215-220.

[50] Sandu N, Sadr-Eshkevari P, Schaller BJ (2011) Usefulness of case reports to improve medical knowledge regarding trigemino-cardiac reflex in skull base surgery. J Med Case Rep.;5:149.

[51] Nöthen C, Sandu N, Prabhakar H, Filis A, Arasho BD, Buchfelder M, Schaller BJ (2010) Trigemino-cardiac reflex and antecedent transient ischemic attacks. Expert Rev Cardiovasc Ther;8(4):509-512.

[52] Sandu N, Schaller B (2010) The trigemino-cardiac reflex: a view to the future. Arch Med Sci;6(1):138-139.

[53] Schaller B, Cornelius JF, Prabhakar H, Koerbel A, Gnanalingham K, Sandu N, Ottaviani G, Filis A, Buchfelder M (2009) The trigemino-cardiac reflex: an update of the current knowledge. J Neurosurg Anesthesiol. 2009 Jul;21(3):187-195.

[54] Schaller B, Filis A, Sandu N, Buchfelder M (2009) Peripheral trigemino-cardiac reflex. Acta Neurochir (Wien);151(12):1727.

[55] Schaller B, Cornelius JF, Sandu N, Ottaviani G, Perez-Pinzon MA (2009) Oxygen-conserving reflexes of the brain: the current molecular knowledge. J Cell Mol Med;13(4): 644-647.

[56] Schaller BJ, Sandu N, Cornelius JF, Filis A, Perez-Pinzon MA (2009) Oxygen-conserving implications of the trigemino-cardiac reflex in the brain: the molecular basis of neuroprotection? Mol Med;15(5-6):125-126.

[57] Schaller B, Filis A, Sandu N, Rasper J, Noethen C, Buchfelder M (2008) Trigemino-cardiac reflex may be refractory to conventional management in adults. Acta Neurochir (Wien);150(9):929-930.

[58] Schaller BJ, Filis A, Buchfelder M (2008) Trigemino-cardiac reflex in humans initiated by peripheral stimulation during neurosurgical skull-base operations. Its first description. Acta Neurochir (Wien).;150(7):715-717.

[59] Schaller BJ, Rasper J, Filis A, Buchfelder M (2008) Difference in functional outcome of ipsilateral tinnitus after intraoperative occurrence of the trigemino-cardiac reflex in surgery for vestibular schwannomas. Acta Neurochir (Wien);150(2):157-160.

[60] Schaller BJ, Weigel D, Filis A, Buchfelder M (2007) Trigemino-cardiac reflex during transsphenoidal surgery for pituitary adenomas: methodological description of a prospective skull base study protocol. Brain Res. 1149:69-75.

[61] Schaller BJ, Buchfelder M (2006) Trigemino-cardiac reflex in skull base surgery: from a better understanding to a better outcome? Acta Neurochir (Wien);148(10): 1029-1031.

[62] Schaller BJ, Buchfelder M, Knauth M (2006) Trigemino-cardiac reflex during skull base surgery: a new entity of ischaemic preconditioning? The potential role of imaging. Eur J Nucl Med Mol Imaging.;33(3):384-385.

[63] Schaller B (2005) Trigemino-cardiac reflex during transsphenoidal surgery for pituitary adenomas. Clin Neurol Neurosurg;107(6):468-474.

[64] Schaller B (2005) Trigemino-cardiac reflex during microvascular trigeminal decompression in cases of trigeminal neuralgia. J Neurosurg Anesthesiol;17(1): 45-48.

[65] Spiriev T, Sandu N, Kondoff S, Tzekov C, Schaller B (2012) Tic and autonomic symptoms. J Neurosurg.;116(6):1397-1398.

[66] Hiebert, SM, Burch E (2003) Simulated human diving and heart rate: Making the most of the diving response as a laboratory exercise. Adv Physiol Educ 2003; 27:130-145.

[67] Esposito E Desai R, Ji, Lo HE (2015) Pharmacologic pre- und postconditioning for stroke: basic mechanisms and translational opportunity. Brain Circ 1: 104-113.

Section 2

Basic Science

Chapter 2

Excitotoxicity and Oxidative Stress in Acute Stroke

Ramon Rama and Julio César García

Additional information is available at the end of the chapter

http://dx.doi.org/10.5772/64991

Abstract

Excitotoxicity, defined as cell death resulting from the toxic actions of excitatory amino acids, is actually considered as a major factor contributing to the early stage of ischemic cell death in stroke. In stroke, once vessel occlusion is produced, the disruptions to the blood flow in the affected areas decrease the delivery of oxygen and metabolic substrates to neurons. Consequently, the lack of oxygen interrupts oxidative phosphorylation by the mitochondria and drastically reduces cellular ATP production, which results in a rapid decline in cellular ATP. After several minutes, inhibition of the Na^+/K^+-ATPase function causes a profound loss of ionic gradients and depolarization of regulated neurons, which leads to excessive release of excitatory amino acids—particularly glutamate—to the extracellular compartment. The presence of excessive amounts of glutamate into the synapses and extrasynaptic sites can lead eventually to neuronal death. Excitotoxicity leads to a number of deleterious consequences, including impairment of cellular calcium homeostasis, generation of free radicals and oxidative stress, mitochondrial damage, and activation of several transcription factors and their genes expression. All these mechanisms' acting synergy can cause neuron death by apoptosis. Oxidative stress induced by excitotoxicity is considered to be the main event leading to brain damage after stroke. On the basis of experimental models, there is ample evidence of the role of oxidative stress in ischemic brain damage.

Keywords: stroke, ischemia, excitotoxicity, NMDAR, calcium, oxidative stress, mitochondrial dysfunction, apoptosis

1. Introduction

Cerebral ischemia is defined as insufficient blood flow to the brain to supply an adequate amount of oxygen and nutrients. Cerebral ischemia accounts for about 80% of all strokes; the other 20% are due to intracranial hemorrhage. Cerebral ischemia occurs when blood flow to the brain or any of its areas is insufficient to supply the oxygen and glucose that the tissue needs to maintain their metabolic activity. Ischemic stroke is the result of total or partial interruption of cerebral arterial blood supply (ischemia) by a thrombus or embolism, which leads to oxygen and glucose deprivation of the tissue that ultimately results in apoptotic and necrotic cell death. Cerebral ischemia may be either permanent (the thrombus occluding the vessel is not removed) or transient (followed by reperfusion). In all cases, a stroke causes dysfunction and death of brain neurons and neurological damage that reflects the location and size of the brain area affected [1, 2]. Brain tissue is very sensitive to ischemia because neurons obtain almost all energy using oxidative metabolism via mitochondrial oxidative phosphorylation where oxygen is the final electron acceptor.

In stroke, once the vessel occlusion is produced, if cerebral arterial blood flow is not restored within a short period, ischemic stroke is the usual result, with subsequent neuron death within the perfusion territory of the vessels affected. Acute ischemic stroke results from acute occlusion of cerebral arteries. Ischemic stroke is characterized by complex sequence of spatial and temporal events evolving over hours and days [1, 2].

Focal ischemia is characterized by an ischemic core surrounded by a "penumbra" region that has partial reduction in blood flow due to the presence of collateral arteries. Lesser reductions in blood flow, which do not lead to apparent functional or metabolic disturbances, are called benign oligemia and do not produce tissue injury [3]. In the ischemic core, a significant reduction of blood flow causes severe deprivation of oxygen and glucose and consequent total bioenergetics failure and neurons are unable to maintain the ionic gradients. As a result, a number of mechanisms that cause altered lipid and protein structural component of cellular membrane are triggered [4]. Neurons are killed rapidly within minutes and the tissue in the ischemic core is irreversibly damaged even if blood flow is reestablished [5].

In the penumbra, neurons become functionally impaired because the ability to fire action potentials is lost but remain metabolically active. Neurons in the penumbra maintain enough energy to sustain their resting membrane potentials, and when collateral blood flow improves, action potential and function are restored. Thus, ischemic penumbra refers to areas of the brain that are damaged during stroke but not killed [6]. In the absence of early reperfusion, the death of neurons in the ischemic penumbra due to ischemic injury progresses, leading to a reduction in penumbra area and expansion of the infarcted core. Tissue injury in the penumbra is the outcome of a complex series of genetic, molecular, and biochemical mechanisms, which contribute either to protecting and repairing the penumbra tissue and recovery of the functional activity or to damaging and then the penumbra area becomes necrotic. The ischemic core is generally considered unsalvageable, whereas the penumbra may be rescued by timely intervention and poses a target for the development of therapeutic treatment.

Results from the recent studies using imaging show that in the early minutes and hours after ischemia onset, the core ischemic contains pockets of injury, which were characterized as "minicores," and surrounded by "minipenumbras" that are heterogeneously distributed. The architecture and reversibility of the penumbra depend on time and location of rCBF reduction in the ischemic brain territory. Depending on the rCBF time, "minicores" coalesce with "micropenumbras." In this way, if unimpeded, the "minicores" can grow into their respective "minipenumbras" to encompass a larger injury region [7].

2. Pathophysiology of neuron death in the stroke

In the last 20 years, experimental and clinical studies have allowed to identify and characterize the multiple mechanisms that injure the brain tissue in a stroke [1, 2, 5, 8]. Brain damage in ischemic stroke is the result of multiple mechanisms acting synergistically at physiological, biochemical, molecular, and genetic level, which impair neurological functions and may cause neuronal death [1, 8, 9] via mechanisms that promote rupture, lysis, phagocytosis or involution, and shrinkage [10]. Knowledge of the molecular mechanisms that underlie neuron death following a stroke is important if we are to devise effective neuroprotective strategies.

A severe transient or permanent reduction of CBF in a restricted vascular territory causes acute ischemic injury. Physiological values of CBF are between 45 and 60 ml blood/100 g/min. It is well documented that in response to reduced CBF time-dependent neuronal events are triggered [11]. Oxygen supply to the brain below a critical level reduces and eventually blocks the oxidative phosphorylation, drastically decreasing cellular ATP production leading to dysfunction of ATPase pumps and to the collapse of ionic gradients. The neuron activity ceases and if oxygen level is not restored quickly, cells die [12].

The brain is highly vulnerable to ischemia. In part, the vulnerability of brain tissue to ischemia reflects its high metabolic demands. The brain has a relatively high energy consumption and depends almost exclusively on the oxidative phosphorylation for energy production. Although the weight of the human brain is only about 2% of the total body weight, it has high metabolic activity and uses 20% of the oxygen and 25% of the glucose consumed by the entire body [13].

Brain activity involves a high metabolic activity by brain neurons, which require to have large amounts of oxygen and glucose. And since the brain has no oxygen storage capacity, the proper functioning of the brain depends on an abundant and continuous supply of oxygen.

Energy in the brain is mainly formed when glucose is oxidized to CO_2 and water through mitochondrial oxidative phosphorylation. The brain requires large amounts of oxygen to generate sufficient ATP to maintain and restore ionic gradients, although demands due to the activity of inhibitory interneurons [14], astrocytes [15], and other brain cells [16], just like the constant rebuilding of each neuron from its constituent proteins, are also a significant factor in the energy cost of brain function [17, 18].

3. Basic mechanisms of ischemic cell injury

Since the severity of ischemia is heterogeneous, the mechanisms involved in ischemic neuronal damage differ according to the severity of ischemia. Thus, in neurons located in the ischemic "core" the ischemia leads to the inability of neuron to generate the energy needed to maintain the cell structure with the activation of mechanisms that cause cell death by necrosis, whereas neurons of the ischemic penumbra are able to maintain cell structure and the possibility of recovering the function. The brain injury in acute ischemic stroke is the result of multiple mechanisms acting synergistically [1, 5, 8].

After the onset of a stroke, ischemic stroke begins with the occlusion of a brain artery, with the consequent restriction in the delivery of basic nutrients to a cerebral region. The affected area of the brain receives insufficient oxygen and glucose. Severe deficit of oxygen and glucose due to disruption of blood flow leads to dysfunction in mitochondrial oxidative phosphorylation resulting in insufficient production of ATP and irreversible failure of energy metabolism [19] and an increase in the formation of superoxide radical [4]. Insufficient ATP leads to the inability of the neuron to maintain the ionic homeostasis; the increase in the formation of superoxide radical attached to a decrease in antioxidant activity can lead to an oxidative stress. The rise of the free radicals leads the mitochondria to increase the production of free radicals and an oxidative stress in the cell, resulting in the oxidation of proteins and lipids components of the structure of the cell membrane and DNA fragmentation. The result is necrotic cell death [20, 21]. It could be said that under these conditions of severe ischemia, neurons die by the direct action of the lack of oxygen and glucose, independently of the influence of neighboring cells. The situation is more complex when it comes to the penumbra zone.

Within the ischemic penumbra, multiple mechanisms have been identified that irreversibly damage brain tissue. After ischemic onset, while there are potential reserves of alternative substrates to glucose, such as glycogen, lactate, and fatty acids, for both glycolysis and respiration, there is no alternative capable of assuming the lack of oxygen and maintain mitochondrial oxidative phosphorylation, the main source of ATP in neurons. Consequently, in situations of severe oxygen deficit, as in the ischemic penumbra, ATP production by mitochondria is insufficient to maintain the activity of ATPase responsible for maintaining ionic gradients. Reduced ATP stimulates the glycolytic metabolism of residual glucose and glycogen, causing an accumulation of protons and lactate, which leads to rapid intracellular acidification and increases the depletion of ATP [4]. After several minutes, inhibition of the Na^+/K^+-ATPase function causes a profound loss of ionic gradients and the depolarization of neurons and astrocytes [1]. This leads to an uncontrolled depolarization of neurons affected in the penumbra, activation of voltage-gated calcium channels and to excessive release of neurotransmitters excitatory amino acids—particularly glutamate—in the presynaptic terminal (**Figure 1**). Simultaneously, neurotransmitter reuptake from the extracellular space is reduced [22, 23]. The presence of excessive amounts of excitatory amino acids into the synapses and extrasynaptic sites can eventually lead to neuronal death, in a process known as excito-toxicity [24], and it is defined as cell death resulting from the toxic actions of excitatory amino acids. Because glutamate is the major excitatory neurotransmitter in the mammalian central nervous system (CNS) where it plays important roles in neuronal growth and axon guidance, in brain development and maturation, and in synaptic plasticity, and constitutes the basis of synaptic transmission in about 10^{14} synapses in the human brain, excitotoxicity usually refers to the injury and death of neurons arising from prolonged intense exposure to glutamate [25–

http://dx.doi.org/10.5772/64991

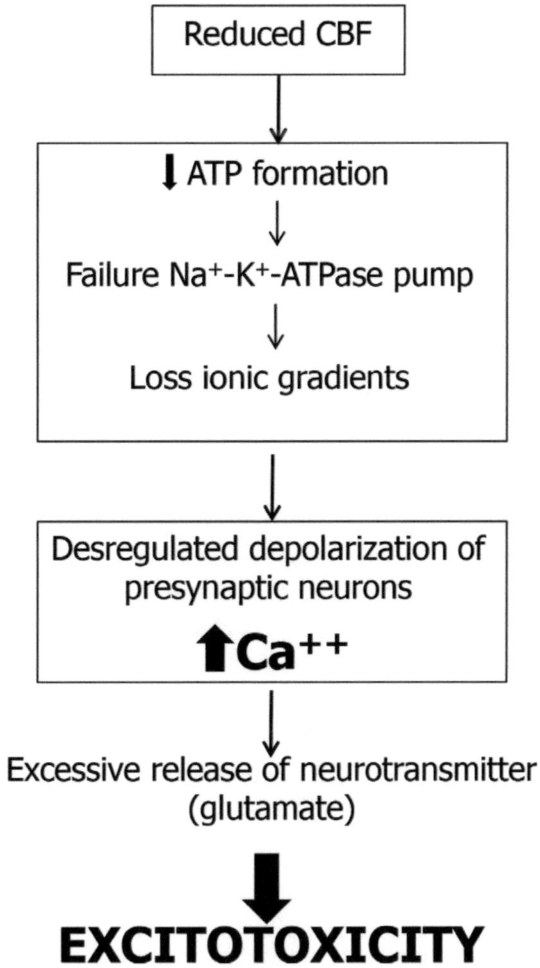

Figure 1. Excessive glutamate release by neurons in stroke. In neuron, the lack of oxygen and glucose due at reduced cerebral blood flow interrupts oxidative phosphorylation by mitochondria and reduces the cellular ATP production. Low ATP levels cause inhibition of the ATPase pump leading to profound loss of cellular membrane ionic gradient, cellular membrane depolarization, and the excessive glutamate release.

27], although other cells such as astrocytes may also suffer damage as a result of excessive levels of glutamate [28].

4. Excitotoxicity and acute ischemic stroke

Excitotoxicity is actually considered as a major factor contributing to the early stage of ischemic cell death in stroke [27, 29–31]. Excitotoxic death requires the excessive influx of the extracellular Ca^{2+} via receptor-operated channels or voltage-sensitive Ca^{2+} channels [32, 33]. The excessive intracellular Ca^{2+} initiates a series of molecular events that culminate in neuronal death [25, 34].

The rise in the extracellular glutamate concentration initiates a positive feedback loop, with further activation of glutamate receptors in neighboring neurons, and as a result, more Na^+ inflow to neurons via monovalent ion channels that decrease ionic gradients and consume ATP, both of which promote further release of glutamate [30]. A marked and prolonged rise in the extracellular glutamate concentration kills central neurons [2, 10]. Excessive glutamate in the synapses leads to glutamate receptors, at a pathophysiological level, triggering a cascade of events that can result in neuronal dysfunction and death.

Excitotoxicity leads to a number of deleterious consequences, including impairment of cellular calcium homeostasis, generation of free radicals and oxidative stress, activation of the mitochondrial permeability transition, secondary excitotoxicity, and activation of several transcription factors and their genes expression.

4.1. Overactivation of glutamate receptors and calcium overload by excitotoxicity

The excitatory effects of glutamate are mediated through two kinds of glutamate receptors: ionotropic receptors, the ligand and the ion channel are part of the same molecular receptor complex, and metabotropic receptors linked to G-protein [35]. They are located in the pre- and postsynaptic neuron membranes of the central nervous system. Glutamate ionotropic receptors are ligand-gated cation channels permeable to Ca^{2+}. Although practically all glutamate receptors are involved in excitotoxic processes, the N-methyl-D-aspartate receptor (NMDAR) is the key initiator of excitotoxic damage [36]. The glutamate overload leads to prolonged stimulation of AMPA and NMDA ionotropic receptor subtypes, which enhance the excessive influx of calcium, sodium, and water into neurons.

NMDAR consist of four subunits: two GluN1 (NR1) and two regulatory subunits that can be GluN2A (NR2A) through GluN2D (NR2D) and GluN3A (NR3A) or GluN3B (NR3B) [37, 38]. Subunit NR1 contains the site where the glutamate is united to the receptor, whereas subunit NR2 contains the site where the glycine is united [39]. The subunit combination and alternative splicing determine the functional properties of the receptors. The pharmacological and biochemical properties mediated by NMDA receptors are largely determined by the type of NR2 subunits incorporated into the heteromeric NR1/NR2 complex [40, 41]. Specific NR2 subtypes appear to play a pivotal role in strokes [42].

The blocking NMDARs containing NR2A enhanced neuron death and prevented the induction of ischemic tolerance, whereas inhibiting NMDARs that contained NR2B attenuated ischemic cell death and enhanced preconditioning-induced neuroprotection in an occlusion model of transient global ischemia in rats [43]. It has been suggested that excitotoxicity is triggered by the selective activation of NMDARs containing the NR2B subunit [43, 44].

Because NR2A and NR2B are the predominant NR2 subunits in the adult forebrain, NMDA receptors that contain NR2A and NR2B may play different roles. NMDARs that contain NR2A subunit would be involved in supporting neuronal survival, whereas NMDAR containing NR2B subunit would be involved in neuron death, and hence have opposing impacts on excitotoxic brain damage after acute brain insults, such as a stroke or brain trauma [42, 43].

NMDARs are found at synaptic or extrasynaptic sites [45, 46]. NMDARs are trafficked to the synapse throughout development and in adulthood, but a significant proportion remain extrasynaptic. The locations of NMDARs in different parts on cellular membrane of neurons that perform different functions suggest that it could be a determining factor in excitotoxicity after a stroke [45, 47]. Thus, participation of NMDARs in synaptic activity plays an important role in neuron survival, whereas activation of NMDARs in extrasynaptic activity appears to be associated with neuronal death [42]. In this regard, it has been observed that stimulation of synaptic NMDAR induces the expression of prosurvival proteins, such as brain-derived neurotrophic factor (BDNF), whereas activation of extrasynaptic NMDAR leads to expression of proapoptotic proteins and suppression of survival pathways [46, 48]. However, it has also been suggested that the apparent differences in excitotoxicity mediated by NMDARs could be due to differences in molecular composition between synaptic/extrasynaptic NMDARs as opposed to the location of the receptors *per se*. In adult brain, NMDARs located in synapses predominantly contain the NR2A subtype while extrasynaptic NMDARs predominantly contain NR2B [49, 50]. Although there is little evidence that differences in subunit composition explain the different effects of glutamate in the functioning of the synaptic or extrasynaptic location of the NMDAR, the activation of NMDARs containing NR2B subunits tends to promote neuron death, irrespective of the location, whereas activation of NMDARs containing NR2A subunits promotes survival [42]. However, NR2A-NMDARs are capable of mediating excitotoxicity [51] and NR2B-NMDARs are capable of mediating both prosurvival and prodeath signaling, depending on the stimulation paradigm [49]. In older neurons expressing comparable levels of NR2A- and NR2B-containing NMDARs, amelioration of Ca^{2+} overload required the inhibition of extrasynaptic receptors containing both NR2 subunits [52].

NMDARs interact with multiple intracellular synaptic and cytoskeletal proteins, mainly through the cytoplasmatic C-termini of the NR1 and NR2 subunits [53, 54]. NMDARs exit in multiprotein complexes that determine the efficiency with which their activation leads to specific signaling events into neuron. It has further been proposed that lethal Ca^{2+} signaling trough NMDARs is determined by interacting between the molecular complex and the NMDARs [55]. At the synapse, NMDAR receptors are found localized within electron-dense structures known as the postsynaptic densities (PSDs) where they form large and dynamic multiprotein signaling complexes [56, 57]. The PSD is a multiprotein complex that includes a group of proteins called membrane-associated guanylate kinases (MAGUKs) [53, 54]. The MAGUK proteins contain several PDZ (postsynaptic density-95/large/area occludens-1 disks) domains. These domains consist of 80–90 amino acids, which involved in the formation of large protein complexes in cells [57]. One PDZ domain, the PSD-95 (postsynaptic density-95), is involved in the formation of NMDAR complex intracellular signaling proteins and enzymes [53, 54]. The scaffolding of protein PSD-95 causes the translocation of nNOS from cytosol to membrane where it is linked to NMDAR through the complex NMDAR-PSD95-nNOS [58]. In ischemic brain, excessive Ca^{2+} influx through NMDAR activates nNOS, which leads to the production of excessive levels of nitric oxide (NO) [56]. This excessive NO together with the hydrogen peroxide produced from Superoxide dismutase (SOD) enzyme cause the production of the highly reactive free radicals peroxynitrites, which promote cellular damage and ultimately neuron death [59, 60]. Thus, during ischemia, Ca^{2+} influx through NMDARs promotes cell death more efficiently than through other Ca^{2+} channels [61], suggesting that NMDAR ion channel is involved in excitotoxicity. The efficiency by which calcium ions activate excitotoxic signals through molecules such as nNOS can be reduced by disruption of the NMDAR-PSD-95 or nNOS-PSD-95 complexes. Suppression of PSD-95 selectively blocks NO production induced by glutamate in NMDARs without affecting NOS expression in cortical neurons [56]. In experimental animals, the use of small peptides that disrupted the interaction of NMDARs with PSD-95 improves the resistance of neurons to focal cerebral ischemia [62]. The importance of the interaction of NMDAR/PSD-95 complex in cerebral ischemia is reinforced by results showing that the inhibition of binding of PSD-95 with NMDAR prevents ischemic brain damage, while the physiological function of the NMDAR remains intact [63]. In neuron cultures, the block of protein-protein interactions of NMDAR/PSD-95 using small peptides that bind to the PDZ domains of PSD-95 modifying their molecular structure protected neurons from excitotoxicity. When these small peptides are used in rats subjected to transient focal cerebral ischemia, a dramatically reduced cerebral infarction and effectively improved their neurological function in rats was observed. The treatment was effective when applied either before or 1 h after the onset of excitotoxicity both *in vitro* as *in vivo* cerebral ischemia [63]. The vulnerability of neurons to excitotoxicity and ischemia was reduced when the NMDAR/PSD-95 interactions were disturbed using small peptides that comprise the NR2B subunit. Proteomic and biochemical analysis of all the human PDZs examined shows that only neurons lacking PSD-95 or nNOS exhibited reduced excitotoxic vulnerability. Only PSD-95 and nNOS participated significantly in excitotoxicity signaling. Thus, it has been shown that despite the ubiquity of proteins that contain the PDZ domain, PSD-95 and nNOS play a more important role in mediating NMDAR-dependent excitotoxicity than any other PDZ proteins [51, 64].

The consideration of the activation of NMDARs, regardless of whether their participation in excitotoxic mechanisms is based on the type of subunit [42, 50] or by their different location [45, 46], as the main responsible mechanism of the disruption of calcium homeostasis in ischemic neurons is perhaps oversimplistic since others mechanisms may be involved [65]. TRP channels inhibitors reduce calcium entry into neurons exposed to excitotoxicity. Members of the TRP family [66], TRPM7 and TRPM2 are membrane channels that are activated during ischemia and contribute to the rise in intracellular calcium [65, 67]. Also, cerebral ischemia increases the calcium permeability about 18-folds in the AMPA glutamate receptors, contributing to the increase in the cytosol Ca^{2+} levels [68]. Other pathways involved in calcium influx into neurons that contribute to the accumulation of calcium in the cytosol of ischemic neurons include Ca^{2+} entry through gated voltage-channels, Ca^{2+}-permeable acid-sensing ion channels [69], activation of metabotropic glutamate receptors via the release of Ca^{2+} from endoplasmic reticulum, and via a cleavage of Na^{+}/ Ca^{2+} exchangers [70]. These data suggest that the main factor involved in the neuron death in stroke is the disruption of Ca^{2+} homeostasis leading to the accumulation of free cytosolic Ca^{2+} and not the route of entry.

In short, the main effect of excessive extracellular glutamate accumulation on the membrane of the neuron is caused by excessive accumulation of calcium in the cytosol and increased NOS activity leading to an increase in intracellular levels of NO.

4.2. The role of the cytoplasmic calcium overload in excitotoxicity

Calcium plays a critical role in the excitotoxic cascade. Thus, excitotoxic cascade does not occur when the Ca^{2+} is removed from extracellular medium [71] or preventing Ca^{2+} release from mitochondria by uncouplers [72]. It is now widely accepted that disturbance of cellular Ca^{2+} homeostasis is key in the death of neurons following a stroke [61, 64, 73]. It is well established that there is a close relationship between the neuronal damage initiated by the excessive release of glutamate during stroke with an excessive calcium influx into the injured neurons [2, 8, 74]. After ischemia, cytoplasmic Ca^{2+} levels in the ischemic neurons rise to 50–100 μM. Such excessive Ca^{2+} levels can trigger many downstream neurotoxic cascades, including the activation and overstimulation of proteases, lipases, phosphatases, and endonucleases [71, 73, 74]. The results include the activation of several signaling pathways, mainly causing an overproduction of free radicals, mitochondrial damage, cell membrane disruption, and DNA fragmentation, which synergistically cause neuron death [1, 2, 64, 75] (**Figure 2**).

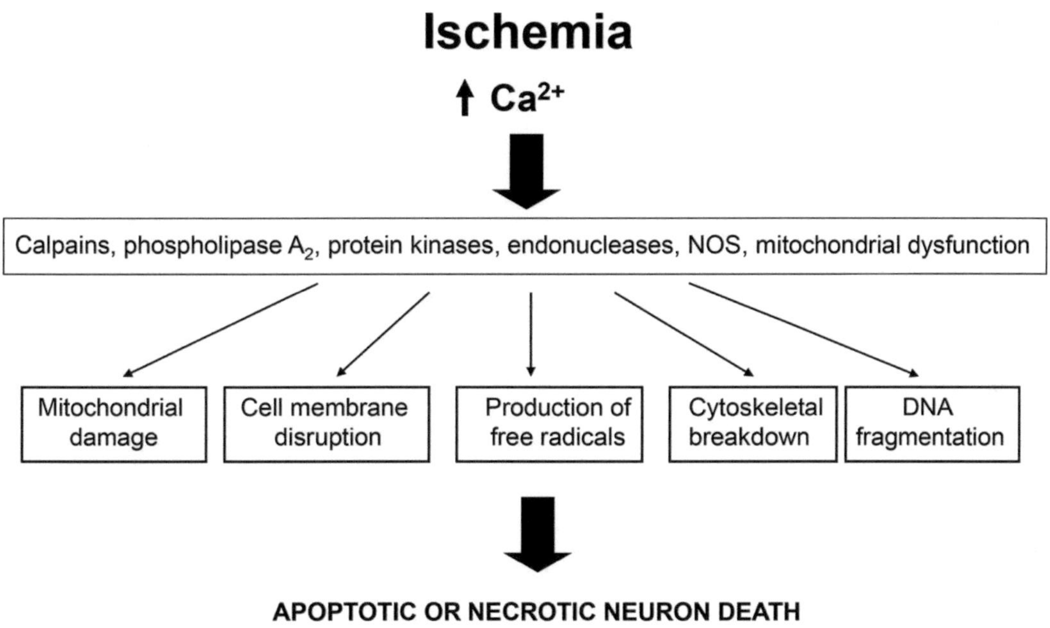

Figure 2. Effects of excessive accumulation of free cytosolic calcium in neurons. Calcium overload induced by excitotoxicity leads to the activation and overstimulation of proteases, lipases, phosphatases, and endonucleases that mainly results in mitochondrial damage, cell membrane disruption, and excessive production of free radicals, which act synergistically causing apoptotic or necrotic neuron death.

4.3. Oxidative stress in acute ischemia damage

Major excitotoxic events promoted by cytoplasmic Ca^{2+} overload due to massively activated glutamate receptors include oxidative/nitrosative stress, calpain activation, and mitochondrial damage, although each of these may individually cause cell death, in ischemia they act synergistically (**Figure 3**).

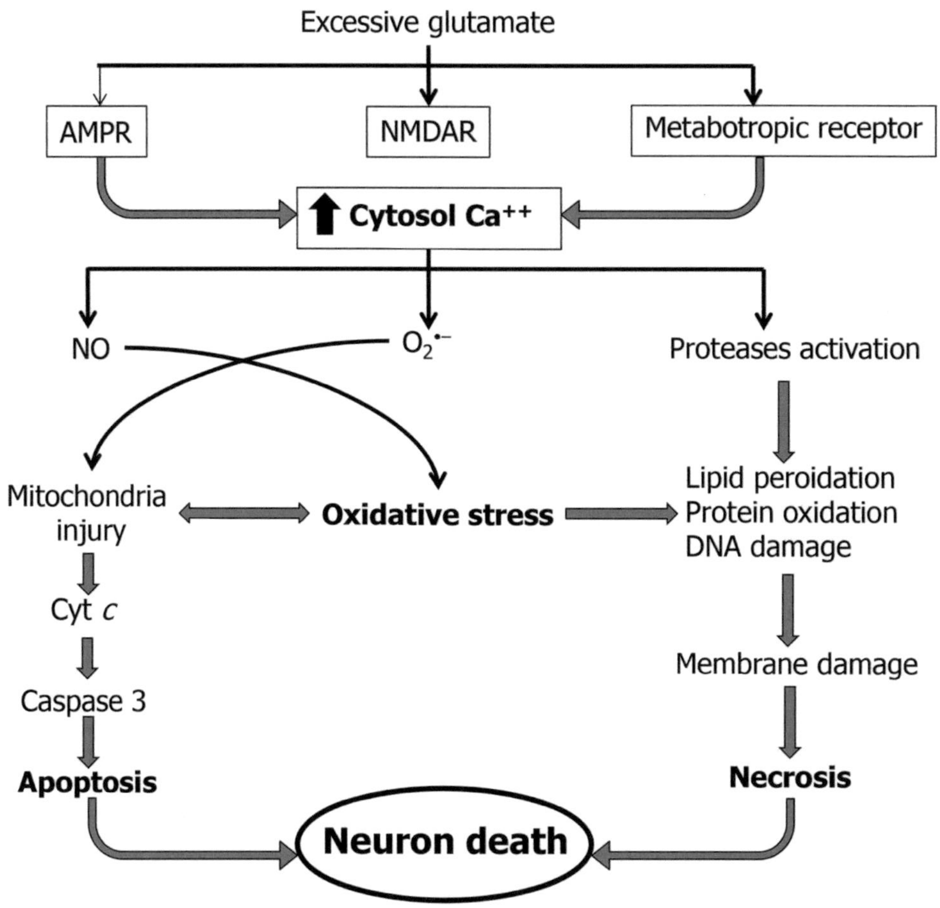

Figure 3. Major cellular mechanisms induced by overstimulation of glutamate receptors in neurons. As a result of excessive activation of glutamate receptors, there is an excessive Ca^{2+} accumulation in the cytosol of neurons leading to oxidative stress and mitochondrial dysfunction. Both situations trigger processes that ultimately cause the death of the neuron.

Oxidative stress is generally defined as an imbalance that favors the production of free radicals over their inactivation by antioxidant defense systems [76, 77]. Oxidative stress describes a condition in which cellular antioxidant defense are insufficient to keep the levels of free radicals below a toxic threshold. This may be either due to excessive production of "free radicals," loss of antioxidant defenses, or both. A "free radical" is any chemical species (atom, molecule) capable of independent existence having one or more unpaired electrons. Free radicals are highly reactive and can directly oxidize and damage macromolecules such as proteins [78], lipids [79], and DNA [80]. Through such interactions, free radicals may irreversibly destroy or alter the function of the target molecule and to worsen the cellular structural architecture and ultimately to cell death. Indirectly, free radicals may also initiate reactions, which may finally lead to neuron death. These reactions include mainly mitochondrial dysfunction [81], cascade apoptotic activation [82], and signal transduction pathways activation [83].

Many lines of evidence demonstrate that free radicals play a pivotal role in excitotoxic death in the brain after stroke [1, 81, 84–86]. The most common free radicals induced by excitotoxicity are molecular derived from oxygen and nitric oxide, called reactive oxygen species (ROS) and reactive nitrogen species (RNS), respectively. Several ROS, including the superoxide radical ($O_2^{\bullet}-$), hydroxyl radical ($OH^{\bullet}$), and certain nonradicals that are either oxidizing agents or easily converted into radicals, such as hydrogen peroxide (H_2O_2) and RNS nitrogen-derived molecules, such as nitric oxide ($NO^{\bullet}$) and peroxynitrite ($ONOO^{-}$), are generated after stroke. Although NO itself is not a radical, it has not been reported that high levels of NO are toxic; however, in the presence of H_2O_2 and $O_2^{\bullet}-$, NO reacts spontaneously leading to the formation of $OH^{\bullet}$ and peroxynitrite acid, which are very cytotoxic.

Although initially free radicals have been identified as major contributors to damage in biological organisms, under physiology conditions free radicals are continuously generated during oxidative metabolism and homeostatic levels are maintained because they play an important role in physiological control of the cell function [87–89]. Intracellular sources of ROS include the mitochondrial electron transport chain (ETC), NADPH oxidases, xanthine oxidase, and arachidonic acid.

Healthy mitochondria use oxygen to generate ATP by oxidative phosphorylation at the mitochondrial respiratory chain. While passing through the mitochondrial electron transport chain, some electrons escape from the mitochondrial ETC, especially from complexes I and III, and react with O_2 to form superoxide anion radicals ($O_2^{\bullet}-$) in the mitochondrial matrix [90–93]. $O_2^{\bullet}-$ is rapidly converted to H_2O_2 either spontaneously, particularly at low pH, or by the superoxide dismutase [90]. In normally respiring (uninhibited) mitochondria, the formation of superoxide and hydrogen peroxide is barely detectable [94–96].

Other important source of ROS is through NADPH oxidase (NOX), an enzyme that uses NADPH to reduce O_2, thus generating large amounts of $O_2^{\bullet}-$. NOX was originally discovered in neutrophils, and subsequently identified in many other cell types including neurons [97]. NOX is a multisubunit complex composed of membrane-associated subunits, cytosolic subunits, and one small rho GTP-binding proteins. In its active form, the NOX transports electrons from NADPH complex in cytosol to the extracellular space. In general, the electron acceptor is oxygen and the product of the electron transfer reaction is $O_2^{\bullet}-$. Thus, overactivation of NOX is a main source of $O_2^{\bullet}-$ in stroke [97]. NOX behaves as an important pro-oxidant enzyme. Protein expression and NOX activity rise after ischemia increasing oxidative stress in the brain tissue in the mice [98]. The postischemic $O_2^{\bullet}-$ generation in neurons was reduced when NOX is inhibited. This reduction of the $O_2^{\bullet}-$ levels due to NOX inhibition was associated with a decrease in the amount of lipid peroxidation or DNA fragmentation [98].

RNS are molecules derived from the nitric oxide ($NO^{\bullet}$). It is now well established that NO is a physiological messenger in the central nervous system and is synthesized by the NO synthase (NOS)-catalyzed reaction [99]. At least three isoforms of NOS have been characterized in brain cells. Neurons produce $NO^{\bullet}$ mainly by Ca^{2+}-dependent activation of neuronal NOS (nNOS or NOS1), which is constitutively expressed in these cells [100]. $NO^{\bullet}$ has a relatively long half-life (approx. 1 s) and whose reactions with biological molecules are slow due to its very rapid diffusion into the blood and consequent removing by reacting with oxyhemoglobin to form nitrate. Along with its important physiological functions, excessive production of $NO^{\bullet}$ is an important pro-oxidant radical because of its ability to combine with $O_2^{\bullet}-$ and H_2O_2 to form $OH^{\bullet}$ and peroxynitrite ($ONOO^{-}$). The latter is readily protonated at cellular pH to peroxynitrous acid (ONOOH), which is very cytotoxic [99, 101].

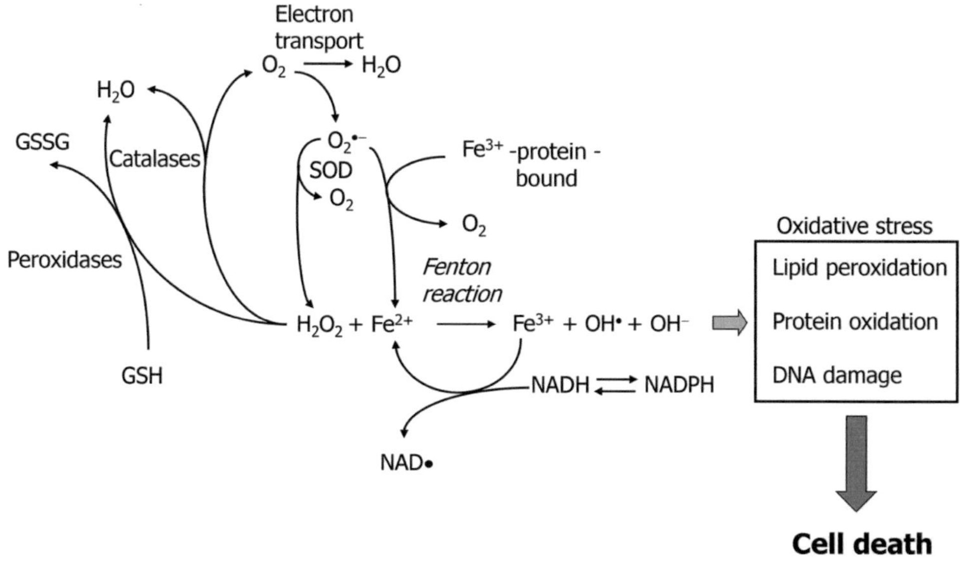

Figure 4. Endogenous antioxidant enzyme systems. Cellular reactions that cause oxidative damage to lipids, proteins, and DNA via Fenton reaction and cell protection by the endogenous antioxidant enzymes principles (SOD, catalases, and peroxidases). Homeostatic level of $O_2^{\bullet}-$ is regulated by SOD isoforms to O_2 and H_2O_2. The latter is a potential source of $OH^{\bullet}$ via Fenton reaction. Catalases and peroxidases regulate the levels of H_2O_2.

To maintain the homeostatic balance and cope with the continuous production of free radicals, cells are equipped with a sophisticated system of enzymes and nonenzymatic antioxidants [76]. Enzymatic components mainly comprise superoxide dismutase (SOD) [102] that converts $O_2^{\bullet}-$ to H_2O_2, the catalase [67] that converts H_2O_2 to H_2O and O_2, and the glutathione peroxidases (GPX) that converts H_2O_2 to H_2O in a reaction that oxidizes glutathione (GSH) to its disulphide form (GSSG). In turn, GSH is regenerated from GSSG by glutathione reductase [103, 104] (**Figure 4**). Also, small molecular nonenzymatic antioxidants, including ascorbic acid, pyruvate, α-tocopherol, and glutathione (GSH), are important in the detoxification of free radicals, provision of antioxidant defense, and prevention of tissue damage [76, 77]. The cell can also combat oxidative stress by regulating ROS generation by eliminating ROS with the help of neutralizing enzymes and scavenger molecules [105], and by repairing those lipids, proteins, or DNA that have been affected by oxidative stress [106].

Oxidative stress induced by excitotoxicity is considered the main event leading to brain damage after cerebral ischemia [73, 81, 82, 107]. Several lines of research indicate that oxidative stress is a primary mediator of neurologic injury following cerebral ischemia [84, 85, 107]. After cerebral ischemia and particularly reperfusion, robust oxidants are generated including superoxide and hydroxyl radicals, which overwhelm endogenous scavenging mechanisms

[108, 109] and are directly involved in the damage of cellular macromolecules, such as lipids, proteins, and nucleic acids, eventually leading to cell death [1, 2, 110] (**Figure 5**). Reperfusion provides oxygen to sustain neuronal viability and also as a substrate for numerous enzymatic oxidation reactions that produce reactive oxidants. During reperfusion to the vessel, oxygen replenished is crucial for neuron survival in the ischemic tissue. However, oxygen can also be used by the mitochondria and by pro-oxidant enzymes to produce more free radicals. The presence of a situation of oxidative stress in the perfused ischemic brain tissue results in several detrimental processes, including overproduction of oxygen radicals, and consumption and failure to adequately replenish the antioxidant systems [108–110].

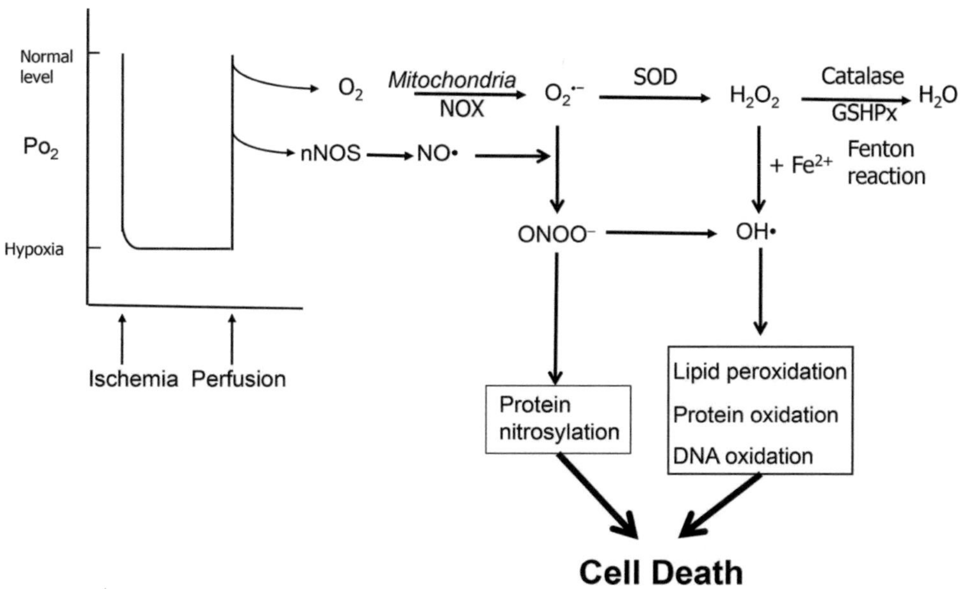

Figure 5. Major sources of ROS and RNS and antioxidant systems during cerebral ischemia and reperfusion. Generated reactive oxygen species by mitochondria and reactive nitrogen species by nitric oxide synthase. SOD converts superoxide radical to H_2O_2 which is converted to H_2O by catalase or GSHPx. Formation of peroxynitrite ($ONOO^-$) and subsequent hydroxyl radical production can directly damage lipids, proteins, and DNA and lead to cell death.

During the ischemic phase, some Ca^{2+}-dependent enzymes, such as phospholipase A_2 (PLA_2) and cyclooxygenase (COX), produce oxygen-free radicals. The activation of PLA_2 by Ca^{2+} results in the generation of arachidonic acid from the phospholipids, which are metabolized by cyclooxygenase to thromboxane and leukotrienes. Both eicosanoids activate NOX and thus contribute to increased free radical formation [111]. COX induces the prostaglandin PGG_2 production from arachidonic acid, which in turn is rapidly peroxidized to PGH_2 with a simultaneous release of $O_2^{\bullet-}$. In the ischemic tissue, activation of PLA_2 and cyclooxygenase generates free radical species, which contribute to lipid peroxidation and membrane damage [111]. However, mitochondrial dysfunction and NOX as sources of RNS are considered the main source of free radical production causing oxidative stress during ischemia/perfusion [107, 112].

4.4. The role of calpains in excitotoxicity

It is now well established that the induced Ca^{2+} overload in neurons after ischemia causes a massive activation of calpains, proteins belonging to the family of calcium-dependent, cysteine proteases, which contribute to excitotoxic cell death [47]. All calpains can act in two modes: under physiological conditions they undergo controlled activation (involving only a few molecules of calpain), whereas during sustained calcium overload under pathological conditions they undergo hyperactivation (involving all the available calpain molecules) [47]. Calpains in the CNS play an important role in the synaptic function and memory formation [47]. In models of stroke in animals, the use of Ca^{2+}-dependent calpain protease inhibitors showed neuroprotective effect [113, 114]. The main mechanism by which calpains contribute to excitotoxic damage is by their ability to cleavage the Na^{+}/Ca^{2+} exchangers (NCX), which is critical to regulate the concentration of calcium into neurons [115]. Thus, calpains contribute to the accumulation of calcium during ischemia [70, 116].

4.5. Mitochondrial dysfunction

The excitotoxicity can contribute to neuron death by altering the functions of mitochondria. Mitochondrial disturbance is the result of both oxidative-nitrosative stress and a direct effect of excessive Ca^{2+} intracellular levels [75, 117, 118]. In ischemia, the excess of cytosolic-free Ca^{2+} caused by overstimulation of glutamate receptors may overload the mitochondrial proton circuit, which leads to the failure in oxidation and an increase in ROS into mitochondria [81, 91]. In mitochondria, surpassed antioxidant protection and oxidative stress ROS can lead to

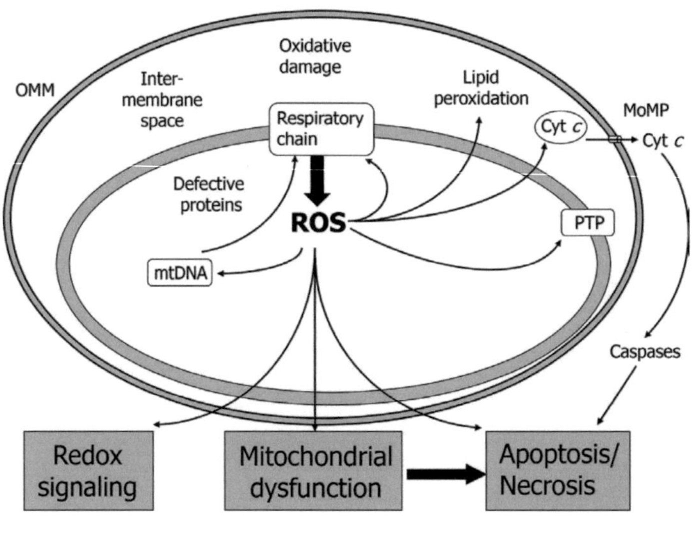

Figure 6. Excessive ROS production by mitochondria leads to direct oxidative damage of mitochondrial proteins, membranes, and DNA, causing mitochondrial dysfunction and finally death neuron by apoptosis or necrosis. Excessive ROS within mitochondria can also induce changes in the mitochondrial permeability transition pore mPTP, which renders the inner membrane permeable to small molecules including cytochrome *c* (cyt *c*). Activation of proapoptotic proteins Bcl-2 produces a pore in the outer membrane of mitochondria that allows the release of cytochrome *c* to the cytosol where it triggers the apoptotic cascade of caspases (modified from Ref. [91]).

oxidative damage to mitochondrial proteins, membranes, and DNA, impairing the ability of mitochondria to synthesize ATP and to carry out their wide range of metabolic functions. Mitochondrial oxidative damage can also enhance the release of proteins located in the mitochondrial inner membrane, including cytochrome *c*, to the intermembrane space. Activation of proapoptotic proteins Bcl-2 enhance the formation of permeability pore in the outer membrane of mitochondria that allows the release of cytochrome *c* to the cytosol where it activates the apoptotic machinery of the cell [91] (**Figure 6**).

During stroke, electron microscope analyses show that Ca^{2+} accumulates in mitochondria very soon after global ischemia and this state persists for several hours [119]. Two events seem to play an important role in the death of neurons in the brain stroke due to the mitochondrial dysfunction induced by the cytosol-free Ca^{2+} accumulation: The oxidative stress due to antioxidant/pro-oxidant imbalance in favor of the second [107, 112], and the activation of the intrinsic apoptotic pathway of caspases [120, 121].

5. Apoptosis

In stroke, neuron death is the result of apoptosis or necrosis [82, 122]. That neuronal death occurs by one or another mechanism depending mainly on the time elapse since the onset of stroke, the severity of blood flow reduction, and the level of metabolic activity that produce the energy in the neuron.

Neuronal cell death by necrosis occurs mainly when the decrease or absence of blood flow implies a severe deficit or absence of oxygen and glucose (OGD) in ischemic brain area and leads to the formation of the ischemic core [20, 21, 123]. Death of neurons by apoptosis occurs mainly in ischemic areas when the existence of a certain level of blood flow provides insufficient oxygen and glucose to maintain the functional activity in the neuron but sufficient to maintain the survival of neurons and leads to the formation of ischemic penumbra. If the blood flow is not restored in this area, excitotoxicity may induce neuronal death by apoptosis [120].

Apoptosis is one of the fundamental mechanisms of cell death that occur during ischemic brain injury [2, 120, 124]. There are two general pathways for activation of apoptosis: the "extrinsic apoptosis," initiated by the ligation of cell surface death receptors such as tumor necrosis factor receptors and FAS receptor, and "intrinsic/mitochondrial apoptosis" pathways [125]. The mitochondrial dysfunction plays a central role in the apoptotic pathway in stroke [120, 126, 127]. Studies of tissue from patients and of animal models have shown that mitochondria-mediated apoptosis is the mode by which many neurons die after an acute stroke [121, 127]. Oxidative stress and cytotoxic accumulation of intracellular Ca^{2+} initiate a series of cytoplasmic and cellular events, including the triggering of the intrinsic apoptotic pathway [2, 34, 115, 121]. Increased ROS/RNS and intracellular-free Ca^{2+} levels mediate induction/activation of proapoptotic proteins leading to changes in the mitochondrial membrane permeability (MMP) [128]. The family Bcl-2 proteins determine the integrity of mitochondria in the face of apoptotic insult [127]. The complex interplay between Bcl-2 proteins regulates the integrity of the mitochondrial outer membrane. Thus, the mitochondrial integrity may be protected by antiapoptotic members of the Bcl-2 family (Bcl-2 and Bcl-xl) together with antiapoptotic kinases Akt and ERK, which inhibit the proapoptotic members of the Bcl-2 family (Bid, Bim, Bax, Bak, and Bad). In cerebral ischemia, proapoptotic stimuli activate the intrinsic apoptotic pathway breaking the antiapoptotic/proapoptotic balance leading to mitochondrial network damage in the neuron [127, 129].

Two members of Bcl-2 family, Bcl-2-associated X protein (BAX) or Bcl-2-associated killer (BAK) seem crucial to cell death. Without them, cells are resistant to majority of apoptotic stimuli [130]. BAX is a cytosolic protein that actively translocates to the mitochondrial outer membrane during apoptosis to participate in membrane damage while that BAK is constitutively expressed at the mitochondrial outer membrane [131]. More recent studies propose that BAX is actively trafficked to the cytosol, a process termed "retrotranslocation" [132, 133]. A differential mitochondrial retrotranslocation has also been proposed by BAK [134].

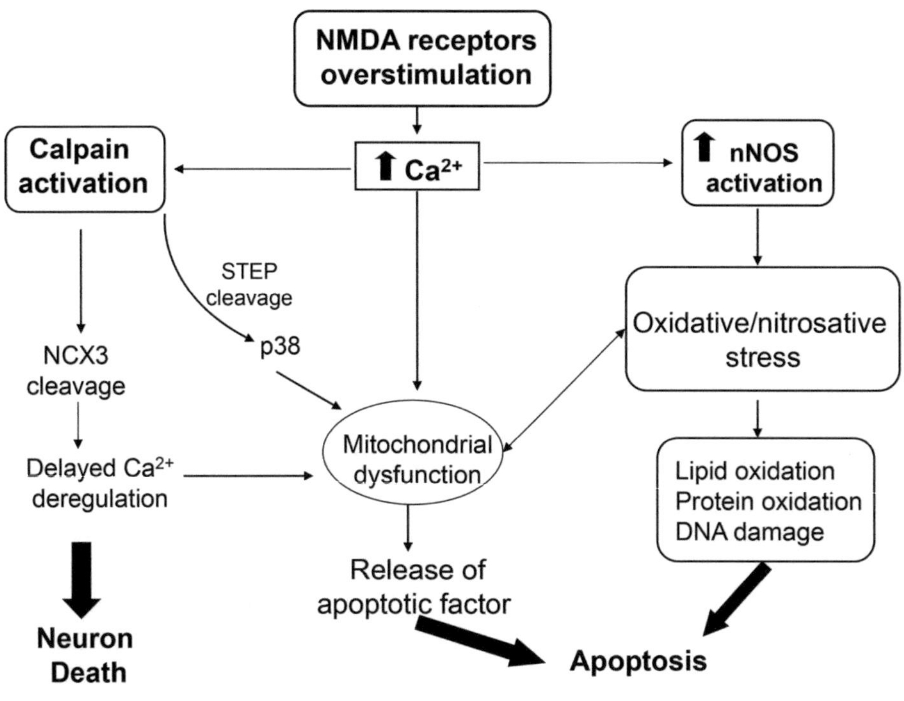

Figure 7. Schematic overview of excitotoxic events during ischemic stroke in the neurons. Overstimulation of NMDAR by glutamate causes excessive increase in calcium concentration in the cytosol. Disruption of intracellular calcium homeostasis leads to calpain and nNOS activation, and mitochondrial dysfunction. Activation of these mechanisms causes a state of oxidative stress. The presence of excess ROS and RNS directly damages essential macromolecules of the cell membrane and otherwise contribute to produce mitochondrial dysfunction. This, in turn, leads to increase oxidative stress and trigger the chain apoptotic events causing neuronal death and contribute to ischemic brain damage.

One of the decisive steps of the apoptotic cascade involves the mitochondrial permeability transition pores (mPTPs) [135, 136]. Under oxidative stress conditions, transient opening of mPTPs in the mitochondrial inner membrane produces the fall of the mitochondrial transmembrane potential and elicits the release of cytochrome *c* as well as other proapoptotic molecules that together initiate the apoptotic cascade. Once released into the cytosol from the mitochondrial intermembrane space, cytochrome *c* binds with apoptotic protease-activating factor-1 (Apaf-1) and procaspase-9 to form an "apoptosome," which actives caspase-9 and subsequently caspase-3. There is a large body of evidence suggesting that cerebral ischemia can cause activation of aspartate-specific proteases, the caspases, which can cleave a larger number of cellular substrates [120, 121]. Caspases are cysteine proteases constitutively presents in cells as zymogens and require proteolytic cleavage into the catalytic active heterodimer. Inhibiting the activation of caspases suppresses the ability of cells to undergo apoptosis or causes a switch from apoptosis to necrosis [137]. Upregulation and activation of caspase-3 have been found to precede neuron death in focal and global cerebral ischemia [120]. Activated caspase-3 cleavage the endonuclease inhibitor ICAD freeing CAD (caspase-activated DNAase), which can cleave the nuclear DNA causing DNA damage and the neuron death [138].

In summary, numerous studies report the important involvement of excitotoxicity and oxidative stress in the complex processes that cause neuronal death in acute ischemic stroke [139]. The hypoxia and the low glucose levels caused by the blood flow reduction in the penumbra zone lead to oxidative stress and excessive release of glutamate. Oxidative stress can cause death of neurons by oxidation of structural macromolecules of the membranes, such as lipids and proteins, and DNA. Mediated by NMDA receptor and by the homeostasis calcium deregulation, excitotoxicity contributes not only to injury of neuron death, but also to transduction of apoptotic signals. Mitochondrial dysfunctions occur as a consequence of cerebral ischemia and promote ischemia-induced neuronal cell death, especially by apoptotic intrinsic pathway (**Figure 7**).

Acknowledgements

This chapter builds upon and is partly reproduced from [139].

Author details

Ramon Rama[1*] and Julio César García[2]

*Address all correspondence to: rrama@ub.edu

1 Department of Cellular Biology, Physiology and Immunology, University of Barcelona, Spain

2 Havana Medical University, La Habana, Cuba

References

[1] Dirnagl U, Iadecola C, Moskowitz MA. Pathobiology of ischaemic stroke: an integrated view. Trends Neurosci 1999; 22: 391–397.

[2] Lo EH, Dalkara T, Moskowitz MA. Mechanisms, challenges and opportunities in stroke. Nat Rev Neurosci 2003; 4: 399–415.

[3] Kidwell CS, Alger JR, Saver JL. Evolving paradigms in neuroimaging of the ischemic penumbra. Stroke 2004; 35: 2662–2665.

[4] Martin RL, Lloyd HGE, Cowan AI. The early events of oxygen and glucose deprivation: setting the scene for neuronal death? Trends Neurosci 1994; 17: 251–257.

[5] Hossmann K-A. The two pathophysiologies of focal brain ischemia: implications for translational stroke research. J Cereb Blood Flow Metab 2012; 32: 1310–1316.

[6] Astrup J, Siesjö BK, Symon L. Thresholds in cerebral ischemia — the ischemic penumbra. Stroke 1979; 12: 723–725.

[7] Del Zoppo GJ, Sharp FR, Heiss W-D, et al. Heterogeneity in the penumbra. J Cereb Blood Flow Metab 2011; 31: 1836–1851.

[8] Moskowitz MA, Lo EH, Iadecola C. The science of stroke: mechanisms in search of treatments. Neuron 2010; 67: 181–198.

[9] Woodruff TM, Thundyil J, Tang S-C, et al. Pathophysiology, treatment, and animal and cellular models of human ischemic stroke. Mol Neurodegener 2011; 6: 11.

[10] Lipton P. Ischemic cell death in brain neurons. Physiol Rev 1999; 79: 1431–1568.

[11] Heiss WD, Sobesky J, Hesselmann V. Identifying thresholds for penumbra and irreversible tissue damage. Stroke 2004; 35: 2671–2674.

[12] Erecińska M, Silver IA. Tissue oxygen tension and brain sensitivity to hypoxia. Respir Physiol 2001; 128: 263–276.

[13] Zauner A, Daugherty WP, Bullock MR, et al. Brain oxygenation and energy metabolism: Part I—Biological function and pathophysiology. Neurosurgery 2002; 51: 289–302.

[14] Raichle ME, Mintun MA. Brain work and brain imaging. Annu Rev Neurosci 2006; 29: 449–476.

[15] Magistretti PJ, Chatton JY. Relationship between L-glutamate-regulated intracellular Na+ dynamics and ATP hydrolysis in astrocytes. J Neural Transm 2005; 112: 77–85.

[16] Fünfschilling U, Supplie LM, Mahad D, et al. Glycolytic oligodendrocytes maintain myelin and long-term axonal integrity. Nature 2012; 485: 517–521.

[17] Marder E, Goaillard J-M. Variability, compensation and homeostasis in neuron and network function. Nat Rev 2006; 7: 563–574.

[18] Locasale JW, Cantley LC. Metabolic flux and the regulation of mammalian cell growth. Cell Metabol 2011; 14: 443–451.

[19] Lo EH. A new penumbra: transitioning from injury into repair after stroke. Nat Med 2008; 14: 497–500.

[20] Nicotera P, Leist M, Manzo L. Neuronal cell death: a demise with different shapes. Trends Pharmacol Sci 1999; 20: 46–51.

[21] Ünal-Çevik I, Kilinç M, Can A, et al. Apoptotic and necrotic death mechanisms are concomitantly activated in the same cell after cerebral ischemia. Stroke 2004; 35: 2189–2194.

[22] Rossi DJ, Oshima T, Attwell D. Glutamate release in severe brain ischaemia is mainly by reversed uptake. Nature 2000; 403: 316–321.

[23] Camacho A, Massieu L. Role of glutamate transporters in the clearance and release of glutamate during ischemia and its relation to neuronal death. Archives Med Res 2006; 37: 11–18.

[24] Olney JW. Brain lesions, obesity, and other disturbances in mice treated with monosodium glutamate. Science 1969; 164: 719–721.

[25] Choi DW. Glutamate neurotoxicity and diseases of the nervous system. Neuron 1988; 1: 623–634.

[26] Dong X, Wang Y, Qin Z. Molecular mechanisms of excitotoxicity and their relevance to pathogenesis of neurodegenerative diseases. Acta Pharmacol Sin 2009; 30: 379–387.

[27] Lai TW, Zhang S, Wang YT. Excitotoxicity and stroke: identifying novel targets for neuroprotection. Prog Neurobiol 2014; 115: 157–188. DOI: 10.1016/j.pneurobio.2013.11.006.

[28] Kritis AA, Stamoula EG, Paniskaki KA, et al. Researching glutamate - induced cytotoxicity in different cell lines: a comparative/collective analysis/study. Front Cell Neurosci 2015; 9: 91.

[29] Rothman SM, Olney JW. Glutamate and the pathophysiology of hypoxic–ischemic brain damage. Ann Neurol 1986; 19: 105–111.

[30] Choi DW, Rothman SM. The role of glutamate neurotoxicity in hypoxic-ischemic neuronal death. Annu Rev Neurosci 1990; 13: 171–182.

[31] Hazell AS. Excitotoxic mechanisms in stroke: an update of concepts and treatment strategies. Neurochem Int 2007; 50: 941–953.

[32] Choi DW. Glutamate neurotoxicity in cortical cell culture is calcium dependent. Neurosci Lett 1985; 58: 293–297.

[33] Garthwaite G, Garthwaite J. Neurotoxicity of excitatory amino acid receptor agonists in rat cerebellar slices: dependence on calcium concentration. Neurosci Lett 1986; 66: 193–198.

[34] Berliocchi L, Bano D, Nicotera P. Ca2+ signals and death programmes in neurons. Philos Trans R Soc Lond B Biol Sci 2005; 360: 2255–2258.

[35] Nakanishi S. Molecular diversity of glutamate receptors and implications for brain function. Science 1992; 258: 597–603.

[36] Waxman EA, Lynch DR. N-methyl-D-aspartate receptor subtypes: multiple roles in excitotoxicity and neurological disease. Neuroscientist 2005; 11: 37–49.

[37] Madden DR. The structure and function of glutamate receptor ion channels. Nat Rev Neurosci 2002; 3: 91–101.

[38] Paoletti P, Neyton J. NMDA receptor subunits: function and pharmacology. Curr Opin Pharmacol 2007; 7: 39–47.

[39] Clements JD, Westbrook GL. Activation kinetics reveal the number of glutamate and glycine binding sites on the N-methyl-D-aspartate receptor. Neuron 1991; 7: 605–613.

[40] Lynch DR, Guttmann RP. NMDA receptor pharmacology: perspectives from molecular biology. Curr Drug Targets 2001; 2: 215–231.

[41] Furukawa H, Singh SK, Mancusso R, et al. Subunit arrangement and function in NMDA receptors. Nature 2005; 438: 185–192.

[42] Liu Y, Wong TP, Aarts M, et al. Neurobiology of disease NMDA receptor subunits have differential roles in mediating excitotoxic neuronal death both in vitro and in vivo. J Neurosci 2007; 27: 2846–2857.

[43] Chen M, Lu T-J, Chen X-J, et al. Differential roles of NMDA receptor subtypes in ischemic neuronal cell death and ischemic tolerance. Stroke 2008; 39: 3042–3048.

[44] Zhou M, Baudry M. Developmental changes in NMDA neurotoxicity reflect developmental changes in subunit composition of NMDA receptors. J Neurosci 2006; 26: 2956–2963.

[45] Sattler R, Xiong Z, Lu WY, et al. Distinct roles of synaptic and extrasynaptic NMDA receptors in excitotoxicity. J Neurosci 2000; 20: 22–33.

[46] Hardingham GE, Bading H. Synaptic versus extrasynaptic NMDA receptor signalling: implications for neurodegenerative disorders. Nat Rev Neurosci 2010; 11: 682–696.

[47] Liu J, Liu MC, Wang KKW. Calpain in the CNS: from synaptic function to neurotoxicity. Sci Signal 2008; 1: 1–7.

[48] Léveillé F, El Gaamouch F, Gouix E, et al. Neuronal viability is controlled by a functional relation between synaptic and extrasynaptic NMDA receptors. FASEB J 2008; 22: 4258–4271.

[49] Martel MA, Wyllie DJA, Hardingham GE. In developing hippocampal neurons, NR2B-containing N-methyl-d-aspartate receptors (NMDARs) can mediate signaling to neuronal survival and synaptic potentiation, as well as neuronal death. Neuroscience 2009; 158: 334–343.

[50] Tu W, Xu X, Peng L, et al. DAPK1 interaction with NMDA receptor NR2B subunits mediates brain damage in stroke. Cell 2010; 140: 222–234.

[51] von Engelhardt J, Coserea I, Pawlak V, et al. Excitotoxicity in vitro by NR2A- and NR2B-containing NMDA receptors. Neuropharmacology 2007; 53: 10–17.

[52] Stanika RI, Pivovarova NB, Brantner CA, et al. Coupling diverse routes of calcium entry to mitochondrial dysfunction and glutamate excitotoxicity. Proc Natl Acad Sci U S A 2009; 106: 9854–9859.

[53] Kornau H-C, Schenker LT, Kennedy MB, et al. Domain interaction between NMDA receptor subunits and the postsynaptic density protein PSD-95. Source Sci New Ser 1995; 269: 1737–1740.

[54] Niethammer M, Kim E, Sheng M. Interaction between the C terminus of NMDA receptor subunits and multiple members of the PSD-95 family of membrane-associated guanylate kinases. J Neurosci 1996; 16: 2157–2163.

[55] Sattler R, Charlton MP, Hafner M, et al. Distinct influx pathways, not calcium load, determine neuronal vulnerability to calcium neurotoxicity. J Neurochem 1998; 71: 2349–2364.

[56] Sattler R, Xiong Z, Lu WY, et al. Specific coupling of NMDA receptor activation to nitric oxide neurotoxicity by PSD-95 protein. Science 1999; 284: 1845–1848.

[57] Kim E, Sheng M. PDZ domain proteins of synapses. Nat Rev Neurosci 2004; 5: 771–781.

[58] Brenman JE, Chao DS, Gee SH, et al. Interaction of nitric oxide synthase with the postsynaptic density protein PSD-95 and α1-syntrophin mediated by PDZ domains. Cell 1996; 84: 757–767.

[59] Iadecola C. Bright and dark sides of nitric oxide in ischemic brain injury. Trends Neurosci 1997; 20: 132–139.

[60] Bolaños JP, Almeida A. Roles of nitric oxide in brain hypoxia-ischemia. Biochim Biophys Acta - Bioenerg 1999; 1411: 415–436.

[61] Arundine M, Tymianski M. Molecular mechanisms of calcium-dependent neurodegeneration in excitotoxicity. Cell Calcium 2003; 34: 325–337.

[62] Aarts M, Liu Y, Li L. Treatment of ischemic brain damage by perturbing NMDA receptor-PSD-95 protein interactions. Science 2002; 298: 846–850.

[63] Sun HS, Doucette TA, Liu Y, et al. Effectiveness of PSD95 inhibitors in permanent and transient focal ischemia in the rat. Stroke 2008; 39: 2544–2553.

[64] Szydlowska K, Tymianski M. Calcium, ischemia and excitotoxicity. Cell Calcium 2010; 47: 122–129.

[65] Tymianski M. Emerging mechanisms of disrupted cellular signaling in brain ischemia. Nat Neurosci 2011; 14: 1369–1373.

[66] Venkatachalam K, Montell C. TRP channels. Annu Rev Biochem 2007; 76: 387–417.

[67] Nazıroğlu M. Molecular role of catalase on oxidative stress-induced Ca(2+) signaling and TRP cation channel activation in nervous system. J Recept Signal Transduct Res 2012; 32: 134–141.

[68] Formisano L, Saggese M, Secondo A, et al. The two isoforms of the Na +/Ca2+ exchanger, NCX1 and NCX3, constitute novel additional targets for the prosurvival action of Akt/protein kinase B pathway. Mol Pharmacol 2008; 73: 727–737.

[69] Xiong ZG, Zhu XM, Chu XP, et al. Neuroprotection in ischemia: blocking calcium-permeable acid-sensing ion channels. Cell 2004; 118: 687–698.

[70] Bano D, Young KW, Guerin CJ, et al. Cleavage of the plasma membrane Na+/Ca2+ exchanger in excitotoxicity. Cell 2005; 120: 275–285.

[71] Sattler R, Tymianski M. Molecular mechanisms of calcium-dependent excitotoxicity. J Mol Med (Berl) 2000; 78: 3–13.

[72] Stout AK, Raphael HM, Kanterewicz BI, et al. Glutamate-induced neuron death requires mitochondrial calcium uptake. Nat Neurosci 1998; 1: 366–373.

[73] Siesjo BK, Zhao Q, Pahlmark K, et al. Glutamate, calcium, and free radicals as mediators of ischemic brain damage. Ann Thorac Surg 1995; 59: 1316–1320.

[74] Orrenius S, Zhivotovsky B, Nicotera P. Regulation of cell death: the calcium-apoptosis link. Nat Rev Mol Cell Biol 2003; 4: 552–565.

[75] Nicholls DG. Mitochondrial calcium function and dysfunction in the central nervous system. Biochim Biophys Acta 2009; 1787: 1416–1424.

[76] Yu BP. Cellular defenses against damage from reactive oxygen species. Physiol Rev 1994; 74: 139–162.

[77] Halliwell B. Oxidative stress and neurodegeneration: where are we now? J Neurochem 2006; 97: 1634–1658.

[78] Berlett BS, Stadtman ER. Protein oxidation in aging, disease, and oxidative stress. J Biol Chem 1997; 272: 20313–20316.

[79] Sakamoto A, Ohnishi ST, Ohnishi T, et al. Relationship between free radical production and lipid peroxidation during ischemia-reperfusion injury in the rat brain. Brain Res 1991; 554: 186–192.

[80] Cui J, Holmes EH, Greene TG, et al. Oxidative DNA damage precedes DNA fragmentation after experimental stroke in rat brain. FASEB J 2000; 14: 955–967.

[81] Lin MT, Beal MF. Mitochondrial dysfunction and oxidative stress in neurodegenerative diseases. Nature 2006; 443: 787–795.

[82] Chen H, Yoshioka H, Kim GS, et al. Oxidative stress in ischemic brain damage: mechanisms of cell death and potential molecular targets for neuroprotection. Antioxid Redox Signal 2011; 14: 1505–1517.

[83] Ferrer I, Planas AM. Signaling of cell death and cell survival following focal cerebral ischemia: life and death struggle in the penumbra. J Neuropathol Exp Neurol 2003; 62: 329–339.

[84] Chan PH. Reactive oxygen radicals in signaling and damage in the ischemic brain. J Cereb Blood Flow Metab 2001; 21: 2–14.

[85] Sugawara T, Chan PH. Reactive oxygen radicals and pathogenesis of neuronal death after cerebral ischemia. Antioxid Redox Signal 2003; 5: 597–607.

[86] Valko M, Leibfritz D, Moncol J, et al. Free radicals and antioxidants in normal physiological functions and human disease. Int J Biochem Cell Biol 2007; 39: 44–84.

[87] Droge W. Free radicals in the physiological control of cell function. Physiol Rev 2002; 82: 47–95.

[88] Nathan C. Specificity of a third kind: Reactive oxygen and nitrogen intermediates in cell signaling. J Clin Investig 2003; 111: 769–778.

[89] D'Autréaux B, Toledano MB. ROS as signalling molecules: mechanisms that generate specificity in ROS homeostasis. Nat Rev Mol Cell Biol 2007; 8: 813–824.

[90] Turrens JF. Superoxide production by the mitochondrial respiratory chain. Biosci Rep 1997; 17: 3–8.

[91] Murphy MP. How mitochondria produce reactive oxygen species. Biochem J 2009; 417: 1–13.

[92] Drose S, Brandt U. Molecular mechanisms of superoxide production by the mitochondrial respiratory chain. Adv Exp Med Biol 2012; 748: 145–169.

[93] Lenaz G. Mitochondria and reactive oxygen species. Which role in physiology and pathology? Adv Exp Med Biol 2012; 942: 93–136.

[94] Staniek K, Nohl H. Are mitochondria a permanent source of reactive oxygen species? Biochim Biophys Acta—Bioenerg 2000; 1460: 268–275.

[95] St-Pierre J, Buckingham JA, Roebuck SJ, et al. Topology of superoxide production from different sites in the mitochondrial electron transport chain. J Biol Chem 2002; 277: 44784–44790.

[96] Andreyev AY, Kushnareva YE, Starkov AA. Mitochondrial metabolism of reactive oxygen species. Biochemistry (Mosc) 2005; 70: 200–214.

[97] Bedard K, Krause K-H. The NOX family of ROS-generating NADPH oxidases: physiology and pathophysiology. Physiol Rev 2007; 87: 245–313.

[98] Chen H, Song YS, Chan PH. Inhibition of NADPH oxidase is neuroprotective after ischemia-reperfusion. J Cereb Blood Flow Metab 2009; 29: 1262–1272.

[99] Pacher P, Beckman JS, Liaudet L. Nitric oxide and peroxynitrite in health and disease. Physiol Rev 2007; 87: 315–424.

[100] Knowles RG, Moncada S. Nitric oxide synthases in mammals. Biochem J 1994; 298: 249–258.

[101] Moncada S, Bolaños JP. Nitric oxide, cell bioenergetics and neurodegeneration. J Neurochem 2006; 97: 1676–1689.

[102] Fridovich I. Superoxide anion radical, superoxide dismutases, and related matters. J Biol Chem 1997; 272: 18515–18517.

[103] Dringen R, Gutterer JM, Hirrlinger J. Glutathione metabolism in brain: metabolic interaction between astrocytes and neurons in the defense against reactive oxygen species. Eur J Biochem 2000; 267: 4912–4916.

[104] Rhee SG, Kang SW, Jeong W, et al. Intracellular messenger function of hydrogen peroxide and its regulation by peroxiredoxins. Curr Opin Cell Biol 2005; 17: 183–189.

[105] Watson SN, Nelson MA, Wildering WC. Redox agents modulate neuronal activity and reproduce physiological aspects of neuronal aging. Neurobiol Aging 2012; 33: 149–161.

[106] Liu D, Croteau DL, Souza-Pinto N, et al. Evidence that OGG1 glycosylase protects neurons against oxidative DNA damage and cell death under ischemic conditions. J Cereb Blood Flow Metab 2011; 31: 680–692.

[107] Niizuma K, Endo H, Chan PH. Oxidative stress and mitochondrial dysfunction as determinants of ischemic neuronal death and survival. J Neurochem 2009; 109 Suppl : 133–138.

[108] Nakashima M, Niwa M, Iwai T, et al. Involvement of free radicals in cerebral vascular reperfusion injury evaluated in a transient focal cerebral ischemia model of rat. Free Radic Biol Med 1999; 26: 722–729.

[109] Schaller B, Graf R. Cerebral ischemia and reperfusion: the pathophysiologic concept as a basis for clinical therapy. J Cereb Blood Flow Metab 2004; 24: 351–371.

[110] Granger DN, Kvietys PR. Reperfusion injury and reactive oxygen species: the evolution of a concept. Redox Biol 2015; 6: 524–551.

[111] Muralikrishna AR, Hatcher JF. Phospholipase A2, reactive oxygen species, and lipid peroxidation in cerebral ischemia. Free Radic Biol Med 2006; 40: 376–387.

[112] Piantadosi CA, Zhang J. Mitochondrial generation of reactive oxygen species after brain ischemia in the rat. Stroke 1996; 27: 327–332.

[113] Rami A, Ferger D, Krieglstein J. Blockade of calpain proteolytic activity rescues neurons from glutamate excitotoxicity. Neurosci Res 1997; 27: 93–97.

[114] Ray SK. Currently evaluated calpain and caspase inhibitors for neuroprotection in experimental brain ischemia. Curr Med Chem 2006; 13: 3425–3440.

[115] Bano D, Nicotera P. Ca2+ signals and neuronal death in brain ischemia. Stroke 2007; 38: 674–676.

[116] Pignataro G, Gala R, Cuomo O, et al. Two sodium/calcium exchanger gene products, NCX1 and NCX3, play a major role in the development of permanent focal cerebral ischemia. Stroke 2004; 35: 2566–2570.

[117] Schinder AF, Olson EC, Spitzer NC, et al. Mitochondrial dysfunction is a primary event in glutamate neurotoxicity. J Neurosci 1996; 16: 6125–6133.

[118] Duchen MR. Mitochondria, calcium-dependent neuronal death and neurodegenerative disease. Pflugers Archiv Eur J Physiol 2012; 464: 111–121.

[119] Zaidan E, Sims NR. The calcium content of mitochondria from brain subregions following short-term forebrain ischemia and recirculation in the rat. J Neurochem 1994; 63: 1812–1819.

[120] Broughton BRS, Reutens DC, Sobey CG. Apoptotic mechanisms after cerebral ischemia. Stroke 2009; 40: e331–9.

[121] Niizuma K, Yoshioka H, Chen H, et al. Mitochondrial and apoptotic neuronal death signaling pathways in cerebral ischemia. Biochimica et Biophysica Acta—Mol Basis Dis 2010; 1802: 92–99.

[122] Wang Y, Qin Z-H. Molecular and cellular mechanisms of excitotoxic neuronal death. Apoptosis 2010; 15: 1382–1402.

[123] Bonfoco E, Krainc D, Ankarcrona M, et al. Apoptosis and necrosis: two distinct events induced, respectively, by mild and intense insults with N-methyl-D-aspartate or nitric oxide/superoxide in cortical cell cultures. Proc Natl Acad Sci U S A 1995; 92: 7162–7166.

[124] Nakka VP, Gusain A, Mehta SL, et al. Molecular mechanisms of apoptosis in cerebral ischemia: multiple neuroprotective opportunities. Mol Neurobiol 2008; 37: 7–38.

[125] Gupta S. Molecular signaling in death receptor and mitochondrial pathways of apoptosis (Review). Intl J Oncol 2003; 22: 15–20.

[126] Chan PH. Mitochondria and neuronal death/survival signaling pathways in cerebral ischemia. Neurochem Res 2004; 29: 1943–1949.

[127] Li MX, Dewson G. Mitochondria and apoptosis: emerging concepts. F1000Prime Rep 2015; 7: 42.

[128] Green DR, Kroemer G. The pathophysiology of mitochondrial cell death. Science 2004; 305: 626–629.

[129] Sedlak TW, Oltvai ZN, Yang E, et al. Multiple Bcl-2 family members demonstrate selective dimerizations with Bax. Proc Natl Acad Sci U S A 1995; 92: 7834–7838.

[130] Wei MC, Zong WX, Cheng EH, et al. Proapoptotic BAX and BAK: a requisite gateway to mitochondrial dysfunction and death. Science 2001; 292: 727–730.

[131] Hsu YT, Wolter KG, Youle RJ. Cytosol-to-membrane redistribution of Bax and Bcl-X(L) during apoptosis. Proc Natl Acad Sci U S A 1997; 94: 3668–3672.

[132] Edlich F, Banerjee S, Suzuki M, et al. Bcl-xL retrotranslocates Bax from the mitochondria into the cytosol. Cell 2011; 145: 104–116.

[133] Schellenberg B, Wang P, Keeble JA, et al. BAX exists in a dynamic equilibrium between the cytosol and mitochondria to control apoptotic priming. Mol Cell 2013; 49: 959–971.

[134] Todt F, Cakir Z, Reichenbach F, et al. Differential retrotranslocation of mitochondrial Bax and Bak. EMBO J 2015; 34: 67–80.

[135] Hirsch T, Marzo I, Kroemer G. Role of the mitochondrial permeability transition pore in apoptosis. Biosci Rep 1997; 17: 67–76.

[136] Bagci EZ, Vodovotz Y, Billiar TR, et al. Bistability in apoptosis: roles of bax, bcl-2, and mitochondrial permeability transition pores. Biophys J 2006; 90: 1546–1559.

[137] Thornberry NA, Lazebnik Y. Caspases: enemies within. Science 1998; 281: 1312–1316.

[138] Elmore S. Apoptosis: a review of programmed cell death. Toxicol Pathol 2007; 35: 495–516.

[139] R Rama and J C García (2012). Excitotoxicity and Oxidative Stress in Acute Ischemic Stroke, pp 29–58, In: Acute Ischemic Stroke, Prof. Julio Cesar Garcia Rodriguez (Ed.), ISBN: 978-953-307-983-7, InTech.

Chapter 3

Cerebral Ischemia Induces Neuronal Vulnerability and Astrocytic Dysfunction in Stroke-Prone Spontaneously Hypertensive Rats

Kazuo Yamagata

Additional information is available at the end of the chapter

http://dx.doi.org/10.5772/64258

Abstract

Stroke-prone spontaneously hypertensive (SHRSP) rats develop severe hypertension, and more than 95% of them die of cerebral stroke. Cerebral ischemia or hypoxia and/or subsequent oxygen reperfusion strongly induces neuronal damage in SHRSP rats. The biochemical features of brain cells such as neuronal cells and astrocytes of SHRSP rats might contribute to the strong tendency of SHRSP rats to suffer strokes. In SHRSP rats, the production of hydroxyl radicals was strongly elevated after reperfusion. Neuronal expression of thioredoxin (*Txn1*) and *Bcl2* genes was significantly reduced in SHRSP rats compared with Wistar Kyoto (WKY) rats. In SHRSP rats, the susceptibility of neuronal cells to death is partly due to an insufficiency of mitochondrial redox regulation and a deficiency of the apoptosis-inhibitory protein Bcl-2. Antioxidant vitamin E may regulate the expression of redox and apoptosis-related proteins in neuronal damage. In astrocytes isolated from SHRSP rats, the cells' proliferative ability and expression of vascular cell adhesion molecule-1 (VCAM-1) and high-mobility group box 1 (HMGB1) are strongly increased compared with those in the WKY rat strain. Astrocytic lactate production, an energy source for neuronal cells, was reduced in SHRSP rats in comparison with the WKY rat strain. SHRSP astrocytes reduced their production of glial cell line–derived neurotrophic factor (GDNF) and L-serine compared to WKY astrocytes during hypoxia and reoxygenation (H/R). Furthermore, sphingosine-1-phosphate (S1P) reduced the expression of GDNF in primary SHRSP rat astrocytes. On the other hand, production of L-serine and the expression of alanine/serine/cysteine/threonine transporter (ASCT1) were lower in SHRSP than in WKY rat astrocytes after exposure to arginine vasopressin (AVP). In this chapter, we describe the neuronal vulnerabilities and astrocytic dysfunctions of SHRSP rats induced by cerebral ischemia.

Keywords: astrocyte, apoptosis, GDNF, neuronal cell death, SHRSP

1. Introduction

Stroke involves cerebral infarction and hemorrhaging and is associated with very high mortality. Stroke causes a loss of brain function due to an insufficient blood supply to the brain. The stroke-prone spontaneously hypertensive (SHRSP) rat is an experimental model of human malignant hypertension (>200 mm Hg), and this rat strain has a high incidence of cerebrovascular disease [1, 2]. Namely, SHRSP rats develop severe hypertension of more than 200 mm Hg, and more than 95% die of stroke [1, 2]. In SHRSP rats, the increase of sodium intake accelerates the rise of blood pressure (BP), and cerebral ischemia induces the appearance of cerebral vasogenic edema [3]. Therefore, SHRSP rats are widely used as a model of human stroke [2].

Studies of SHRSP rats may provide considerable useful information regarding human strokes and should indicate genetic susceptibility of particular types of cerebrovascular diseases [4]. Indeed, this strain shares features with human lacunar stroke [5]. Twenty minutes of cerebral ischemia in SHRSP rats induced a large efflux of glutamate, causing strong delayed neuronal death in region CA1 of the hippocampus, whereas the parental strain of SHRSP rats, Wistar Kyoto (WKY) rats, lacked these characteristics under the same conditions [6]. The hippocampal neurons of SHRSP rats were innately vulnerable to ischemic stimulation, and the Ca^{2+} channel blockers prevented neuronal cell death in SHRSP rats [7]. The production of hydroxyl radicals by neurons was strongly elevated after reperfusion of SHRSP rats. In neuronal cells, expression of the thioredoxin gene (*Txn1*) and the *Bcl2* gene was significantly reduced in SHRSP rats compared with WKY rats [8]. We showed that SHRSP rat neurons were more vulnerable than WKY rat neurons during cerebral ischemia-hypoxia [9, 10]. In these findings, we noticed that unknown factors other than a hereditary weakness in the neurons themselves played additional roles in accelerating cell death in SHRSP rats during cerebral ischemia [9, 10]. On the other hand, lactate production from astrocytes (an energy source for neuronal cells) was reduced in SHRSP rat cells in comparison with the WKY rat strain [11]. Moreover, astrocytes from SHRSP rats reduced lactate production, glial cell line–derived neurotrophic factor (GDNF), and L-serine in comparison with WKY rat astrocytes during hypoxia and reoxygenation (H/R) [12]. In addition, the release of L-serine and the expression of lactate transporter were lower in SHRSP rats than in WKY rat astrocytes after exposure to arginine vasopressin (AVP) [13].

Cerebral ischemia promotes blood-brain barrier (BBB) destruction, increases edema, and increases nervous system cell death. In particular, the reperfusion after cerebral ischemia rapidly generates a large quantity of reactive oxygen species (ROS), but the pathogenic mechanism of SHRSP rats in stroke is not well understood. In SHRSP rats, endothelial injury is induced at multiple sites following BBB leakage. Ultimately, this results in vessel rupture [14, 15]. Thus, we asked whether there were significant differences between the functions of WKY and SHRSP rat neurons and astrocytes during cerebral ischemia. Here, we present an overview of the cellular characteristic of SHRSP rat and WKY rat neurons and astrocytes during cerebral ischemia.

2. Cerebral ischemic stress induces neuronal vulnerability in SHRSP rats

2.1. Cell death of neuronal cells isolated from SHRSP rats during ischemia

In SHRSP rats, cerebral ischemia of 20 min duration enhances the production of large amounts of glutamate, causing delayed neuronal cell death in the CA1 region of the hippocampus [6]. Briefly, the neurons of SHRSP rats are more susceptible to H/R states than those of WKY rats [7, 9, 10]. We examined cultured neuronal cells isolated from the brains of SHRSP rats and WKY rats. The cells were cultured for 6–24 h under hypoxic conditions (1% O_2) and subsequently for 1.5–5 h in a reoxygenated state to assess cell viability [9]. None of the neuronal cells were stainable by trypan blue, indicating the absence of cell death in both strains. The majority (65–85%) of neuronal cells survived even after 36 h of hypoxic culture. Following hypoxia, after 1.5 h of reoxygenation, only 10–30% of neurons survived. The percentages of neuronal cell deaths in WKY rats and SHRSP rats were 41% (necrosis, 12%; apoptosis, 29%) and 78% (necrosis, 15%; apoptosis, 63%), respectively. Following hypoxia, 3 h of reoxygenation led to 68% cell death in WKY rats, whereas 99% of the neuronal cells from SHRSP rats were dead. Using the TdT-mediated dUTP nick end labeling (TUNEL) method, we found little or no DNA fragmentation in SHRSP rat neuronal cells after culture in 20% oxygen. In contrast, following 36 h of hypoxia and 3 h of reoxygenation, we noted a markedly increased fragmentation of DNA that was generally localized to areas containing many lipid droplets [9]. We classified the levels of apoptosis in H/R status by a morphological analysis of neuronal cell death [9, 10]. Briefly, we showed the characteristics of neuronal apoptosis in SHRSP rats in **Figure 1**. In the initial stage of apoptosis, neuronal cell axons and dendrites were lost, and many lipid droplets appeared in the neuronal cell body (A). In the next stage of apoptosis, cell shrinkage was

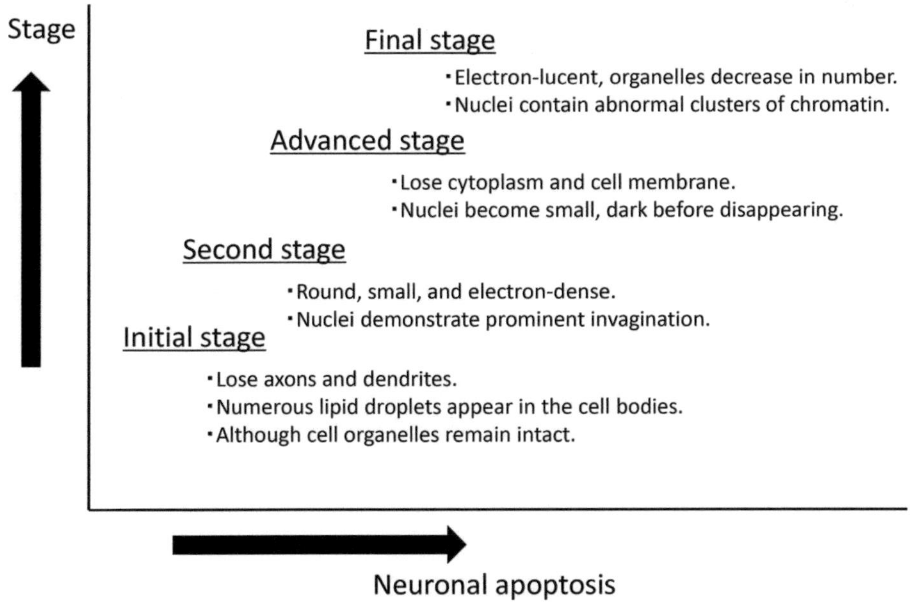

Figure 1. Characteristics of apoptosis in neuronal cells during H/R in SHRSP rats.

observed (B) and, next, continued development of apoptotic morphology (C). Finally, the neuronal cell membrane was lost and the nucleus disappeared (D). These processes eventually led to neuronal cell death. In SHRSP rats, a report demonstrated that the angiotensin II type 1 receptor-activated caspase-3 in the rostral ventrolateral medulla and was involved in sympathoexcitation [16]. These features may be associated with stroke pathogenic mechanisms of SHRSP rats.

2.2. Oxidative stress-induced neuronal cell death and redox changes in SHRSP rats

In the brain, ischemia leads to the rapid generation of a large amount of ROS and induces neuronal cell injury through self-perpetuating reactions. Cerebral ischemia increases the intracellular level of calcium ions and activates calcium-dependent proteases. These reactions activate xanthine dehydrogenase (XDH) and generate xanthine oxidase (XOD). The superoxide anion radicals generated via this pathway cause neuronal cell death in the brain [17]. Free radicals are generated by reoxygenation after cerebral ischemia, and they enhance the injury of brain neuronal cells [18]. These findings suggest that reducing the ROS (such as hydroxyl radicals produced during H/R) would be beneficial for preventing neuronal injury [19]. This might be achieved by increasing the level of antioxidant substances such as vitamin E.

Ischemic stimulation is considered to be the process that most strongly enhances cell death in cerebral ischemia in the SHRSP rat stroke model. In SHRSP rats, ischemic stimulation, i.e., the reoxygenation that occurs after hypoxia, generates a large amount of ROS that lead directly to neuronal death [20]. The expression of the thioredoxin gene (*Txn1*) was significantly reduced in neurons isolated from SHRSP rats compared with WKY rats [8]. Txn protein acts against ROS via its SH group. Furthermore, Txn proteins have many functions that are involved in intracellular signal transduction. For that reason, reduced expression of *Txn1* is associated with an attenuation of the defense system during oxidative stress in SHRSP rats. This in turn causes H/R-induced neuronal cell death. These findings indicated that redox regulatory functions in SHRSP rat neurons were markedly reduced by oxygen stimulation after hypoxia, and such changes may be involved in neuronal vulnerability. From these results, we suggested that the susceptibility of neurons to apoptosis in SHRSP rats is partly due to an insufficiency of mitochondrial thioredoxin and apoptosis-inhibitory proteins.

2.3. Protective effects of antioxidant vitamin E in neuronal cell death of SHRSP rats

Vitamin E, which is present in biological membranes, contains a hydroxyl group that reacts with unpaired electrons and can be reduced to form peroxyl radicals. The main antioxidant effect of vitamin E is to rapidly add alkoxy radicals (RO·) and hydrogen to peroxy radicals (ROO·). This is the mechanism of a chain-breaking antioxidant that blocks reactive oxygen metabolic cascades [21, 22].

We demonstrated the preventive effects of vitamin E against neuronal cell death associated with cerebral ischemia-reperfusion, particularly apoptosis, in WKY and SHRSP rat strains [9, 19]. Hypoxic stimuli followed by oxygen reperfusion induced strong neuronal damage in both WKY and SHRSP rats [9, 10]. The rate of neuronal cell death (mainly apoptosis) occurring during H/R was markedly higher in the neurons of SHRSP rats than in those of WKY rats. Vitamin E is mostly enriched in microsomal cell membranes of mitochondria of the liver and heart. Transport of vitamin E to mitochondria or the microsomes is achieved by vitamin E binding to proteins [23]. Reports demonstrated that the α-tocopherol-binding protein, afamin, transported α-tocopherol across an in vitro model of the BBB. The model consisted of porcine brain capillary endothelial cells and cultured astrocytoma cells [24]. Thus, afamin might function to maintain α-tocopherol homeostasis at the BBB in vivo. Furthermore, scavenger receptor class B type I (SR-BI) facilitates selective uptake of HDL-related α-tocopherol at the BBB [25]. Damage related to oxidative stress alters traffic to neuronal cells and changes the levels of vitamin E in mitochondria. The addition of vitamin E almost completely inhibited neuronal death in SHRSP and WKY rat lines. Vitamin E decreased neuronal cell death in a dose-dependent manner over the range of 10–50 μg/mL. With vitamin E at 50–300 μg/mL, neuronal death was almost completely prevented [9]. In SHRSP rat neurons, we used HPLC to investigate the vitamin E levels in neuronal mitochondria after vitamin E supplementation (20–300 μg/mL) [9]. The accumulation of vitamin E in mitochondria of neuronal cells after 36 h of hypoxia was confirmed. Vitamin E accumulated most effectively into the mitochondria of neuronal cells at 50 μg/mL. When neuronal cell death was induced by reoxygenation for 3 h after 36 h of hypoxia, vitamin E prevented neuronal cell death at 50 μg/mL. Vitamin E prevented stroke and loss of both memory and cognition functions [26]. Vitamin E might have a marked inhibitory effect against neuronal damage after being incorporated into biological membranes, particularly mitochondrial membranes, and capturing the reactive oxygen and free radicals formed.

2.4. Regulation of the Bcl-2 family proteins in neuronal cell death

We pointed out that apoptosis is the likely mechanism responsible for ischemic neuronal death in SHRSP rats [9, 27]. The expression of apoptosis-inducing molecules such as Bax was

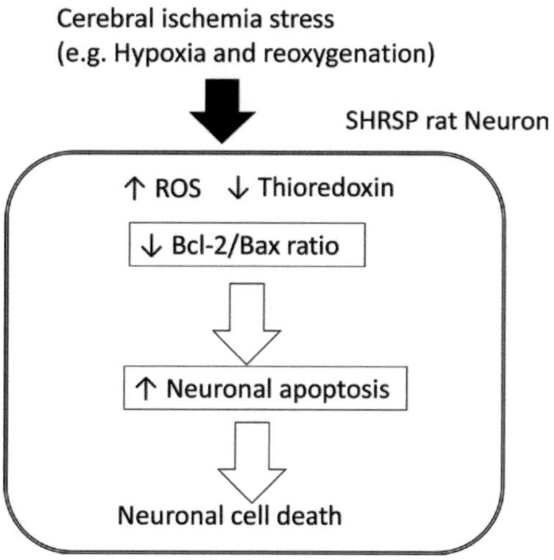

Figure 2. Apoptosis of neuron in SHRSP rats by cerebral ischemia stimulation.

enhanced in injured neuronal cells [8]. On the other hand, in surviving neurons, expression of apoptosis-inhibiting molecules such as Bcl-2 and Bcl-XL was elevated in rat brains following global ischemia [28]. The expression of *Bcl2* mRNA after H/R was investigated by quantitative reverse transcriptase-polymerase chain reaction (RT-PCR) using cultured neuronal cells isolated from SHRSP and WKY rats [8]. An analysis of *Bcl2* mRNA expression in SHRSP and WKY rats showed that the most remarkable difference occurred after 30 min of reoxygenation. The expression of *Bcl2* mRNA was significantly decreased in SHRSP compared to WKY rats. The vulnerability of neuronal cells to ischemic stress promotes neuronal cell death during stroke in SHRSP rats (**Figure 2**) [8].

3. Characteristics of astrocytes in SHRSP rats during stroke

3.1. Gliosis and the proliferation rate of astrocytes in SHRSP rats

After brain injury, the number of reactive astrocytes increases [29]. These reactive astrocytes have prominent characteristics of growing cells [30]. The growth state of astrocytes in vitro reflects the physiological abnormalities occurring in brain damage. In astrocytes cultured from SHRSP rat brains in 10% fetal bovine serum (FBS), the cell growth rate was faster than astrocytes from WKY rats. For example, the doubling time of cultured astrocytes isolated from SHRSP rats was 21 h, whereas that of WKY rat astrocytes was 30 h [31]. These results indicated the elevated growth capacity of SHRSP rat astrocytes. The greater increase in the numbers of reactive astrocytes in SHRSP rats may have pathological consequences. In addition, reports have indicated enhanced astrocytic reactivity to epidermal growth factor (EGF). SHRSP rat astrocytes responded more strongly to EGF than WKY rat astrocytes, with larger increases in cell number. In the ischemic brain, proliferative astrocytes were found around the infarcted tissue [32]. Likewise, these proliferating astrocytes were immunoreactive for the EGF receptor (EGFR). The increased growth activity of SHRSP rat astrocytes suggests that cerebral vascular lesions in cerebral ischemia may be due to dysfunctional responses to EGF [32].

3.2. Production of neurotrophic factor by SHRSP astrocytes

Astrocytes modulate several functions such as the uptake of glutamate [33] and the induction of the blood-brain barrier (BBB) [34] and induce production of cytokines [35] and neurotrophic factors [36]. In SHRSP rat strain, astrocytic properties relate to the development of brain disorders [37–39]. For example, neuron regeneration is controlled through the production of neurotrophic factors from astrocytes after brain injury [32].

Neuronal vulnerability of SHRSP rats under ischemic conditions was correlated with reduced GDNF production by SHRSP rat astrocytes [13]. The study focused on the production of GDNF under normal conditions and H/R in cultured astrocytes from WKY and SHRSP rat strains. SHRSP rat astrocytes released higher levels of GDNF than did WKY rats under normal oxygen concentrations [13] (**Figure 3**). On the other hand, after hypoxia and 1.5 or 6 h reoxygenation, the expression of GDNF was significantly lower in astrocytes from the SHRSP rat strain than the WKY rat strain [13]. Furthermore, sphingosine-1-phosphate (S1P) [40] and adenosine [41] reduced the expression of GDNF in primary SHRSP rat astrocytes. S1P is a lysophospholipid released by activated platelets [42, 43], and it enhances the apoptosis of neuronal cells in the central nervous system (CNS) [44]. A report demonstrated that GDNF is a potent factor for the survival of neuronal cells [45]. Thus, in SHRSP rats, upregulation of S1P attenuates GDNF production by astrocytes (**Figure 4**). This reduces neuronal protection mediated by the neurotrophic factor, GDNF. In traumatic injury of the CNS, the attenuated release of GDNF by astrocytes may be involved in neuronal vulnerability in the SHRSP rat strain. Adenosine enhances the levels of several growth factors in ischemic brain tissues, likely as part of a preventive response. In the CNS, adenosine in the extracellular space acts as an intercellular signaling molecule, and at high levels, it induces apoptosis [46]. Briefly, adenosine has both immediate effects such as neurotransmission and neurotrophic effects that enhance changes in cell metabolism and structure and has neuroprotective function [47, 48]. The expression of GDNF was regulated differently in cultured astrocytes from SHRSP compared to WKY rats. The amount of GDNF produced was lower in astrocytes of adenosine-treated SHRSP rats compared with WKY rats. These results indicate that GDNF production is regulated dynamically during reoxygenation and ischemic conditions by S1P and adenosine. Under postischemic reoxygenation conditions, the production of GDNF, neurturin (NTN), and its receptor increases in the brain tissue [49]. The pathogenesis of GDNF released by SHRSP rats is unknown. However, the specific metabolic properties of SHRSP rats may be associated with increased expression of GDNF [13].

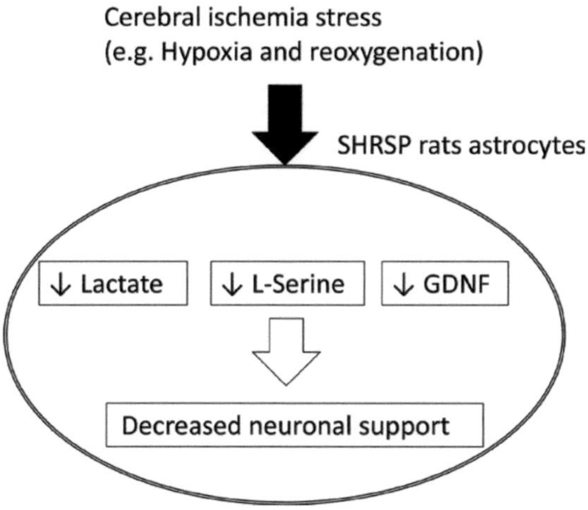

Figure 3. Alteration of astrocytes in SHRSP rats by cerebral ischemia stimulation.

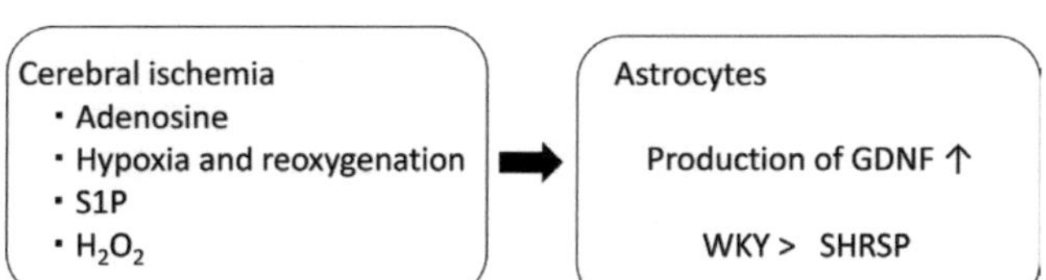

Figure 4. Regulation of GDNF in astrocytes of SHRSP rats by cerebral ischemia status.

3.3. Hypoxia and arginine vasopressin (AVP) induce astrocytic dysfunction in SHRSP rats

3.3.1. Altered regulation of L-serine in SHRSP astrocytes

In the CNS, L-serine is generated by astrocytes, and it accelerates neurite outgrowth from ganglion neurons and enhances neuronal survival [50]. L-Serine is synthesized by 3-phosphoglycerate dehydrogenase (3-PGDH) in glial cells but not in neurons [51]. L-Serine released from astrocytes is transported to the extracellular space by neural amino acid transporter alanine/serine/cysteine/threonine transporter (ASCT1) proteins and becomes available to neuronal cells [52]. Induces outgrowth of ganglion neurons and neuronal survival by L-serine from astrocytes. Hence, L-serine synthesis and the expression of ASCT1 protein were essential for neuronal survival and differentiation [53]. On the other hand, the expression of 3-PGDH and ASCT1 proteins is enhanced by excitotoxic damage in the mouse brain hippocampus [54]. In astrocytes isolated from SHRSP rats, glutamate-induced stimulation of L-serine production was reduced [55]. The production of L-serine was regulated by astrocytes in response to molecules such as glutamate, kainic acid (KA), and free radicals and others that induced neurodegenerative disorders [54, 56, 57].

Arginine vasopressin (AVP) induced the effects of inflammatory molecules in traumatic neuronal injury [58]. Furthermore, ischemic conditions such as hypoxia and AVP affect cerebral cell volume [59, 60], ion uptake by cerebral cells via Na/H exchange (NHE) [61], and Na-K-Cl cotransporter (NKCC) activities [62, 63]. AVP and hypoxia contribute to ischemia-induced astrocyte swelling [64]. During cerebral ischemia, astrocyte swelling leads to ischemic neuronal cell death. AVP might contribute to astrocyte swelling induced by hypoxia and reperfusion in SHRSP rats. On the other hand, L-serine generation might be regulated by astrocytes in response to a variety of molecules such as AVP that enhance brain edema in SHRSP rats [12].

3.3.2. Inflammatory regulation and expression of HMGB1 and adhesion molecules in SHRSP astrocytes

High-mobility group box 1 (HMGB1) regulates nucleosomal structure stabilization, modulates inflammation, and is involved in recovery after stroke [65–67]. Hypoxia induces HMGB1 expression in neurons and astrocytes [68]. Furthermore, after hypoxia, HMGB1 enhances breakdown of the blood-brain barrier (BBB) during ischemic injury [69]. These results indicate that HMGB1 is involved in inflammatory responses associated with stroke after ischemia [70]. One report demonstrated that HMGB1 is produced by neuronal cells and glial cells and aggravates ischemic neurodegeneration [68]. In reactive astrocytes, production of HMGB1 accelerates endothelial progenitor cell-mediated neurovascular remodeling during stroke recovery [71]. On the other hand, in oxygen-glucose deprivation or reperfusion, HMGB1 produced from astrocytes induces endogenous neural stem or progenitor cell proliferation [67, 72]. One study examined the expression of AVP-induced HMGB1 in cultured primary astrocytes isolated from WKY, SHR, SHRSP, and SHRpch1_18 rats [12]. AVP induced HMGB1 expression at 50 and 100 nM, and it was significantly higher in SHR, SHRSP, and SHRpch1_18 rat astrocytes than in WKY rat astrocytes. HMGB1 may relate to early stages of the inflammatory response [69]. Reports have indicated that myelin loss is associated with neuroinflammation [73] and that it induces inflammation after MCA occlusion [74] in the SHRSP rat strain. This characteristic of SHRSP, SHR, and SHRpch1_18 rats is likely an important contributor to enhanced inflammation in astrocytes and could explain how AVP augments the inflammatory reaction and induces neuronal cell death [12].

Following exposure to tumor necrosis factor-alpha (TNF-α), the expression of vascular cell adhesion molecule-1 (VCAM-1) by SHRSP rat astrocytes was increased compared with those from WKY rats. Expression of TNF-α and adhesion molecules are related to the presence of early neurological exacerbation and infarct volume in stroke [75, 76]. TNF-α is generated by microglial cells and infiltrating macrophages following ischemic stroke [77]. In H/R treatment of SHRSP rat astrocytes, the expression of monocyte chemotactic protein-1 (MCP-1) was increased compared with that under normal oxygen. Inhibition or genetic lack of these adhesion molecules decreased infarct volume, edema, and/or mortality in different animal models of ischemic stroke [78]. These enhanced levels of adhesion molecules in H/R and TNF-α treatment may be induced by stroke in SHRSP rats. In SHRSP rats, alteration and attenuation of astrocyte functions promote neuronal cell death during stroke [79].

4. Conclusions

The level of neuronal cell death in SHRSP rats is significantly higher than in the WKY rat strain [9, 10]. In cerebral ischemia, the properties of SHRSP rat neuronal cells, unlike those of WKY rats, might be a factor in the elevated frequency of stroke. Vitamin E reduces neuronal cell damage caused by ROS generated in cerebral ischemia. Thus, antioxidants such as vitamin E could be used as a treatment for oxidative stress-mediated diseases. These antioxidants may regulate redox potential and apoptosis-related proteins. Furthermore, in SHRSP rats, astrocyte properties contribute to the development of brain disorders. In SHRSP rat astrocytes, attenuation and loss of several functions such as GDNF and L-serine were demonstrated under cerebral ischemic stroke conditions (**Figure 4**). In addition, after ischemic reperfusion, generation of MCP-1 is strongly enhanced in SHRSP rat astrocytes [80]. The expression of VCAM-1 and MCP-1 [81] is markedly elevated in SHRSP astrocytes compared with WKY rat astrocytes. Taken together, neuronal vulnerability and altered regulation of the neuronal supportive functions of astrocytes increase the risk of stroke in SHRSP rats.

Supply of oxygen is critical to neuronal cells viability. On the other hand, oxygen reperfusion induces cellular dysfunction, apoptosis, and necrosis. From several animal experiment data, clinical therapy by single-drug treatment may have little effect [82].

Conflict of interest

None declared.

Acknowledgements

The work was supported by grants from the Nihon University Multidisciplinary Research Grant for 2014. We thank Prof. Yukio Yamori (Mukogawa Women's University, Japan), Prof. Yasuo Nara (Mukogawa Women's University, Japan), and Dr. Motoki Tagami (Sanraku Hospital, Japan) for their enormous support and for discussions in studies of astrocytes of the SHRSP/Izm rat.

Abbreviations

BBB	blood-brain barrier
CNS	central nervous system
GDNF	glial cell line–derived neurotrophic factor
ROS	reactive oxygen sepsis
HMGB1	high-mobility group box 1
NHE	Na/H exchange
NKCC	Na-K-Cl cotransporter
S1P	sphingosine 1-phosphate
SHRSP	stroke-prone spontaneously hypertensive
VCAM-1	vascular cell adhesion molecule-1
WKY	Wister Kyoto

Author details

Kazuo Yamagata

Address all correspondence to: kyamagat@brs.nihon-u.ac.jp

Department of Food Bioscience and Biotechnology, College of Bioresource Sciences, Nihon University (NUBS), Fujisawa, Kanagawa, Japan

References

[1] Okamoto K, Yamori Y, Nagaoka K. Establishment of the stroke-prone spontaneously hypertensive rats (SHR). Circ Res 1974: 35 (suppl 1); 1143–53.

[2] Yamori Y, Nagaoka A, Okamoto K. Importance of genetic factors in hypertensive cerebrovascular lesions: an evidence obtained by successive selective breeding of stroke-prone and-resistant SHR. Jpn Circ J 1974: 38; 1095–100.

[3] Nagaoka A, Iwatsuka H, Suzuoki Z, Okamoto K. Genetic predisposition to stroke in spontaneously hypertensive rats. Am J Physiol 1976: 230; 1354–59.

[4] Nabika T, Cui Z, Masuda J. The stroke-prone spontaneously hypertensive rat: how good is it as a model for cerebrovascular diseases? Cell Mol Neurobiol 2004: 24; 639–46.

[5] Bailey EL, Smith C, Sudlow CL, Wardlaw JM. Is the spontaneously hypertensive stroke prone rat a pertinent model of sub cortical ischemic stroke? Int J Stroke 2011: 6; 434–4.

[6] Gemba T, Matsunaga K, Ueda M. Changes in extracellular concentration of amino acids in the hippocampus during cerebral ischemia in stroke-prone SHR, stroke-resistant SHR and normotensive rats. Neurosci Lett 1992: 135; 184–8.

[7] Yasui M, Kawasaki K. Vulnerability of CA1 neurons in SHRSP hippocampal slices to ischemia, and its protection by Ca^{2+} channel blockers. Brain Res 1994: 642; 146–52.

[8] Yamagata K, Tagami M, Ikeda K, et al. Altered gene expressions during hypoxia and reoxygenation in cortical neurons isolated from stroke-prone spontaneously hypertensive rats. Neurosci Lett 2000: 284; 131–4.

[9] Tagami M, Yamagata K, Ikeda K, et al. Vitamin E prevents apoptosis in cortical neurons during hypoxia and oxygen reperfusion. Lab Invest 1998: 78; 1415–29.

[10] Tagami M, Ikeda K, Yamagata K, et al. Vitamin E prevents apoptosis in hippocampal neurons caused by cerebral ischemia and reperfusion in stroke-prone spontaneously hypertensive rats. Lab Invest 1999: 79; 609–15.

[11] Yamagata K, Tagami M, Ikeda K, et al. Reduced production of lactate during hypoxia and reoxygenation in astrocytes isolated from stroke-prone spontaneously hypertensive rats. Neurosci Lett 2000: 296; 113–16.

[12] Yamagata K, Yamamoto M, Kawakami K, et al. Arginine vasopressin regulated ASCT1 expression in astrocytes from stroke-prone spontaneously hypertensive rats and congenic SHRpch1_18 rats. Neuroscience 2014: 267; 277–85.

[13] Yamagata K, Tagami M, Ikeda K, et al. Differential regulation of glial cell line-derived neurotrophic factor (GDNF) mRNA expression during hypoxia and reoxygenation in astrocytes isolated from stroke-prone spontaneously hypertensive rats. Glia 2002: 37; 1–7.

[14] Braun H, Bueche CZ, Garz C, et al. Stases are associated with blood-brain barrier damage and a restricted activation of coagulation in SHRSP. J Neurol Sci 2012; 322: 71–6.

[15] Schreiber S, Bueche CZ, Garz C, Braun H. Blood brain barrier breakdown as the starting point of cerebral small vessel disease?—new insights from a rat model. Exp Transl Stroke Med 2013: 5;4.

[16] Kishi T, Hirooka Y, Konno S, et al. Angiotensin II type 1 receptor-activated caspase-3 through ras/mitogen-activated protein kinase/extracellular signal-regulated kinase in the rostral ventrolateral medulla is involved in sympathoexcitation in stroke-prone spontaneously hypertensive rats. Hypertension 2010: 55; 291–7.

[17] Thompson-Gorman SL, Zweier JL. Evaluation of the role of xanthine oxidase in myocardial reperfusion injury. J Biol Chem 1990: 265; 6656–63.

[18] Bolli R. Oxygen-derived free radicals and myocardial reperfusion injury: an overview. Cardiovasc Drugs Ther 1991: 5 (Suppl 2); 249–68.

[19] Yamagata K, Tagami M, Yamori Y. Neuronal vulnerability of stroke-prone spontaneously hypertensive rats to ischemia and its prevention with antioxidants such as vitamin E. Neuroscience 2010: 170; 1–7.

[20] Negishi H, Ikeda K, Nara Y, Yamori Y. Increased hydroxyl radicals in the hippocampus of stroke-prone spontaneously hypertensive rats during transient ischemia and recirculation. Neurosci Lett 2001: 306; 206–08.

[21] Packer L, Landvik S. Vitamin E in biological systems. Adv Exp Med Biol 1990: 264; 93–103.

[22] Chow CK. Vitamin E and oxidative stress. Free Radic Biol Med 1991: 11; 215.

[23] Manor D, Morley S. The alpha-tocopherol transfer protein. Vitam Horm 2007: 76; 45–65.

[24] Kratzer I, Bernhart E, Wintersperger A, et al. Afamin is synthesized by cerebrovascular endothelial cells and mediates alpha-tocopherol transport across an in vitro model of the blood-brain barrier. J Neurochem 2009: 108; 707–18.

[25] Balazs Z, Panzenboeck U, Hammer A, Sovic A, et al. Uptake and transport of high-density lipoprotein (HDL) and HDL-associated alpha-tocopherol by an in vitro blood-brain barrier model. J Neurochem 2004: 89; 939–50.

[26] Murad LB, Guimaraes MR, Paganelli A, et al. Alpha-tocopherol in the brain tissue preservation of stroke-prone spontaneously hypertensive rats. J Physiol Biochem 2014: 70; 49–60.

[27] Yamagata K, Ichinose S, Tagawa C, et al. Vitamin E regulates SMase activity, GSH levels, and inhibits neuronal death in stroke-prone spontaneously hypertensive rats during hypoxia and reoxygenation. J Exp Stroke Transl Med 2009: 1; 41–8.

[28] Chen J. Apoptosis repressor genes Bcl-2 and Bcl-x-long are expressed in the rat brain following global ischemia. J Cereb Blood Flow Metab 1997: 17; 2–10.

[29] Bramanti V, Tomassoni D, Avitabile M, et al. Biomarkers of glial cell proliferation and differentiation in culture. Front Biosci 2010: 2; 558–70.

[30] Pekny M, Nilsson M. Astrocyte activation and reactive gliosis. Glia 2005: 50; 427–34.

[31] Yamagata K, Nara Y, Tagami M, et al. Demonstration of hereditarily accelerated proliferation in astrocytes derived from spontaneously hypertensive rats. Clin Exp Pharmacol Physiol 1995: 22; 605–9.

[32] Planas AM, Justicia C, Soriano MA, Ferrer I. Epidermal growth factor receptor in proliferating reactive glia following transient focal ischemia in the rat brain. Glia 1998: 23; 120–9.

[33] Gouix E, Leveille F, Nicole O, et al. Reverse glial glutamate uptake triggers neuronal cell death through extrasynaptic NMDA receptor activation. Mol Cell Neurosci 2009: 40; 463–73.

[34] Abbott NJ, Ronnback L, Hansson E. Astrocyte-endothelial interactions at the blood-brain barrier. Nat Rev Neurosci 2006: 7; 41–53.

[35] Suzumura A, Takeuchi H, Zhang G, Kuno R, et al. Roles of glia-derived cytokines on neuronal degeneration and regeneration. Ann N Y Acad Sci 2006: 1088; 219–29.

[36] Muller HW, Junghans U, Kappler J. Astroglial neurotrophic and neurite-promoting factors. Pharmacol Ther 1995: 65; 1–18.

[37] Tagami M, Kubota A, Nara Y, et al. Detailed disease processes of cerebral pericytes and astrocytes in stroke-prone SHR. Clin Exp Hypertens A 1991: 13; 1069–75.

[38] Tagami M, Nara Y, Kubota A, et al. Ultrastructural changes in cerebral pericytes and astrocytes of stroke-prone spontaneously hypertensive rats. Stroke 1990: 21; 1064–71.

[39] Tomassoni D, Avola R, Di Tullio MA, Sabbatini M, Vitaioli L, Amenta F. Increased expression of glial fibrillary acidic protein in the brain of spontaneously hypertensive rats. Clin Exp Hypertens 2004: 26(4); 335–50.

[40] Yamagata K, Tagami M, Torii Y, et al. Sphingosine 1-phosphate induces the production of glial cell line-derived neurotrophic factor and cellular proliferation in astrocytes. Glia 2003: 41; 199–206.

[41] Yamagata K, Hakata K, Maeda A, et al. Adenosine induces expression of glial cell line-derived neurotrophic factor (GDNF) in primary rat astrocytes. Neurosci Res 2007: 59; 467–74.

[42] Yatomi Y, Ruan F, Hakomori S, Igarashi Y. Sphingosine-1-phosphate: a platelet-activating sphingolipid released from agonist-stimulated human platelets. Blood 1995: 86; 193–202.

[43] Yatomi Y, Ohmori T, Rile G, et al. Sphingosine 1-phosphate as a major bioactive lysophospholipid that is released from platelets and interacts with endothelial cells. Blood 2000: 96; 3431–8.

[44] Moore AN, Kampfl AW, Zhao X, Hayes RL, Dash PK. Sphingosine-1-phosphate induces apoptosis of cultured hippocampal neurons that requires protein phosphatases and activator protein-1 complexes. Neuroscience 1999: 94; 405–15.

[45] Lin LF, Doherty DH, Lile JD, Bektesh S, Collins F. GDNF: a glial cell line-derived neurotrophic factor for midbrain dopaminergic neurons. Science 1993: 260; 1130–2.

[46] Fields RD, Burnstock G. Purinergic signalling in neuron-glia interactions. Nat Rev Neurosci 2006: 7; 423–36.

[47] Ciccarelli R, Ballerini P, Sabatino G, et al. Involvement of astrocytes in purine-mediated reparative processes in the brain. Int J Dev Neurosci 2001: 19; 395–14.

[48] Rathbone MP, Middlemiss PJ, Gysbers JW, et al. Trophic effects of purines in neurons and glial cells. Prog Neurobiol 1999: 59; 663–90.

[49] Kokaia Z, Airaksinen MS, Nanobashvili A, et al. GDNF family ligands and receptors are differentially regulated after brain insults in the rat. Eur J Neurosci 1999: 11; 1202–16.

[50] Mitoma J, Furuya S, Hirabayashi Y. A novel metabolic communication between neurons and astrocytes: non-essential amino acid l-serine released from astrocytes is essential for developing hippocampal neurons. Neurosci Res 1998: 30; 195–99.

[51] Yamasaki M, Yamada K, Furuya S, et al. 3-Phosphoglycerate dehydrogenase, a key enzyme for l-serine biosynthesis, is preferentially expressed in the radial glia/astrocyte lineage and olfactory ensheathing glia in the mouse brain. J Neurosci 2001: 21; 7691–704.

[52] Zerangue N, Kavanaugh MP. ASCT-1 is a neutral amino acid exchanger with chloride channel activity. J Biol Chem 1996: 271; 27991–4.

[53] Furuya S, Tabata T, Mitoma J, et al. l-Serine and glycine serve as major astroglia-derived trophic factors for cerebellar Purkinje neurons. Proc Natl Acad Sci U S A 2000: 97; 11528–33.

[54] Jeon GS, Choi DH, Lee HN, et al. Expression of l-serine biosynthetic enzyme 3-phosphoglycerate dehydrogenase (Phgdh) and neutral amino acid transporter ASCT1 following an excitotoxic lesion in the mouse hippocampus. Neurochem Res 2009: 34; 827–34.

[55] Yamagata K, Shoji Y, Terashima T, Yokogoshi H. Glutamate reduces secretion of l-serine in astrocytes isolated from stroke-prone spontaneously hypertensive rats. Neuroscience 2006: 143; 729–37.

[56] Lehmann A, Hansso E. Kainate-induced stimulation of amino acid release from primary astroglial cultures of the rat hippocampus. Neurochem Int 1988;13(4); 557-61.

[57] Mustafa AK, Kumar M, Selvakumar B, et al. Nitric oxide S-nitrosylates serine racemase, mediating feedback inhibition of d-serine formation. Proc Natl Acad Sci U S A 2007: 104; 2950–5.

[58] Szmydynger-Chodobska J, Fox LM, Lynch KM, Zink BJ, Chodobski A. Vasopressin amplifies the production of proinflammatory mediators in traumatic brain injury. J Neurotrauma 2010: 27; 1449–61.

[59] Brillault J, Lam TI, Rutkowsky JM, Foroutan S, O'Donnell ME. Hypoxia effects on cell volume and ion uptake of cerebral microvascular endothelial cells. Am J Physiol Cell Physiol 2008: 294; C88–96.

[60] O'Donnell ME, Duong V, Suvatne J, Foroutan S, Johnson DM. Arginine vasopressin stimulation of cerebral microvascular endothelial cell Na-K-Cl cotransporter activity is V1 receptor and [Ca] dependent. Am J Physiol Cell Physiol 2005: 289; C283–92.

[61] Lam T, Wise PM, O'Donnell ME. Cerebral microvascular endothelial cell Na/H exchange: evidence for the presence of NHE1 and NHE2 isoforms and regulation by arginine vasopressin. Am J Physiol Cell Physiol 2009: 297; C278–89.

[62] Jayakumar AR, Panickar KS, Curtis KM, Tong XY, Moriyama M, Norenberg MD. Na-K-Cl cotransporter-1 in the mechanism of cell swelling in cultured astrocytes after fluid percussion injury. J Neurochem 2011: 117; 437–48.

[63] Foroutan S, Brillault J, Forbush B, O'Donnell ME. Moderate-to-severe ischemic conditions increase activity and phosphorylation of the cerebral microvascular endothelial cell Na^+-K^+-Cl^- cotransporter. Am J Physiol Cell Physiol 2005: 289; C1492–501.

[64] Rutkowsky JM, Wallace BK, Wise PM, O'Donnell ME. Effects of estradiol on ischemic factor-induced astrocyte swelling and AQP4 protein abundance. Am J Physiol Cell Physiol 2011: 301; C204–12.

[65] Kim JB, Sig Choi J, Yu YM, et al. HMGB1, a novel cytokine-like mediator linking acute neuronal death and delayed neuroinflammation in the postischemic brain. J Neurosci 2006: 26; 6413–21.

[66] Hayakawa K, Qiu J, Lo EH. Biphasic actions of HMGB1 signaling in inflammation and recovery after stroke. Ann NY Acad Sci 2010: 1207; 50–7.

[67] Lei C, Lin S, Zhang C, et al. High-mobility group box1 protein promotes neuroinflammation after intracerebral hemorrhage in rats. Neuroscience 2013: 228; 190–9.

[68] Faraco G, Fossati S, Bianchi ME, et al. High mobility group box 1 protein is released by neural cells upon different stresses and worsens ischemic neurodegeneration in vitro and in vivo. J Neurochem 2007: 103; 590–603.

[69] Huang J, Liu B, Yang C, et al. Acute hyperglycemia worsens ischemic stroke-induced brain damage via high mobility group box-1 in rats. Brain Res 2013: 1535; 148–55.

[70] Schulze J, Zierath D, Tanzi P, et al. Severe stroke induces long-lasting alterations of high-mobility group box 1. Stroke 2013: 44; 246–8.

[71] Hayakawa K, Pham LD, Katusic ZS, Arai K, Lo EH. Astrocytic high-mobility group box 1 promotes endothelial progenitor cell-mediated neurovascular remodeling during stroke recovery. Proc Natl Acad Sci USA 2012: 109; 7505–10.

[72] Li M, Sun L, Li Y, Xie C, Wan D, Luo Y. Oxygen glucose deprivation/reperfusion astrocytes promotes primary neural stem/progenitor cell proliferation by releasing high-mobility group box 1. Neurochem Res 2014: 39; 1440–50.

[73] Jalal FY, Yang Y, Thompson J, Lopez AC, Rosenberg GA. Myelin loss associated with neuroinflammation in hypertensive rats. Stroke 2012: 43; 1115–22.

[74] Moller K, Boltze J, Posel C, et al. Sterile inflammation after permanent distal MCA occlusion in hypertensive rats. J Cereb Blood Flow Metab 2014: 34; 307–15.

[75] Rodríguez-Yáñez M, Castillo J. Role of inflammatory markers in brain ischemia. Role of inflammatory markers in brain ischemia. Curr Opin Neurol 2008: 21; 353–7.

[76] Clausen BH, Lambertsen KL, Babcock AA, et al. Interleukin-1beta and tumor necrosis factor-alpha are expressed by different subsets of microglia and macrophages after ischemic stroke in mice. J Neuroinflammation 2008: 5; 46.

[77] Lambertsen KL, Clausen BH, Fenger C, et al. Microglia and macrophages express tumor necrosis factor receptor p75 following middle cerebral artery occlusion in mice. Neuroscience 2007: 144; 934–49.

[78] Yilmaz G, Granger DN. Cell adhesion molecules and ischemic stroke. Neuronal Res 2008: 30; 783–93.

[79] Yamagata K. Pathological alterations of astrocytes in stroke-prone spontaneously hypertensive rats under ischemic conditions. Neurochem Int 2012: 60; 91–98.

[80] Sakurai-Yamashita Y, Shigematsu K, Yamashita K, Niwa M. Expression of MCP-1 in the hippocampus of SHRSP with ischemia-related delayed neuronal death. Cell Mol Neurobiol 2006: 26; 823–31.

[81] Yamagata K, Kitazawa T, Shinoda M, et al. Stroke status evoked adhesion molecule genetic alterations in astrocytes isolated from stroke-prone spontaneously hypertensive rats and the apigenin inhibition of their expression. Stroke Res Treat 2010; 2010. pii: 386389.

[82] Schaller B, Graf R. Cerebral ischemia and reperfusion: the pathophysiologic concept as a basis for clinical therapy. J Cereb Blood Flow Metab 2004: 24(4); 351–371.

Importance of the Arterial Blood Supply to the Rabbit and Guinea Pig Spinal Cord in Experimental Ischemia

David Mazensky and Slavka Flesarova

Additional information is available at the end of the chapter

http://dx.doi.org/10.5772/64352

Abstract

Spinal cord ischemia belongs to the one of the most frequently occurring results of spinal cord damage, with broad range of several symptoms and complications. The superficial position of fine arterial system of the spinal cord predicts the spinal cord ischemic injury. The laboratory animals, such as rabbits and guinea pigs, serve for the study of spinal cord ischemic injury. The aim of this work was to describe the arterial blood supply to the spinal cord in New Zealand White rabbits and English self guinea pigs, using the corrosion and dissecting technique. In both species, we found variations in arrangement and origin of segmental arteries of descending aorta, the basilar artery, the ventral spinal artery, the dorsal spinal arteries, the artery of Adamkiewicz, and the segmental dorsal and ventral branches arising from the arterial spinal branches. The presence of the artery of Adamkiewicz and nearly regular segmental blood supply to the spinal cord are responsible for the use of rabbit and guinea pig as a simple model of ischemic damage to the spinal cord. The understanding of the arterial arrangement to the spinal cord plays a very important role in avoiding the spinal cord ischemia or infarction during surgical interventions to the spine.

Keywords: artery, experiment, guinea pig, rabbit, spinal cord injury

1. Introduction

1.1. Spinal cord injury

Spinal cord injury represents a significant health problem associated with lifelong disability and a broad range of secondary complications. Although spinal cord trauma causes loss of neuronal cell bodies as well as myelinated axons, the dysfunction of the white matter tracts is the factor that determines most of the clinical symptoms. In addition, the management of spinal cord injury patients is challenging. According to the damaged part of the spinal cord, the spinal cord injury can lead to the respiratory insufficiency due to the paralysis of breathing muscles, necessitating mechanical ventilators, phrenic nerve pacing, loss of sensory and motor functions, recurrent kidney stones, urinary tract infection, pressure sores, and cardiac and respiratory dysfunction. In the majority of cases, the spinal cord injury results into the spinal cord ischemia due to the superficial position of fine arterial system of the spinal cord.

1.2. Laboratory animals in experimental spinal cord injury

The advances made so far with the benefit of animal model have been primarily in understanding the cell biology of the injured nervous system. Rodent models are the common type of mammal employed in experimental spinal cord injury studies, and widespread research have been conducted using rats, mice, gerbils, guinea pigs, and hamsters [1]. Other animal experiments include cats, rabbits, and dogs [1, 2]. Of course, larger mammals such as nonhuman primate, goats, and pigs are also used but very rarely and are less experienced models based in spinal cord injury research, requiring expensive aftercare and housing as well as stringent ethical considerations [1–4].

1.2.1. Rabbit

Rabbits are commonly used in biomedical research. Currently, many strains of rabbit are available. Laboratory rabbits belong to the order Lagomorpha and are collectively referred to as lagomorphs [5]. The most popular strain for research purposes is a medium-sized (weighing between 3 and 5 kg), New Zealand White outbred rabbit. A number of advantages make rabbits a widely used animal in biomedical research. Their size, ease of handling, and relative ease of blood collection due to their large ear vessels make them suitable for many types of experiments [6]. The rabbits are suitable for long-term experiments, because most of them live for 5–8 years, but some individuals live to the age of 10 years or more.

1.2.2. Guinea pig

Guinea pigs occupy special place in research. This rodent species, with its unique physiology and anatomy, has come to symbolize all experimental subjects. The special place in research implies that guinea pigs are one of the most commonly used laboratory animals in research. They represent an appropriate animal for several types of experiments because of their small size, cleanliness, docileness, and relatively easy maintenance [7].

1.2.3. Rabbit and guinea pig in experimental spinal cord injury

The two before-mentioned species have been used as experimental models in the study of spinal cord ischemic injury, and the effect of various neuroprotective drugs on such way altered the nervous tissue [8–13]. The more detailed knowledge of anatomy of the spinal cord blood supply with focus on all possible variations can contribute to the protection of the spinal cord. The aim of our study was to describe the arterial blood supply to rabbit and guinea pig spinal

http://dx.doi.org/10.5772/64352

cord using the corrosion and dissecting technique. We described some variations of the principal arteries and the segmental arteries contributing to the arterial blood supply in the corresponding region.

2. Materials and methods

2.1. Experimental animals

2.1.1. Rabbit

Adult New Zealand White rabbits in number of 20, at 140 days of age (weight range 2.5–3 kg) consisting of 10 males and 10 females, were used in this study. The work was performed in an accredited experimental laboratory at the University of Veterinary Medicine and Pharmacy in Košice, Slovak Republic. Standard conditions were ensured to all animals: approved cages, relative humidity (45%), temperature (15–20°C), light period (12 hours), feed (granular mixed, KLASIK, de Heus, Bučovice, Czech Republic), and drinking water (ad libitum). The corrosion technique was used for 10 rabbits, females (n = 5) and males (n = 5), and the dissecting technique for 10 rabbits, females (n = 5) and males (n = 5).

2.1.2. Guinea pig

Adult English self guinea pigs in number of twenty, at 220 days of age (weight range 0.8–1 kg) consisting of 10 males and 10 females, were used in this study. The work was performed in an accredited experimental laboratory at the University of Veterinary Medicine and Pharmacy in Košice, Slovak Republic. Standard conditions were ensured to all animals: approved cages, relative humidity (45%), temperature (15–20°C), light period (12 hours), feed (FANTASIA, Tatrapet, Liptovský Mikuláš, Slovak Republic), and drinking water (ad libitum). The corrosion technique was used for 10 guinea pigs, females (n = 5) and males (n = 5), and the dissecting technique for 10 guinea pigs, females (n = 5) and males (n = 5).

2.2. Casting media

2.2.1. Corrosion technique

In the corrosion technique, Spofacryl (SpofaDental, Czech Republic) was used as a casting medium. It consists of a powdered component (copolymer of methyl methacrylate, copolymer of methacrylate, sodium p-toluenesulfinate, pigments, and fluorescent agent), liquid component (methyl methacrylate, methacrylic acid, ethylene glycol dimethacrylate, stabilizers, and amine), and red pigment (1,2-benzenedicarboxylic acid, bis[2-ethylhexyl ester], epoxidized soybean oil, and 2-naphthalenecarboxylic acid).

2.2.2. Dissecting technique

Batson's No. 17 Plastic Replica and Corrosion Kit (Polysciences Europe GmbH, Germany) was used as a casting medium in the dissecting technique. It consists of base solution A (polymethyl methacrylate; methyl methacrylate; dibutyl phthalate; 2-methyl-, 1,2-ethanediyl ester; and 2-propenoic acid), catalyst (dibutyl phthalate, benzoyl peroxide, and acetone), promoter C (N,N-dimethyl-4-toluidine and dibutyl phthalate), and red pigment (2-naphthalenecarboxylic acid, 1,2-benzenedicarboxylic acid, epoxidized soybean oil, and bis[2-ethylhexyl ester]).

2.3. Methods

2.3.1. Surgical preparation of animals

First step in surgical preparation of animals was the intravenous application of heparin (50,000 UI/kg) 30 minutes before the animals were euthanized using the embutramide (T-61, 0.3 mL/kg) also intravenously. For better manipulation during the dissection and prevention from the hair sticking to the corrosive casts during maceration process was the skin subsequently as far as possibly removed. The entrance into the thoracic cavity was performed from the left side by removing of the parts of the ribs. Before the introduction of a ligature to the initial part of ascending aorta, the pericardial cavity was opened. Plastic cannula was inserted into the ascending aorta through the opened left ventricle. After the cannula was fixed in the ascending aorta, the perfusion started. The decrease of pressure in arteries and veins and performing of good injection were accomplished by opening of the right auricle of the heart. The manual perfusion of the arterial and venous system using the cannula by means of 2.5–3 l of warm (37°C), pH 7.3, and 0.9% NaOH in 0.01 M phosphate took 15–20 min [14].

2.3.2. Casting medium preparation

2.3.2.1. Corrosion technique

Powdered component with a weight of 20 g was added to the red pigment. To this mixture, liquid component in amount of 10 mL was added, and both components were mixed together.

2.3.2.2. Dissecting technique

The red pigment was added to the base solution A prior to mixing the catalyst and promoter C. The pigment was added in the amount of 5% of the base solution A. After mixing of the base solution A and the pigment together, the mixture was divided into two similar parts. Each of them has a volume of 10 mL. The first of these parts was mixed with the catalyst in volume of 6 mL. The second part was mixed with six drops of promoter C. After the initial mixing, these two parts were fused and mixed together.

2.3.3. Casting medium application

The same cannula fixed to the ascending aorta serves for manual filling of the arterial system with the casting medium. The red casting medium in the superficial body vessels determined

http://dx.doi.org/10.5772/64352

the adequate filling of arteries and an even distribution. After the completion of arterial casting, for at least 30 minutes, the bodies must not be manipulated. After this time period, the bodies were submersed in water (40–60°C; 24 hours) to ensure adequate polymerization of the applied casting medium in the arterial system.

2.3.4. Corrosion technique

The variable soft tissues, which surrounded the polymerized casting medium, were dissolved by the potassium hydroxide (KOH) in concentration of 2–4% for 2 days. For the faster corrosion, a constant temperature (40°C) of the used solution must be achieved [15]. Every 12 hours, the corrosion solution was changed. After the dissolution, the rest of the surrounding soft tissues were removed from the corrosion casts in running water. Then, the corrosion casts were dried at the room temperature.

2.3.5. Dissecting technique

By the dissecting technique, 10% formaldehyde was injected into the vertebral canal between the last lumbar vertebra and sacrum, between the last cervical and first thoracic vertebra, and between the occipital bone and the first cervical vertebra to fix the spinal cord. After 1-week fixation, the vertebral canal was opened by removing vertebral arches in sacral, lumbar, thoracic, and cervical regions. Also, the occipital bone was partly removed. The prepared spinal cords were fixed in 10% formaldehyde (Section 1).

3. Results

3.1. Rabbit

3.1.1. Cervical spinal cord

In the cervical spinal cord, we found more complex arterial blood supply in comparison with the rest of the spinal cord. The most cranial section of cervical spinal cord was supplied with blood by means of small branches arising from the posterior inferior cerebellar artery. This artery originated from the vertebral artery bilaterally. The bilateral vertebral arteries entered into the vertebral canal through the lateral vertebral opening of the atlas. The fusion of the bilateral vertebral arteries was located on the caudal border of the dorsal surface of the basilar part of the occipital bone. From this fusion, the basilar artery which participated on the formation of arterial cerebral ring continued cranially. The fusion of vertebral arteries was present in 50% of cases without gap (**Figure 1**) and in 30% of cases with one longitudinal gap (**Figure 2**). In 20% of cases, we found two gaps. At the level of fusion of bilateral vertebral arteries originated the ventral spinal artery. Its origin was from the right-sided vertebral artery, from the left-sided vertebral artery (**Figure 2**), and from the anastomosis of two branches, each coming from the medial surface of the corresponding vertebral artery (**Figure 1**). The frequency of origins of ventral spinal artery is shown in **Table 1**.

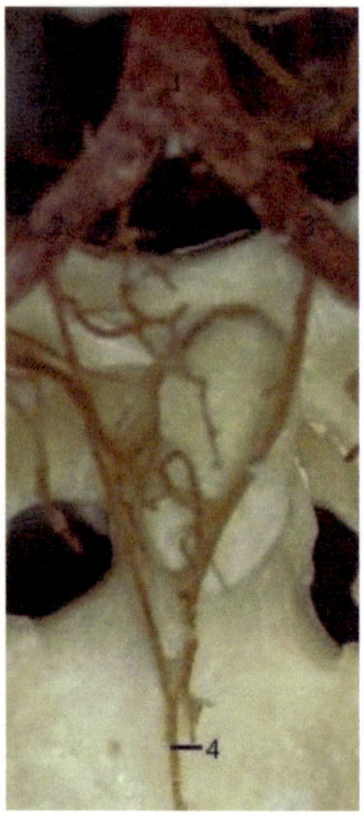

Figure 1. The origin of the ventral spinal artery from the anastomosis of two branches, each coming from the medial surface of the corresponding vertebral artery. (1) Basilar artery, (2) left vertebral artery, (3) right vertebral artery, and (4) ventral spinal artery. Macerated specimen, dorsal view, magnification 8x.

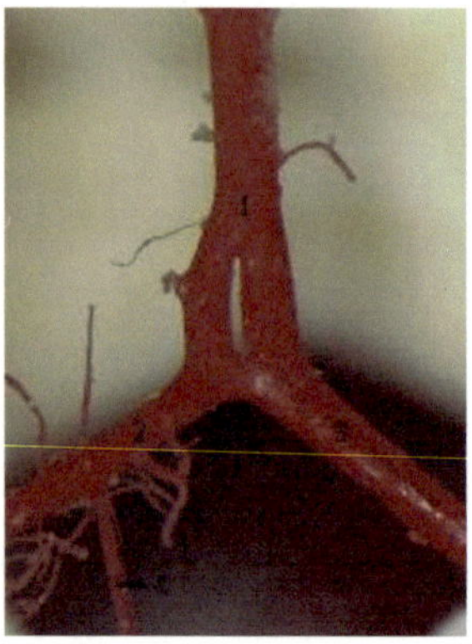

Figure 2. The origin of the ventral spinal artery from the left-sided vertebral artery. The fusion of bilateral vertebral arteries is visible on one longitudinal gap. (1) Basilar artery, (2) left vertebral artery, (3) right vertebral artery, and (4) ventral spinal artery. Macerated specimen, dorsal view, magnification 12.5x.

	Corrosion technique (%)	Dissecting technique (%)	Average (%)
Bilateral origin	20	30	25
Right-sided origin	40	40	40
Left-sided origin	40	30	35

Table 1. Origin of ventral spinal artery using the corrosion technique (10 rabbits) and dissecting technique (10 rabbits).

	Occurrence of spinal branches (%)	
	Right	Left
C 1	0	0
C 2	70	50
C 3	50	30
C 4	50	50
C 5	30	50
C 6	20	70
C 7	30	50
C 8	50	50

C, cervical segment of the spinal cord.

Table 2. Frequency of occurrence of spinal branches in the cervical spinal cord using the dissecting technique (10 rabbits).

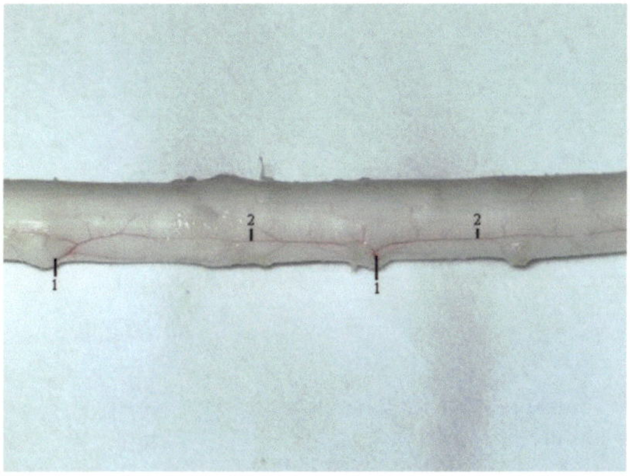

Figure 3. Dorsal branches of the spinal branches joining the irregular dorsal spinal arteries. (1) Dorsal branch of spinal branch and (2) irregular dorsal spinal artery. Dissected specimen, dorsolateral view, magnification 5x.

The ventral spinal artery was located along the ventral median fissure on the ventral surface of the cervical spinal cord. Bilateral vertebral arteries gave off spinal branches which entered the vertebral canal through the intervertebral openings. Inside the vertebral canal, the spinal branches divided into the dorsal and ventral branch with direction to the spinal cord. The ventral branches joined the ventral spinal artery. The frequency of occurrence of individual ventral branches joining the ventral spinal artery is shown in **Table 2**. In the cervical spinal cord, the ventral branches joining the ventral spinal artery were present as right-sided in 46.2% and as left-sided in 53.8% of cases.

We found two irregular longitudinal dorsal spinal arteries receiving dorsal branches of spinal arteries (**Figure 3**) or the absence of the dorsal spinal arteries (**Figure 4**) on the dorsal surface of the spinal cord. In the case of the presence of two longitudinal dorsal spinal arteries, their arrangement was very variable. These two longitudinal dorsal spinal arteries were formed only by fusion of the small cranially and caudally directed branches originating from the dorsal branches. In the case of the absence of dorsal spinal arteries, the dorsal surface of the spinal cord was supplied by means of dorsal branches forming irregular loops between each other on the same and on the opposite side. There was no origin of the dorsal spinal arteries present in the area of fusion of bilateral vertebral arteries. The frequency of occurrence of dorsal branches was the same as of the ventral branches.

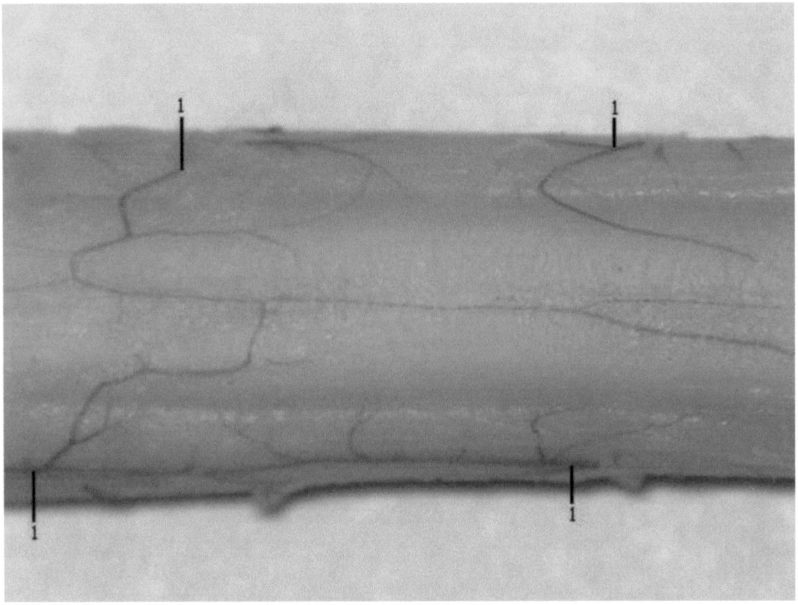

Figure 4. Dorsal branches of the spinal branches in the form of irregular loops. (1) Dorsal branch of spinal branch. Dissected specimen, dorsal view, magnification 12.5x.

3.1.2. Thoracolumbar spinal cord

The thoracic spinal cord received the arterial blood by means of spinal branches originating from the dorsal intercostal arteries which were present in 13 pairs. Dorsal intercostal arteries as paired branches arising from the dorsal surface of the thoracic aorta were present in nine pairs in 70% of cases, in eight pairs in 20% of cases, and in 10 pairs in 10% of cases. The remaining three to five pairs originated from the supreme intercostal artery. The more cranial origin of the left-sided dorsal intercostal arteries than the right-sided was present in 60% of cases (**Figure 5**). The origin of right- and left-sided dorsal intercostal arteries at the same level was present in 20% of cases (**Figure 6**). The origin of first nine pairs at the same level and the more cranial origin of the left-sided arteries than the right-sided by the remaining pairs were present in 10% of cases. The more cranially located origin of the right-sided arteries than the left-sided arteries by the first eight pairs and the origin of the remaining pairs at the same level were found in 10% of cases.

http://dx.doi.org/10.5772/64352

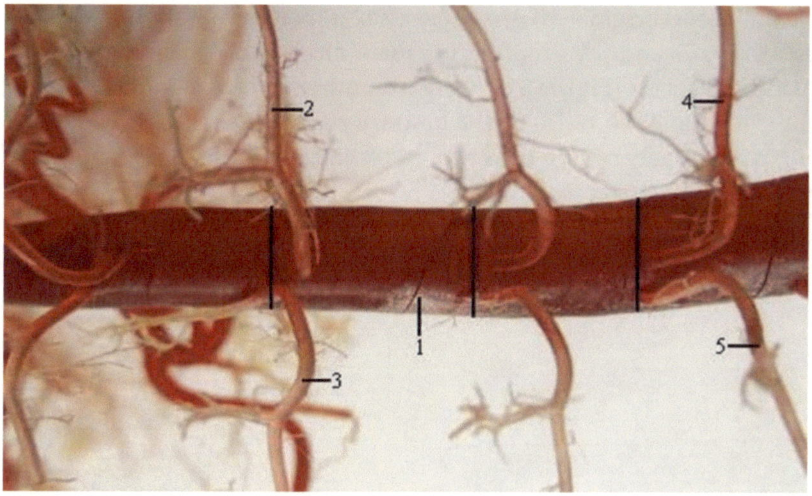

Figure 5. More cranially located origin of the left-sided dorsal intercostal arteries than the right-sided. (1) Thoracic aorta, (2) 10th left dorsal intercostal artery, (3) 10th right dorsal intercostal artery, (4) eighth left dorsal intercostal artery, and (5) eighth right dorsal intercostal artery. The black line indicates the shift of origin of dorsal intercostal arteries. Macerated specimen, dorsal view, macroscopic image.

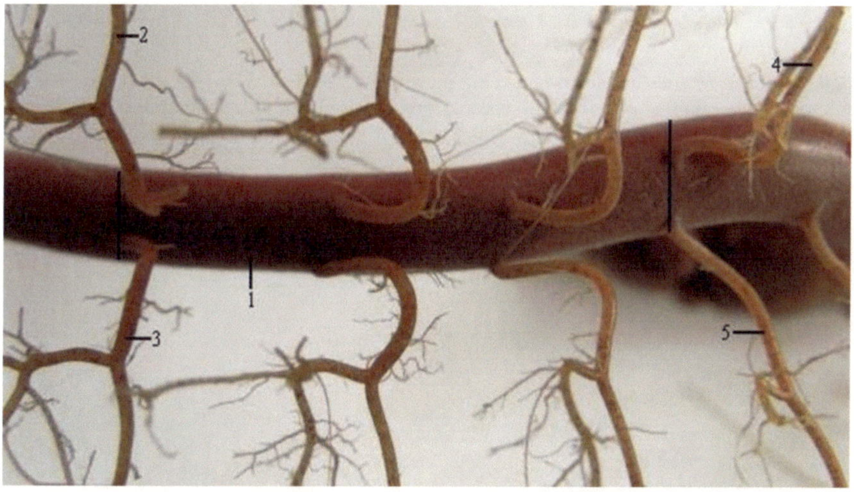

Figure 6. Origin of dorsal intercostal arteries at the same level. (1) Thoracic aorta, (2) 10th left dorsal intercostal artery, (3) 10th right dorsal intercostal artery, (4) seventh left dorsal intercostal artery, and (5) seventh right dorsal intercostal artery. The black line indicates the place of origin of dorsal intercostal arteries. Macerated specimen, dorsal view, macroscopic image.

The paired lumbar arteries originated from the dorsal surface of the abdominal aorta. Their spinal branches represent the arterial blood supply to the lumbar spinal cord. Lumbar arteries in number of six pairs were present in 90% of cases and in five pairs in 10% of cases. The remaining last pair was originating from the median sacral artery. In 60% of cases, the lumbar arteries at the same level originated by means of a common trunk (**Figure 7**). The independent origin of first two pairs and the origin of the remaining pairs by means of a common trunk were present in 30% of cases (**Figure 8**). The more cranial origin of the left-sided lumbar arteries than the right-sided lumbar arteries by the first two pairs and the origin of lumbar arteries by the remaining pairs by means of a common trunk from the dorsal surface of the abdominal aorta were present in 10% of cases.

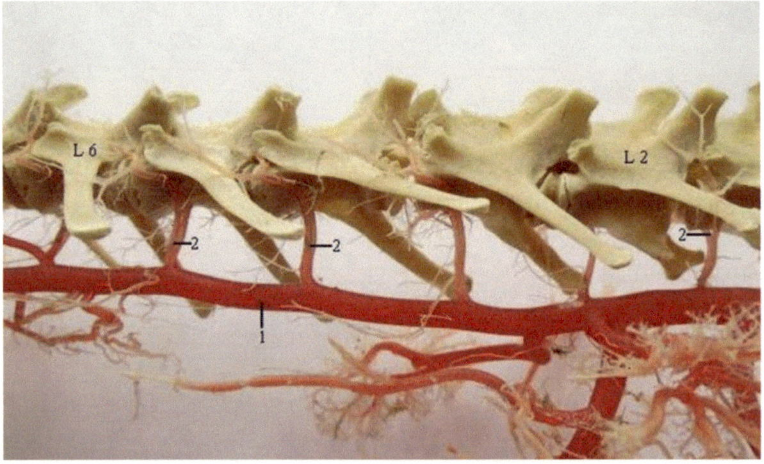

Figure 7. Origin of lumbar arteries by means of a common trunk. (1) Abdominal aorta and (2) the point of division of common trunk for bilateral lumbar arteries. L 2—second lumbar vertebra and L 6—sixth lumbar vertebra. Macerated specimen, lateral view, macroscopic image.

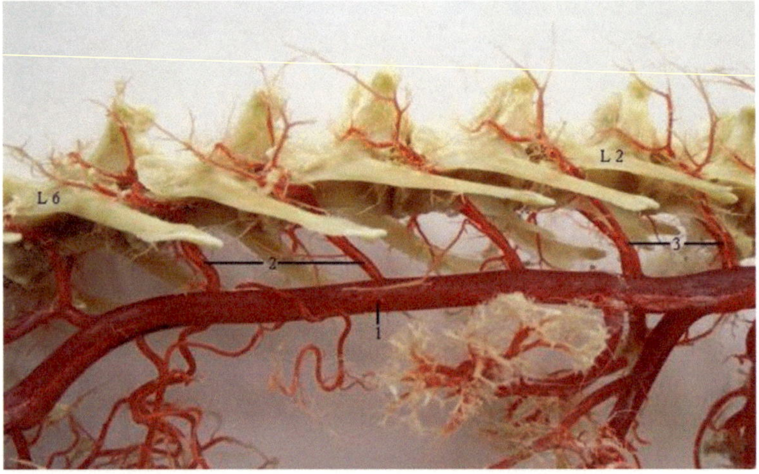

Figure 8. Origin of lumbar arteries by means of a common trunk. The first two pairs originated as independent branches. (1) Abdominal aorta, (2) common trunk for bilateral lumbar arteries, and (3) the separate origin of bilateral lumbar arteries. Macerated specimen, lateral view, macroscopic image.

http://dx.doi.org/10.5772/64352

The spinal branches with origin from the dorsal intercostal and lumbar arteries entered the vertebral canal through the intervertebral openings in association with the respective spinal nerve roots. Inside the vertebral canal, each spinal branch was divided into the dorsal and ventral branches. The ventral branches joined the ventral spinal artery.

Level	Occurrence of spinal branches (%)			
	Ventral		Dorsal	
	Right	Left	Right	Left
Th 1	20	50	40	50
Th 2	60	70	70	40
Th 3	0	30	50	70
Th 4	30	60	70	90
Th 5	0	90	40	100
Th 6	20	100	30	60
Th 7	70	70	100	60
Th 8	20	100	60	100
Th 9	10	30	0	70
Th 10	20	80	60	20
Th 11	30	30	50	80
Th 12	10	40	0	80
Th 13	40	60	30	100
L 1	50	50	50	40
L 2	30	20	40	80
L 3	50	60	60	60
L 4	70	80	30	40
L 5	50	70	60	50
L 6	50	50	50	50

L, lumbar segment of the spinal cord and Th, thoracic segment of the spinal cord.

Table 3. Occurrence of ventral and dorsal branches of arterial spinal branches in the thoracolumbar spinal cord (dissecting technique, 10 rabbits).

The frequency of occurrence of individual ventral branches is shown in **Table 3**. The left-sided ventral branches entering the ventral spinal artery in thoracic spinal cord were present in 71.1% of cases and the right-sided ventral branches in 28.9% of cases. The left-sided ventral branches entering the ventral spinal artery in lumbar spinal cord were present in 52.4% of cases and right-sided in 47.6% of cases. Along the entire thoracolumbar spinal cord, the left-sided ventral branches were present in 64.4% of cases and the right-sided in 35.6% of cases, which is most likely related to left-sided localization of the descending aorta.

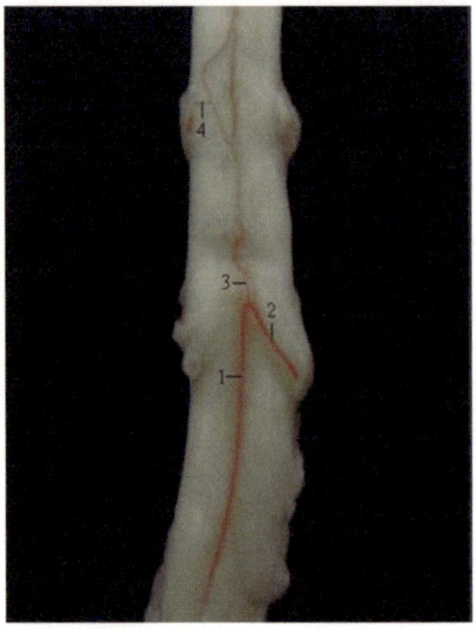

Figure 9. Left-sided localization of the artery of Adamkiewicz. (1) Ventral spinal artery, (2) the artery of Adamkiewicz, (3) branch of the artery of Adamkiewicz running cranially, and (4) ventral branch of spinal branch of the fifth right lumbar artery. Dissected specimen, ventral view, macroscopic image.

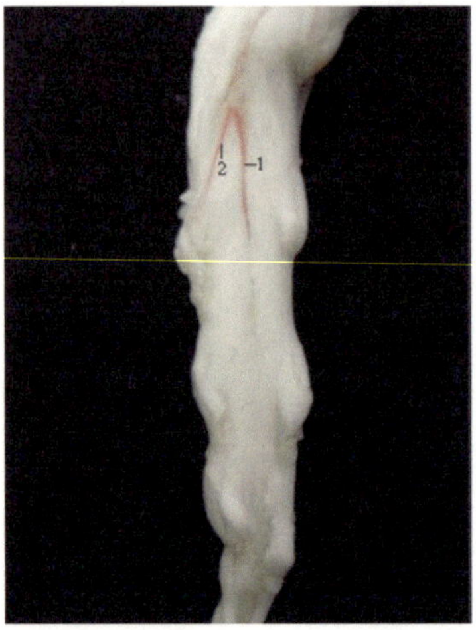

Figure 10. Right-sided localization of the artery of Adamkiewicz. (1) Ventral spinal artery and (2) the artery of Adamkiewicz. Dissected specimen, ventral view, macroscopic image.

A feeding artery with larger diameter entered the ventral spinal artery together with numerous weak spinal branches with smaller diameter. This bigger artery originated from the spinal branch which arose from the sixth lumbar artery. Thereafter, it arose and it ran through the intervertebral foramen to enter the vertebral canal. In all the studied specimens, we found this artery, which is known as the artery of Adamkiewicz or the arteria radicularis magna. It was present as left-sided artery in 50% of cases (**Figure 9**) and as right-sided artery also in 50% of cases (**Figure 10**). The artery of Adamkiewicz represented the arterial blood supply of the lumbar spinal cord caudally from the point of narrowing of the ventral spinal artery. After reaching median ventral fissure, it ran caudally replacing the ventral spinal artery and sent an important thin branch cranially to the thinning ventral spinal artery (**Figure 9**).

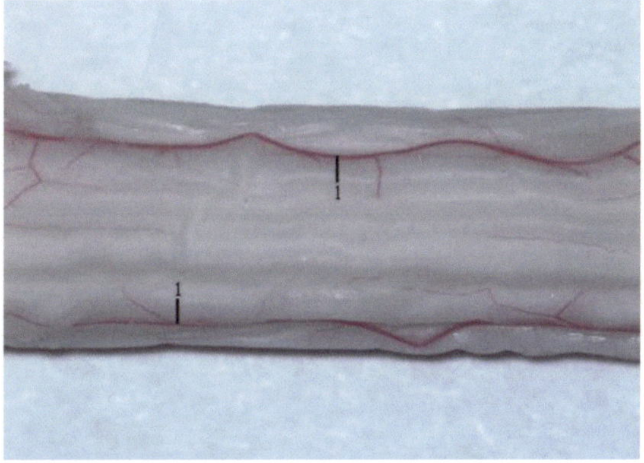

Figure 11. The presence of two irregular longitudinal dorsal spinal arteries. (1) Dorsal spinal artery. Dissected specimen, dorsal view, magnification 12.5x.

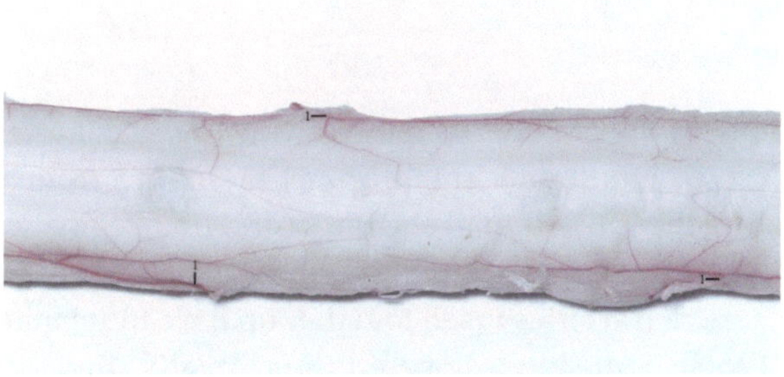

Figure 12. The absence of longitudinal dorsal spinal arteries. (1) Dorsal branch of spinal branch. Dissected specimen, dorsal view, magnification 12.5x.

On the dorsal surface of the thoracolumbar spinal cord, two irregular longitudinal dorsal spinal arteries were present in 70% of cases (**Figure 11**). They were located bilaterally in the lateral dorsal groove. We found the absence of longitudinal dorsal spinal arteries on the dorsal surface of thoracolumbar spinal cord in 20% of cases (**Figure 12**). Three irregular longitudinal dorsal spinal arteries receiving the dorsal branches were present in 10% of cases. The third artery was lying in the median dorsal groove (**Figure 13**). In the cases of the presence of two irregular longitudinal dorsal spinal arteries, these were formed only by the fusion of small cranially and caudally directed branches arising from the dorsal branches of the spinal branches. They formed irregular loops between each other on the same and on the opposite side. The frequency of occurrence of individual dorsal branches is shown in **Table 3**. The dorsal branches in the thoracic spinal cord were present in 60.5% of cases as left-sided and in 39.5% of cases as right-sided. The dorsal branches in the lumbar spinal cord were present in 52.5% of cases as left-sided and in 47.5% of cases as right-sided. Along the entire thoracolumbar spinal cord, the left-sided dorsal branches were present in 58.2% of cases and the right-sided in 41.8% of cases; this is most likely related to the left-sided localization of the descending aorta.

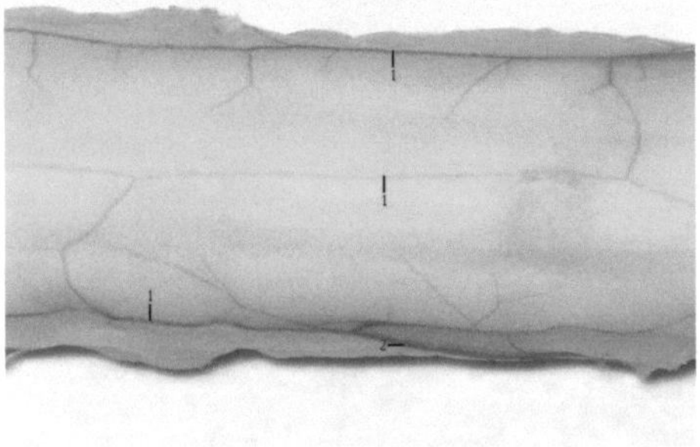

Figure 13. Dorsal branches of spinal branches forming three irregular longitudinal dorsal spinal arteries. (1) Dorsal spinal artery and (2) dorsal branch of spinal artery. Dissected specimen, dorsal view, magnification 12.5x.

3.2. Guinea pig

3.2.1. Cervical spinal cord

The arterial blood supply to the cervical spinal cord was more complex in comparison with the rest of the spinal cord. Numerous small branches arising from the posterior inferior cerebellar artery supplied the most cranial section of the first segment of the cervical spinal cord. Bilateral vertebral arteries entered the vertebral canal through the lateral vertebral opening of the atlas. These two arteries fused together on the caudal margin of the basilar part of the occipital bone. From the fusion originated the cranially directed basilar artery which participated on the formation of the cerebral arterial circle. The fusion of bilateral vertebral arteries has no triangular gap in 60% of cases (**Figure 14**) and one longitudinal gap in 30% of cases. A communicating branch between bilateral vertebral arteries was present in 10% of cases (**Figure 15**). The ventral spinal artery originated at the place of fusion of bilateral vertebral arteries. This origin was from the right-sided vertebral artery (**Figure 15**), from the left-sided vertebral artery, and from the anastomosis of two branches originating from the medial surface of the corresponding vertebral artery (**Figure 14**). The frequency of rostral origins of the ventral spinal artery is shown in **Table 4**.

The ventral spinal artery runs along the ventral median fissure of the cervical spinal cord. Spinal branches originating from the bilateral vertebral arteries entered the vertebral canal through the intervertebral openings. Inside the vertebral canal, they were divided into the dorsal and ventral branches with direction to the spinal cord. Some of the ventral branches joined the ventral spinal artery. The frequency of occurrence of individual ventral branches joining the ventral spinal artery is shown in **Table 5**. The left-sided ventral branches joining the ventral spinal artery were present in 58.2% of cases and the right-sided in 41.8% of cases.

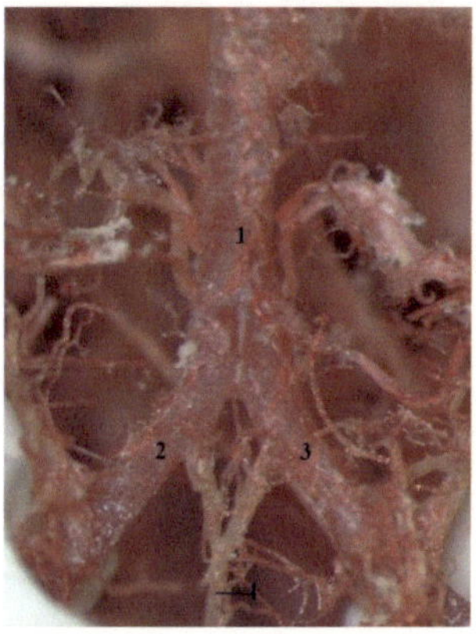

Figure 14. The anastomosis of two branches with origin on the medial surface of bilateral vertebral arteries forming the ventral spinal artery. (1) Basilar artery, (2) left vertebral artery, (3) right vertebral artery, and (4) ventral spinal artery. Macerated specimen, dorsal view, magnification 12.5x.

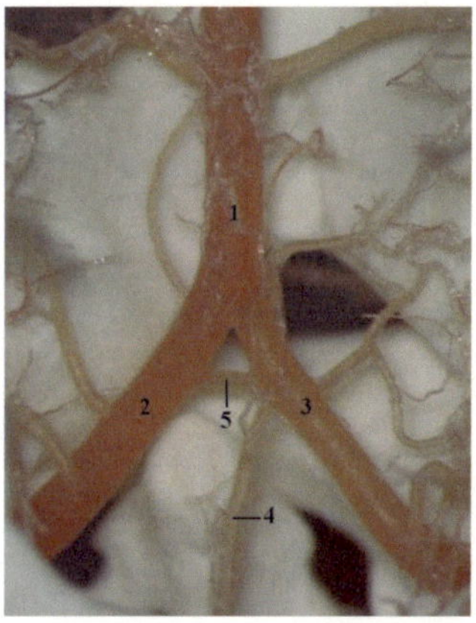

Figure 15. Ventral spinal artery originating from the right vertebral artery. Connection of both vertebral arteries by means of communicating branch. (1) Basilar artery, (2) left vertebral artery, (3) right vertebral artery, (4) ventral spinal artery, and (5) communicating branch. Macerated specimen, dorsal view, magnification 12.5x.

On the dorsal surface of the cervical spinal cord, we found two longitudinal dorsal spinal arteries in 60% of cases (**Figure 16**), three longitudinal dorsal spinal arteries in 30% of cases (**Figure 17**), or they were absent in 10% of cases. The fusion of the small cranially and caudally directed branches originating from the dorsal branches of spinal arteries represents the form of two longitudinal dorsal spinal arteries. In the cases of the absence of the dorsal spinal arteries, the dorsal surface of the cervical spinal cord receives the arterial blood by means of dorsal branches of spinal arteries with very irregular arrangement (**Figure 18**). We found no rostral origins of dorsal spinal arteries in the place of fusion of bilateral vertebral arteries. The frequency of occurrence of individual dorsal branches reaching the cervical spinal cord is shown in **Table 5**. The left-sided dorsal branches were present in 63.3% of cases, and the right-sided dorsal branches were present in 36.7% of cases.

	Corrosion technique (%)	Dissecting technique (%)	Average (%)
Bilateral origin	20	30	25
Right-sided origin	40	40	40
Left-sided origin	40	30	35

Table 4. Rostral origin of ventral spinal artery using the corrosion technique (10 guinea pigs) and dissecting technique (10 guinea pigs).

Level	Occurrence of spinal branches (%)			
	Ventral		Dorsal	
	Right	Left	Right	Left
C 1	0	0	50	50
C 2	30	30	0	50
C 3	0	0	50	60
C 4	30	60	30	90
C 5	50	50	50	50
C 6	90	30	60	100
C 7	0	100	0	50
C 8	30	50	50	50

C, cervical segment of the spinal cord.

Table 5. Frequency of occurrence of ventral branches of spinal branches of the cervical spinal cord using the dissecting technique (10 guinea pigs).

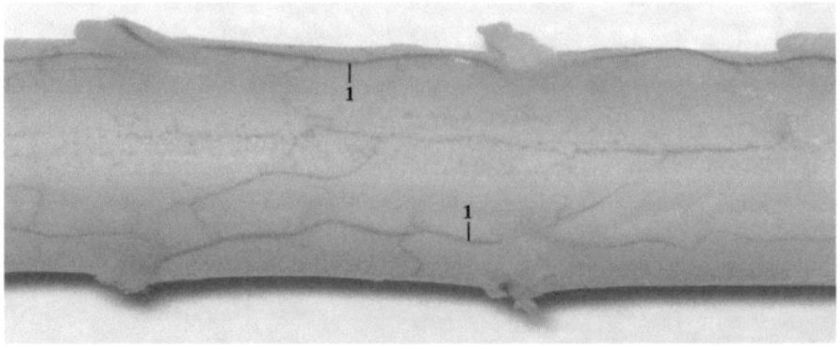

Figure 16. The presence of two dorsal spinal arteries. (1) Dorsal spinal artery. Dissected specimen, dorsal view, magnification 12.5x.

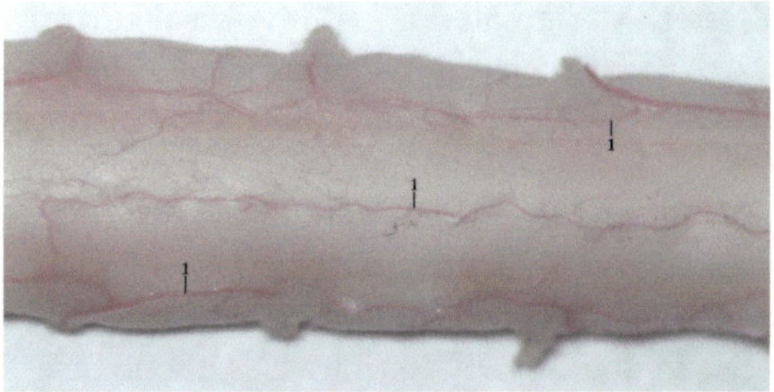

Figure 17. The presence of three dorsal spinal arteries. (1) Dorsal spinal artery. Dissected specimen, dorsal view, magnification 12.5x.

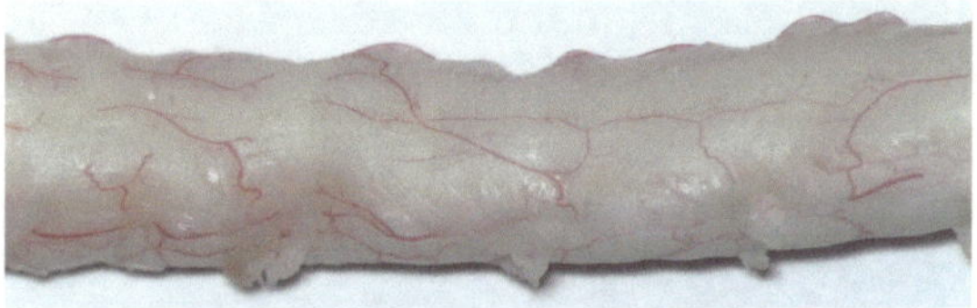

Figure 18. Dorsal branches of spinal branches with irregular arrangement. Dissected specimen, dorsolateral view, magnification 12.5x.

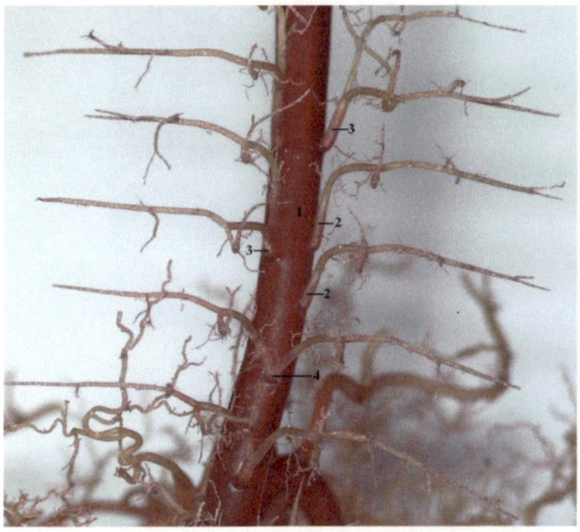

Figure 19. Dorsal intercostal arteries. (1) Thoracic aorta, (2) dorsal intercostal arteries with independent origin, (3) craniocaudal division of a common trunk of dorsal intercostal arteries, and (4) right-left division of common trunk of dorsal intercostal arteries. Macerated specimen, dorsal view, magnification 5x.

3.2.2. *Thoracolumbar spinal cord*

In the thoracic spinal cord, the arterial blood supply is performed by means of spinal branches arising from the dorsal intercostal arteries (**Figure 19**) which were present in number of 12 pairs. Dorsal intercostal arteries originated from the dorsal surface of the thoracic aorta in number of eight pairs in 70% of cases, in number of seven pairs in 20% of cases, and in number of nine pairs in 10% of cases. The remaining three to five pairs arose from the supreme intercostal artery. The origin of dorsal intercostal arteries by means of common trunk was present in 70% of cases. We found the division in right-left direction of common trunk in 60% of cases and in craniocaudal direction in 40% of cases. There was a high degree of variability present in the formation of common trunk. It was formed by two dorsal intercostal arteries in four cases, by three arteries in one case, by four arteries in one case, and by five arteries also in one case. The right- and left-sided arteries at the same level originated independently in 30% of cases.

The lumbar spinal cord received the arterial blood supply by means of spinal branches originating from the paired lumbar arteries. In all the cases, we found seven pairs of lumbar arteries. The first six pairs originated from the dorsal surface of the abdominal aorta, and the last one pair was a branch from the median sacral artery in 80% of cases. The origin of two last pairs from the median sacral artery was present in 10% of cases. Also in 10% of cases, we found the origin of all seven pairs from the abdominal aorta. The origin of lumbar arteries at the same level by means of a common trunk with the division in the right-left direction was present in 60% of cases. The independent origin of the right- and left-sided arteries at the same level was present in 40% of cases (**Figure 20**).

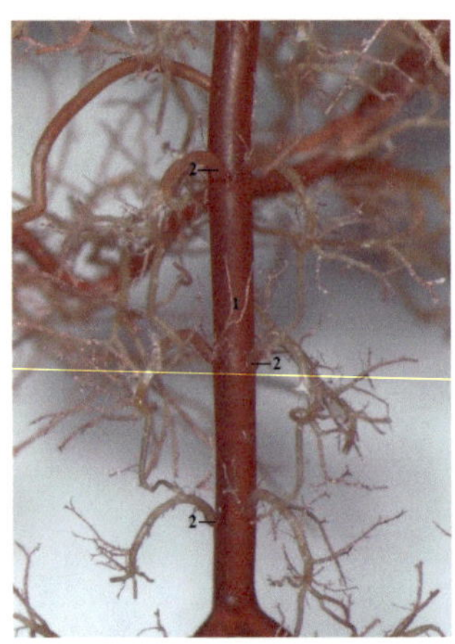

Figure 20. Origin of lumbar arteries. (1) Abdominal aorta and (2) independent origin of lumbar arteries. Macerated specimen, dorsal view, magnification 5x.

Dorsal intercostal arteries and lumbar arteries gave off spinal branches which entered the vertebral canal through the intervertebral openings. The entering was associated with the respective spinal nerve roots. After their entrance into the vertebral canal, the spinal branches divided into the dorsal and ventral branch. The ventral branches joined the ventral spinal artery. The occurrence of individual ventral branches joining the ventral spinal artery is shown in **Table 6**. The ventral spinal artery was located subdurally along the ventral median fissure of the thoracolumbar spinal cord. We found the left-sided ventral branches joining the

http://dx.doi.org/10.5772/64352

ventral spinal artery in the thoracic spinal cord in 69.5% of cases and the right-sided in 30.5% of cases. We found the left-sided ventral branches joining the ventral spinal artery in the lumbar spinal cord in 54.2% of cases and right-sided in 45.8% of cases. Along the entire thoracolumbar spinal cord, the left-sided branches joining the ventral spinal artery were present in 63.8% of cases and right-sided in 36.2% of cases, which is most likely related to the left-sided localization of the descending aorta.

Levell	Occurrence of spinal branches (%)			
	Ventral		Dorsal	
	Right	Left	Right	Left
Th 1	30	60	50	50
Th 2	30	30	50	60
Th 3	30	100	30	30
Th 4	0	30	0	30
Th 5	0	50	30	50
Th 6	50	50	30	30
Th 7	0	30	30	50
Th 8	30	60	30	0
Th 9	0	50	10	30
Th 10	50	50	30	50
Th 11	30	30	30	90
Th 12	0	30	60	30
L 1	0	0	50	30
L 2	0	90	30	30
L 3	30	0	0	30
L 4	60	30	0	30
L 5	50	50	0	60
L 6	50	0	90	100
L 7	30	90	30	100

L, lumbar segment of the spinal cord and Th, thoracic segment of the spinal cord.

Table 6. Occurrence of ventral and dorsal branches of arterial spinal branches in the thoracolumbar spinal cord (dissecting technique, 10 guinea pigs).

In addition to relatively small spinal branches, a bigger feeding artery with origin from the spinal branch of the fifth left lumbar artery in 60% of cases was present (**Figure 21**). The doubled artery of Adamkiewicz with two different levels of origin was present in 30% of cases. The left-sided artery originated from the spinal branch of the fourth lumbar artery and the right-sided from the spinal branch of the fifth lumbar artery (**Figure 22**). The artery of Adamkiewicz with the origin from the spinal branch of the fifth right- and left-sided lumbar artery was present in 10% of cases. These two separated arteries were continuing caudally on the ventral surface of the lumbar spinal cord. These two arteries fused together at the level of the sixth lumbar vertebra. From this point, the single ventral spinal artery continued caudally. A communicating branch connected together with the bilateral spinal branches at the level of the fifth lumbar artery and sent cranially thin branches joining the ventral spinal artery (**Figure 23**). In all the cases, the artery of Adamkiewicz was joining the ventral spinal artery.

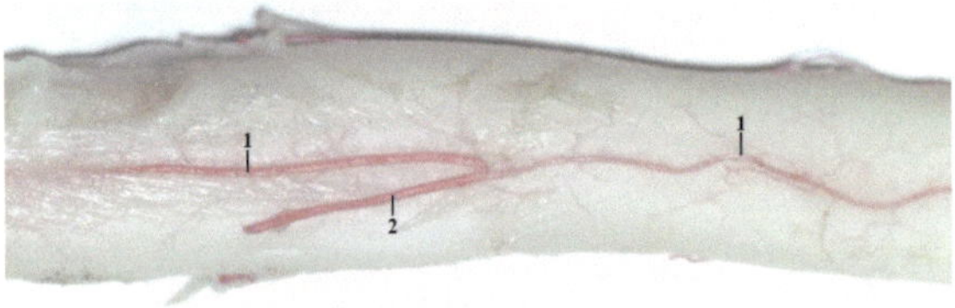

Figure 21. Left-sided localization of artery of Adamkiewicz. (1) Ventral spinal artery and (2) artery of Adamkiewicz. Dissected specimen, ventral view, magnification 8x.

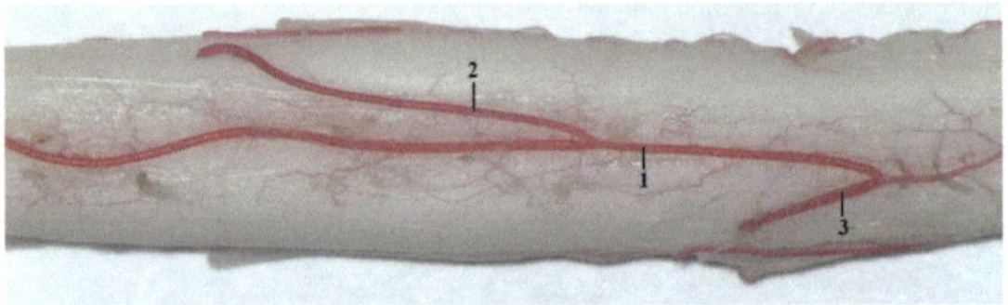

Figure 22. Doubled artery of Adamkiewicz. (1) Ventral spinal artery, (2) right-sided artery of Adamkiewicz, and (3) left-sided artery of Adamkiewicz. Dissected specimen, ventral view, magnification 8x.

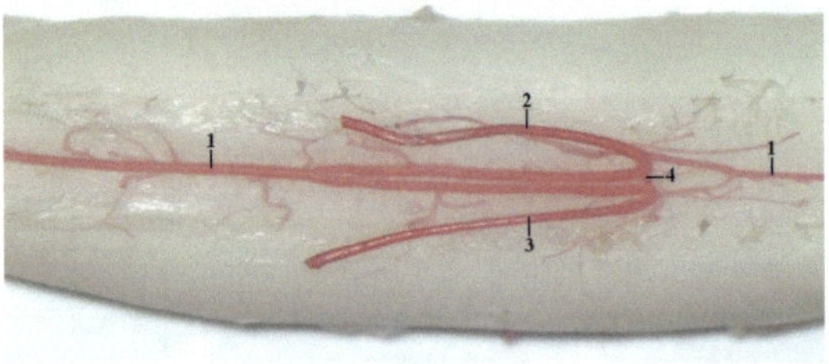

Figure 23. Doubled artery of Adamkiewicz. (1) Ventral spinal artery, (2) right-sided artery of Adamkiewicz, (3) left-sided artery of Adamkiewicz, and (4) communicating branch. Dissected specimen, ventral view, magnification 12.5x.

In 60% of cases, we found two irregular longitudinal dorsal spinal arteries located in lateral dorsal grooves (**Figure 24**). The dorsal branches of spinal branches were joined to the dorsal spinal arteries. Three irregular longitudinal dorsal spinal arteries receiving the dorsal branches of spinal branches were present in 40% of cases (**Figure 25**). The third dorsal spinal artery runs along the median dorsal groove. The occurrence of individual dorsal branches is shown in **Table 6**. In the cases of the presence of two irregular longitudinal dorsal spinal arteries, they were formed only by the fusion of the small cranially and caudally directed branches originating from the dorsal branches. The left-sided dorsal branches in the thoracic spinal cord were present in 56.8% and the right-sided in 43.2% of cases. The left-sided dorsal branches in the lumbar spinal cord were present in 65.5% of cases and right-sided in 34.5% of cases. Along the entire thoracolumbar spinal cord, the left-sided dorsal branches were present in 60.3% of cases and the right-sided in 39.7% of cases.

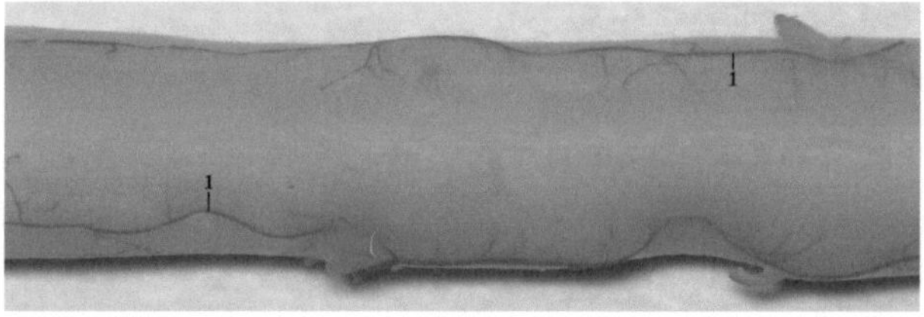

Figure 24. The presence of two longitudinal dorsal spinal arteries. (1) Dorsal spinal artery. Dissected specimen, dorsal view, magnification 12.5x.

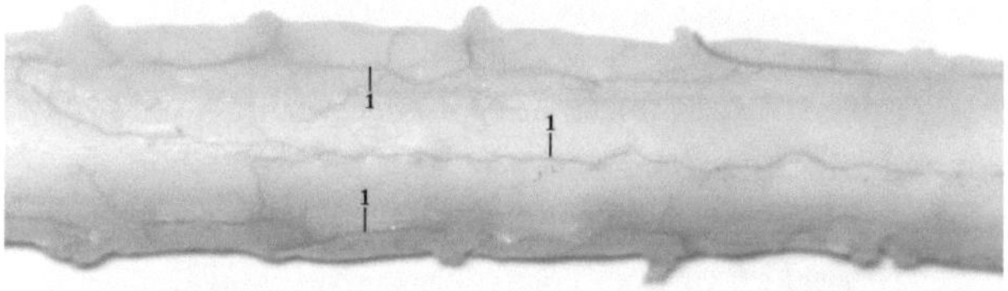

Figure 25. The presence of three longitudinal dorsal spinal arteries. (1) Dorsal spinal artery. Dissected specimen, dorsal view, magnification 12.5x.

4. Discussion

4.1. Cervical spinal cord

Based on our results, it can be concluded that the blood supply of the cervical spinal cord in rabbit and guinea pig has high variability. In contrast with our findings, only uniform origin of the ventral spinal artery in both species was described [16, 17]. Cervical spinal cord injury was studied in several species of experimental animals. The dogs, rats, pigs, rabbits, and guinea pigs belong to the most used species. The arterial arrangement of the cervical spinal cord in the dog was studied in detail with pointing on the variations in formation of the ventral spinal artery and the frequency of occurrence of spinal branches [18]. The rat was also studied in details, but the results of several studies differ [17, 19–21]. In pigs, only variations and the presence of extrasegmental arteries of the spinal cord blood supply were described [22, 23]. The frequency of occurrence of the spinal branches in our study was higher on the left than on the right side, opposite to the dog [18].

The arterial blood supply to the cervical spinal cord in monkeys, dogs, rabbits, and rats was studied by [24]. The origin of the ventral spinal artery was not recorded, and the ventral spinal artery was described as paired vessel. In our specimens, the ventral spinal artery was in a form of a single trunk with different types of origin in the place of fusion of bilateral vertebral arteries. In this work, the origin of dorsal spinal arteries from the posterior inferior cerebellar artery was described. In our specimens, we did not find the origin of the dorsal spinal arteries.

Some reports described the similarity of the arterial blood supply to the cervical spinal cord in rabbits, guinea pigs, and humans [16, 17]. Based on our study, we can conclude that there is partly different arterial pattern compared with human. The fusion of basilar artery is in human without gap [25]. In rabbits and guinea pigs, we found different types and numbers of gaps. In humans, the anterior spinal artery (homologue to the ventral spinal artery in animals) is formed by the fusion of the anterior spinal branches arising from the vertebral arteries [26]. In rabbits and guinea pigs, we found three different types of origin of ventral spinal artery in the place of fusion of vertebral bilateral arteries. In rabbits, we found the right-sided ventral branches joining the ventral spinal artery in 46.2% and left-sided in 53.8% of cases, and in guinea pig, the right-sided ventral branches were present in 41.8% of cases and the left-sided in 58.2% of cases. Only two or three ventral branches joining the anterior spinal artery were described in humans [27].

In rabbits and guinea pigs, we found on the dorsal surface high variability in the arrangement of the dorsal spinal arteries (in human, the posterior spinal arteries). The posterior spinal arteries in human are normally continuous rostral to caudal and supply the posterior third of the spinal cord [28]. The frequency of occurrence of individual dorsal and ventral branches in rabbits and guinea pigs was greater than in the case in humans.

According to our results, it can be concluded that the higher resistance to ischemic damage by the interruption of ventral and dorsal spinal arteries was because of the presence of dorsal and ventral branches reaching the cervical spinal cord in almost every segment. Rabbits and guinea pigs are often used as an experimental model for the study of spinal cord injury. The cervical spinal cord served as experimental model for the study of several types of damage [13, 29, 30].

4.2. Thoracolumbar spinal cord

Based on our results, it can be concluded that the blood supply to the thoracolumbar spinal cord in rabbit and guinea pig has high variability. The anatomical arrangement with regard to the origin of segmental dorsal intercostal and lumbar arteries has a very important role during operations of thoracoabdominal aneurysms [31]. Correctly performed reimplantation of segmental arteries decreases the risk of spinal cord ischemia, which can also lead to the paraplegia [32–34]. Till now in rabbits, the segmental arteries were described as paired branches originating independently from the dorsal surface of descending aorta [35, 36]. In guinea pigs, the presence of dorsal intercostal arteries with the origin from the supreme intercostal artery and the costocervical trunk was very variable. It varies from four to seven arteries on each side. Twelve pairs of dorsal intercostal arteries were present, and the remaining arteries were direct branches with the origin from the thoracic aorta [37]. In guinea pigs, the dorsal intercostal and lumbar arteries were described as paired branches arising independently from the dorsal surface of descending aorta [35, 36]. In guinea pigs, two types of origin of seven pairs of lumbar arteries were found: an independent origin and origin by means of a common trunk of the arteries at the same level [38].

In the study of ischemic injury in the thoracolumbar spinal cord, dogs, rats, pigs, rabbits, guinea pigs, and mice were used as experimental animals. In dogs, high variability in the density of arteries forming the spinal arterial ring and in the spinal branches was described [18]. In rats, the results in the study of arterial supply to the thoracolumbar spinal cord were very different [17, 19–21]. The dorsal spinal arteries were found in number of two [39] or as less constant [19]. In pigs, the studies were concentrated on the extrasegmental blood supply to the thoracolumbar spinal cord [22]. In mice, the spinal cord blood supply was partially described [10, 40].

Only one work dealing with arterial arrangement of the thoracolumbar spinal cord in rabbit and guinea pig was published [17]. But in this work, the artery of Adamkiewicz, the place of its origin, and any other variations were not described. We found variable arrangement of the artery of Adamkiewicz in rabbit and guinea pig, but in both species it was present in all cases. In guinea pig, doubled artery of Adamkiewicz with origin from spinal branch of the third or fourth lumbar artery was found [16]. In our study, the artery of Adamkiewicz was single or doubled with variable level of origin. In dogs, the artery of Adamkiewicz was found only in one half of the studied specimens. In rats, the presence of artery of Adamkiewicz is questionable. Some authors described its presence in all cases [17, 19, 20, 41], but some authors doubt its presence [21, 42]. In pigs, the artery of Adamkiewicz was not described [12, 13]. In mice, it was found in all cases [10] and also in humans [43].

The vascular arrangement of the dorsal spinal arteries in rabbits and guinea pigs was very variable. The dorsal spinal arteries in guinea pigs were described as two smaller anastomotic chains of arteries, running in the lateral dorsal grooves [16]. In our study, the number of dorsal spinal arteries varied from two to three. In humans, the posterior spinal arteries (homologue to the dorsal spinal arteries in animals) were found as normally trunks continuing in the cranial to caudal direction [28]. In dogs, four dorsal spinal arteries were described [18]. In rats, two much less constant dorsal spinal arteries with irregular connections between each other were found [19]. In mice, two spinal arteries [10] or only one single artery were described [40].

Our results indicate high variability in the presence of dorsal and ventral branches supplying the rabbit and guinea pig thoracolumbar spinal cord. On the left side, they occurred in higher numbers. The segmental arteries reaching the spinal cord ensured the blood supply of the ventral and dorsal surface of the respective segments of thoracolumbar spinal cord. In rabbits, the absence or irregularity of dorsal and ventral branches supplying the thoracic spinal cord was higher than that of branches supplying the lumbar spinal cord. The higher risk of ischemic damage to the thoracic spinal cord in rabbit was concluded. In guinea pigs, we found higher absence or irregularity of dorsal and ventral branches supplying the lumbar spinal cord, which allowed us to assume higher risk of irreparable ischemic damage to the lumbar spinal cord.

Based on results of the study, it is possible to conclude that the more appropriate model for the experimental study of ischemic injury of the thoracic spinal cord is the guinea pig and of the lumbar spinal cord is the rabbit, due to a lower incidence of variations of arterial arrangement in the corresponding spinal cord region. This implies that the thoracic spinal cord in guinea pig and lumbar spinal cord in rabbit are the most similar in their arterial arrangement to the homosegmental blood supply of human spinal cord.

5. Conclusion

The principles of blood vessel distribution to the spinal cord can be explained by the studies of arterial arrangements of several animals used as experimental models. In general, these studies can provide the additional information about the vascularization schema of the central nervous system [19].

For the prediction of functional results of neurological injuries and disorders, animal models from which the rodent models have a special place were used. Several clinical symptoms described in human patients are very parallel to the symptoms observed in rodents. The analysis of therapeutic approaches and behavioral sequel will help to determinate the limitations and strengths of animal models. It is very important to respect each aspect before an experimental study is started [44]. It is important to assess goals and expectations of the experiment before choosing a model. The understanding of the arterial arrangement to the spinal cord plays a very important role in avoiding the spinal cord ischemia or infarction during surgical interventions to the spine [45]. The presence of the artery of Adamkiewicz and nearly regular segmental blood supply to the thoracolumbar spinal cord in all studied animals is responsible for the use of rabbit and guinea pig as a simple model of ischemic damage to the thoracolumbar spinal cord.

The determination of appropriate species in the experiments of spinal cord injury requires the detailed study of the spinal cord arteries in all species used in this research area. The biased or erroneous outcomes can be caused by the presence of variation in arterial arrangement.

Author details

David Mazensky* and Slavka Flesarova

*Address all correspondence to: MazenskyD@azet.sk

University of Veterinary Medicine Pharmacy, Kosice, Slovak Republic

References

[1] Blight AR. Animal models of spinal cord injury. Topics in Spinal Cord Injury Rehabilitation. 2000;6:1–13. DOI: org/10.1310/2XNY-A824-UCTF-EN4D

[2] Lukáčová N, Pavel J, Gálik J. Spinal cord injury: the rabbit model. In: Aldskogius H, editor. Animal Models of Spinal Cord Repair. 1st ed. Uppsala: Humana Press; 2012. p. 149–158. DOI: 10.1007/978-1-62703-197-4_7

[3] Kundi S, Bicknell R, Ahmed Z. Spinal cord injury: Current mammalian models. American Journal of Neuroscience. 2013;4:1–12. DOI : 10.3844/amjnsp.2013.1.12

[4] Talac R, Friedman JA, Moore MJ, Lu L, Jabbari E, Windebank AJ, Currier BL, Yaszemski MJ. Animal models of spinal cord injury for evaluation of tissue engineering treatment strategies. Biomaterials. 2004;25:1505–1510. DOI: 10.1016/S0142-9612(03)00497-6

[5] Hrapkiewicz K, Medina L, Holmes DD. Rabbits. In: Hrapkiewicz K, Colby LA, Denison P, editors. Clinical laboratory animal medicine: An introduction. 2nd ed. Chichester: Wiley; 1998. p. 135–172. DOI: 10.1111/j.1748-5827.1998.tb03704.x

[6] Donnelly H. Quality in laboratory animals. In: Tuffery AA, editor. Laboratory Animals —An Introduction for Experimenters. 2nd ed. Chichester: Wiley; 1995. p. 181–203.

[7] Suckow MA, Stevens, KA, Wilson RP. The laboratory rabbit, guinea pig, hamster, and other rodents. 1st ed. Toronto: Elsevier; 2012. 1288 p.

[8] De Girolami U, Zivin JA. Neuropathology of experimental spinal cord ischemia in the rabbit. Journal of Neuropathology and Experimental Neurology. 1982;41:129–149.

[9] Vacanti FX, Kwun BD. Vascular occlusion produced over 24 hours increases spinal cord tolerance to occlusion. Journal of Surgical Research. 1996;62:29–31. DOI: 10.1006/jsre.1996.0168

[10] Lang-Lazdunski L, Matsushita K, Hirt L, Waeber Ch, Vonsattel J-PG, Moskowitz MA. Spinal cord ischemia. Development of a model in the mouse. Stroke. 2000;31:208–213. DOI: 10.1161/01.STR.31.1.208

[11] Luo J, Li N, Robinson JP, Shi R. The increase of reactive oxygen species and their inhibition in an isolated guinea pig spinal cord compression model. Spinal Cord. 2002;40:656–665. DOI: 10.1038/sj.sc.3101363

[12] McBride JM, Smith DT, Byrn SR, Borgens RB, Shi R. 4-Aminopyridine derivatives enhance impulse conduction in guinea-pig spinal cord following traumatic injury. Neuroscience. 2007;148:44–52. DOI: 10.1016/j.neuroscience.2007.05.039

[13] Sun W, Fu Y, Shi Y, Cheng J-X, Cao P, Shi R. Paranodal myelin damage after acute stretch in guinea pig spinal cord. Journal of Neurotrauma. 2012;29:611–619. DOI: 10.1089/neu.2011.2086

[14] Hossler FE, Monson FC. Microvasculature of the rabbit urinary bladder. Anatomical Record. 1995;243:438–448. DOI: 10.1002/ar.1092430406

[15] Kresakova L, Purzyc H, Schusterova I, Fulton B, Maloveska M, Vdoviakova K, Kravcova Z, Boldizar M. Non-standard intracranial connections and alternative pathways between dural venous sinuses and cerebral veins in the rat. Anatomical Science International. 2015;90:172–179. DOI: 10.1007/s12565-014-0241-2

[16] Knox-Macaulay H, Morrell MT, Potts DM, Preston TD. The arterial supply to the spinal cord of the guinea pig. Acta Anatomica. 1960;40:249–255. DOI:10.1159/000141587

[17] Soutoul JH, Gouaz'e A, Castaing J. The spinal cord arteries of experimental animals. 3. Comparative study of the rat, guinea-pig, rabbit, cat, dog, orang-outang, chimpanzee, with man and fetus. Pathologie Biologie. 1964;12:950'962.

[18] Pais D, Casal D, Arantes M, Casimiro M, O'Neill JG. Spinal cord arteries in Canis familiaris and their variations: implications in experimental procedures. Brazilian Journal of Morphological Sciences. 2007;24:224–228.

[19] Woollam DHM, Millen JW. The arterial supply of the spinal cord and its significance. Journal of Neurology, Neurosurgery and Psychiatry. 1955;18:97–102. DOI: 10.1136/jnnp.18.2.97

[20] Brightman MW. Comparative anatomy of spinal cord vasculature. Anatomical Record. 1956;124:264. DOI: 10.1002/ar.1091240209

[21] Schievink WI, Luyendijk W, Los JA. Does the artery of Adamkiewicz exist in the albino rat? Journal of Anatomy. 1988;161:95–101.

[22] Strauch JT, Spielvogel D, Lauten A, Zhang N, Shiang H, Weisz D, Bodian CA, Griepp RB. Importance of extrasegmental vessels for spinal cord blood supply in a chronic porcine model. European Journal of Cardio-thoracic Surgery. 2003;24:817–824. DOI: 10.1016/S1010-7940(03)00460-3

[23] Strauch JT, Lauten A, Zhang N, Wahlers T, Griepp RB. Anatomy of spinal cord blood supply in the pig. The Annals of Thoracic Surgery. 2007;83:2130–2134. DOI:10.1016/j.athoracsur.2007.01.060

[24] Chakravorty BG. Arterial supply of the cervical spinal cord and its relation to the cervical myelopathy in spondylosis. Annals of the Royal College of Surgeons of England. 1969;45:232–251.

[25] Ashwini CA, Shubha R, Jayanthi KS. Comparative anatomy of the circle of Willis in man, cow, sheep, goat, and pig. Neuroanatomy. 2008;7:54–65.

[26] Shajmi MF, Maziak DE, Shajmi FM, Ginsberg RJ, Pon R. Circulation of the spinal cord: an important consideration for thoracic surgeon. Annals of Thoracic Surgery. 2003;76:315–321. DOI: 10.1016/S0003-4975(03)00139-5

[27] Melissano G, Civilini E, Bertoglio L, Calliari F, Campos Moraes Amato A, Chiesa R. Angio-CT imaging of the spinal cord vascularisation. European Journal of Vascular and Endovascular Surgery. 2009;39:436–440. DOI: 10.1016/j.ejvs.2009.11.026.

[28] Cheshire WP, Santos CC, Massey EW, Howard JF. Spinal cord infarction: etiology and outcome. Neurology. 1996;47:321–330. DOI: 10.1212/WNL.47.2.321

[29] Klironomos G, Karadimas S, Mavrakis A, Mirilas P, Savvas I, Papadaki E, Papachristou DJ, Gatzounis G. New experimental rabbit animal model for cervical spondylotic myelopathy. Spinal Cord. 2011;49:1097–1102. DOI: 10.1038/sc.2011.71.

[30] Park J-H. Does small size vertebral or vertebrobasilar artery matter in ischemic stroke? In: Garcia Rodriguez JC, editor. Acute Ischemic Stroke. 1st ed. Rijeka: InTech; 2012. p. 213–224.

[31] David N, Roux N, Douvrin F, Clavier E, Bessou JP, Plissonnier D. Aortic aneurysm surgery: long-term patency of the reimplanted intercostal arteries. The Annals of Vascular Surgery. 2012;26:839–844. DOI: 10.1016/j.avsg.2011.08.026

[32] Grabitz K, Sandmann W, Stühmeier K, Mainzer B, Godehardt E, Ohle B, Hatwich U. The risk of ischemic spinal cord injury in patients undergoing graft replacement for thoracoabdominal aortic aneurysms. Journal of Vascular Surgery. 1996;23:230–240. DOI: 10.1016/S0741-5214(96)70267-7

[33] de Haan P, Kalkman CJ, de Mol BA, Ubags LH, Veldman DJ, Jacobs MJ. Efficacy of transcranial motor-evoked myogenic potentials to detect spinal cord ischemia during operations for thoracoabdominal aneurysms. The Journal of Thoracic and Cardiovascular Surgery. 1997;113:87–101. DOI: 10.1016/S0022-5223(97)70403-3

[34] Etz DC, Halstead JC, Spielvogel D, Shahani R, Lazla, R, Homann TM, Weisz DJ, Plestis K, Griepp RB. Thoracic and thoracoabdominal aneurysm repair: is reimplantation of spinal cord arteries a waste of time? The Annals of Thoracic Surgery. 2006;82:1670–1677. DOI: 10.1016/j.athoracsur.2006.05.029

[35] Nejedly K. Biology and systematic anatomy of laboratory animals. 1st ed. Prague: SPN; 1965. 629 p.

[36] Popesko P, Rajtova V, Horak J. A Colour Atlas of Anatomy of Small Laboratory Animals 1. 1st ed. New York: Saunders; 2003. 256 p.

[37] Shively MJ, Stump JE. The systemic arterial pattern of the guinea pig: the head, thorax, and thoracic limb. American Journal of Anatomy. 1974;139:269–284. DOI: 10.1002/aja.1001390208

[38] Shively MJ, Stump JE. The systemic arterial pattern of the guinea pig: the abdomen. Anatomical Record. 1975;182:355–366. DOI: 10.1002/ar.1091820309

[39] Lazorthes G, Gouaze A, Zadeh JO, Santini JJ, Lazorthes Y, Burdin P. Arterial vascularization of the spinal cord: recent studies of the anastomotic substitution pathways. Journal of Neurosurgery. 1971;35:253–262. DOI: 10.3171/jns.1971.35.3.0253

[40] Bilgen M, Al-Hafez B. Comparison of spinal vasculature in mouse and rat: investigations using MR angiography. Neuroanatomy. 2006;5:12–16.

[41] Gouazé A, Soutoul JH, Santini JJ, Duprey G. Artery of the lumbar nlargement of the 16 cord in some mammals. Proceedings der Association of Anatomists. 1965;49:762–775.

[42] Tveten L. Spinal cord vascularity IV. The spinal cord arteries in the rat. Acta Radiologica: Diagnosis. 1976;17:385–398. DOI: 10.1177/028418517601700401

[43] Milen MT, Bloom DA, Culligan J. Albert Adamkiewicz (1850–1921)—his artery and its significance for the retroperitoneal surgeon. World Journal of Urology. 1999;17:168–170. DOI: 10.1007/s003450050126

[44] Geissler SA, Schmidt CE, Schallert T. Rodent models and behavioral outcomes of cervical spinal cord injury. Journal of Spine. 2013;7 Suppl 4: 001. DOI: 10.4172/2165-7939.S4-001

[45] Gao L, Wang L, Su B, Wang P, Ye J, Shen H. The vascular supply to the spinal cord and its relationship to anterior spine surgical approaches. Spine Journal. 2013;13:966–973. DOI: 10.1016/j.spinee.2013.03.017

Section 3

Translational Science

Chapter 5

Forebrain Ischemic Stroke and the Phenomenon of Ischemic Tolerance: Is Homocysteine Foe or Friend?

Ján Lehotský, Maria Kovalská, Barbara Tothová, Anna Beňová, Dagmar Kalenská and Peter Kaplán

Additional information is available at the end of the chapter

http://dx.doi.org/10.5772/64611

Abstract

Hyperhomocysteinemia (hHCy) is a recognized comorbid risk factor of human brain stroke. We overview here the recent data on the homocysteine (Hcy) metabolism and on the genetic and metabolic causes of hHCy-related neuropathologies. In context of our results which detected an increased oxidative stress in hyperhomocysteinemic rats, we discuss here the role of free radicals in this disorder. Brain ischemia-reperfusion causes delayed neuronal death. Ischemic tolerance evoked by preconditioning (IPC) represents a phenomenon of central nervous system (CNS) adaptation to any subsequent ischemia. The paper describes changes in the mitogen-activated protein kinases (MAPKs) protein pathways, and apoptotic markers were used to follow the degeneration process. Our studies provide evidence for the interplay and tight integration between extracellular signal-regulated kinase (ERK) and p38 MAPKs signaling mechanisms in response to the hHCy and also in association with brain ischemia/IPC challenge. Recognition of the effects of risk factors in the ischemic tolerance would lead to improved therapeutics, especially the brain tissue.

Keywords: hyperhomocysteinemia, ischemic tolerance, oxidative stress, brain, preconditioning

1. Introduction

Comorbidities are widely recognized as possible risk factors for cardiovascular and cerebrovascular diseases [1–4]. Clinically described comorbidities such as earlier incidence of any type of stroke, prior transient ischemic attack (TIA), arterial disease, atrial fibrillation, unproper diet and/or obesity, and physical inactivity are known to elevate risk for ischemic stroke [3, 4]. As it has been proved by several studies, even mild hyperhomocysteinemia (hHCy) increases the incidence of ischemic brain damage, probably due to pleiotropic effect of homocysteine (Hcy) and the impact of venous and arterial atherosclerotic changes [2, 5–7]. In fact, Hcy inhibits NO synthesis by endothelial cells and platelets and stimulates the production of reactive oxygen species (ROS) by the release of arachidonic acid from platelets. In parallel, it also inhibits glutathione peroxidase and therefore stimulates the proliferation of endothelial cells (see [6] for review). In addition, Hcy has been shown to inhibit methyltransferases, to suppress DNA repair, and to facilitate apoptosis when accumulated inside the cells. Auto-oxidation of Hcy metabolites results in H_2O_2 accumulation [8], and long-term incubation of neurons with Hcy metabolites induces necrotic cell death [9]. Consequently, homocysteine level has been shown to be comorbidly elevated in neurodegenerative and acute disorders of the central nervous system (CNS), for example, Alzheimer's disease or Parkinson's disease [10]. Thus, the incorporation of animal models more consistent with the clinical population afflicted by stroke is urgently needed for proper exploration of the disease's etiology such as stroke and other cerebrovascular diseases. In fact, only limited number of literature data can be found to describe the mutual influence of comorbid hyperhomocysteinemia to ischemic damage on animal models of ischemic stroke.

2. Phenomenon of ischemic tolerance evolution

The brain is highly susceptible to hypoxia or ischemia, and numerous endogenous mechanisms exist to protect neural tissue from its effects and to produce a protective state known as ischemic tolerance [3, 4, 11]. It represents an evolutionally conserved endogenous neuroprotection/plasticity, which can be induced by various paradigmas/stressors. Preconditioning is one of the recognized neuroprotective strategies, which is induced prior to stroke as a preventative measure in a high-risk individuals. It also can be used as a precaution against secondary stroke following medical procedures such as aneurysm repair or cardiac surgery [1, 3, 4, 12]. In the clinical settings of human stroke, which is hardly predicted, a novel algorithm of postconditioning may have a very high therapeutic value. Remarkably, it could be used afterward of ictus to stimulate protective and regenerative pathways or as a precaution against stroke recurrence [1, 12, 13]. Clinical studies are needed to test the safety and efficacy of these novel strategies in humans [3, 4]. Although the cascade of molecular processes determining ischemic preconditioning is not fully understood, it has been shown to influence receptor activities, mitogen-activating protein (MAP) and other kinases and apoptotic mechanisms. Additionally, ischemic tolerance in the brain can also be stimulated remotely, for example, by the application of a tourniquet to one of the limbs also in human patients with subarachnoid hemorrhage. More detailed studies are still needed to clinically validate this phenomenon [1, 3, 12, 14–16].

In spite of the high clinical relevance, only limited number of experiments can be found in the literature to describe the mutual influence of comorbid hyperhomocysteinemia to ischemic damage on animal models of human stroke. This paper summarizes current knowledge of the homocysteine metabolism and the genetic and the metabolic causes of hyperhomocysteinemia-related neurotoxicity. Based on results from our laboratory, in this context, we also found that the combination of experimental hyperhomocysteinemia (hHCy) with ischemic insult and/or with the pre-ischemic challenge affects the extent of neuronal degeneration as well as the MAP kinase pathways involved in the preconditioning phenomenon.

3. Toxicity of homocysteine as recognized from its metabolism

Homocysteine (Hcy) is an intermediate sulfhydryl-containing amino acid derived from methionine with recognized toxicity to neural cells and vascular endothelial cells. It originates from a dietary protein through S-adenosyl methionine conversion [17]. Human patients with severe hyperhomocysteinemia (hHcy) are characterized by a perplex of typical clinical cardiovascular manifestations, which include neurological abnormalities, such as cerebral atrophy, dementia, and seizures [18]. A large number of epidemiological investigations have revealed the association of folate deficiency and hyperhomocysteinemia with an increased risk of vascular diseases and brain ischemic stroke [6, 19].

Homocysteine metabolism includes three independent alternative pathways:

i. re-methylation,

ii. transmethylation to methionine, or

iii. transsulfuration to cysteine.

In addition to the already recognized causative role of mutations or polymorphisms in the key genes encoding enzymes of Hcy metabolism to cardiovascular disorders and also stroke, a novel observation already proved that epigenetic mechanisms, such as DNA methylation, chromatin remodeling, RNA editing, noncoding RNAs (ncRNAs), and microRNAs (miRNAs), might be equally relevant in the stroke etiopathogenesis [3, 20]. Earlier genetic studies suggest that polymorphisms of the genes, which encode the metabolic pathways, such as methylenetetrahydrofolate reductase (MTHFR), cystathionine β-synthase (CBS), DNA methyltransferase (DNMT), and nicotinamide N-methyltransferase (NNMT), might play an important role in stroke development during elevated level of Hcy. Additionally, nutritional supplements, for example, folic acid (a cofactor in one-carbon metabolism), can regulate the epigenetic alterations of neuronal cells and may play an important role in the maintenance of neuronal integrity [18, 20].

General Hcy metabolism in liver represents mainly methyl group transfer and re-methylation and requires vitamin B_{12} and folic acid for N-5-methyltetrahydrofolate-homocysteine methyltransferase. Additionally, the transsulfuration reaction of Hcy depends on the presence of vitamin B_6. Remarkably in the CNS, the Hcy metabolism differs from other organs. The transsulfuration pathway is practically absent and the re-methylation pathway using betaine is not present [6, 21]. Thus, the effectivity to metabolize or convert homocysteine mostly relies on externally delivered folate and cobalamine in the form of vitamins. The glial cells contain very low deposits of vitamin $B_{12,}$ which is exhausted rather quickly during its negative balance.

The harmful effect of the homocysteine to CNS neurons is quite well known. It has an influence to both the neuronal survival rate and the functionality of neurons to the signal transmission. As a consequence, it also affects the formation of functional neural networks with the effect surpassing simple neuronal survival.

In our laboratory, we have analyzed the neurotoxic properties of Hcy on glial cells, using a glioblastoma cell line as a study model. The viability of cells was assayed both biochemically and cytologically. As proved, Hcy concentration around 50 μmol/l induced cell death. It is worth noting that Hcy induces cell death of human glial cells at concentrations which corresponds to the mild clinically occurred hyperhomocysteinemia. We propose that Hcy-induced impairment of neuronal functions along with the damage of glial cells may contribute to the etiopathogenesis of neurological disorders associated with hyperhomocysteinemia [22]. As shown in clinical studies, an elevated Hcy level associates with CNS disorders, such as stroke, Alzheimer's disease, dementia, as well as with classical homocystinuria [2, 6].

In humans, plasma Hcy concentration varies from 5 to 10 μmol/l and its elevated level is classified as hyperhomocysteinemia (hHcy) with mild, moderate, intermediate, and severe (for concentrations higher than 100 μmol/l), manifested also with homocystinuria [19]. As generally believed, homocysteine is produced merely in all tissues. On the other hand, its metabolic inactivation proceeds only in the liver/kidney, mainly through the transsulfuration pathway. As the outcome, in tissues such as the blood vessels and the brain, where re-methylation enzymes are merely absent, the reduction of MTHFR activity leads to homocysteine accumulation. As analyzed in various genetic cohorts, the MTHFR C677T polymorphism has been established as a risk factor for ischemic stroke in different laboratories [23].

Selective neurotoxic effect of Hcy includes various pathomechanisms such as glutamate receptor-mediated neurotoxicity [2, 24]. Notably, glutamatergic excitotoxicity is also associated with the brain damage caused by ischemic insult. Hcy was shown as an inductor of caspase-dependent neuronal apoptosis, by a mechanism involving several detrimental steps, such as the DNA damage, poly-ADP-ribose polymerase (PARP) dysregulation, and mitochondrial dysfunction by caspase-3 activation. Hcy appears to also be critically involved in the glial-vascular interface communications as part of the blood-brain barrier. The important role of astrocytes in the regulation of overall brain metabolism and in particular in the brain energy metabolism has already been proved [4, 22]. As generally believed, the elevation of the Hcy activates an excitatory glutamatergic neurotransmission in different brain areas, which stimulates neuronal damage derived from an excessive Ca^{2+} influx and reactive oxygen species generation.

Principally, dysbalance in redox state and oxidative stress has been proposed as one of the primary etiologies for hHCy-related pathogenesis [6, 19]. Previous observations proved that dysequilibrium in redox balance may be a key factor in the pathogenesis of vascular hypertrophy, thrombosis, and atherosclerosis in hyperhomocysteinemic animals [25]. In fact, reactive oxygen species (ROS) are side products of the Hcy-free thiol group oxidation, mainly when Hcy binds via a disulfide bridge with plasma proteins—mainly albumin— or with other low-molecular plasma thiols, or secondarily with other Hcy molecule.

Already proposed reactions responsible for Hcy-induced oxidative stress include:

i. inhibition of the activity of cellular antioxidant enzymes,

ii. Hcy auto-oxidation,

iii. nitric oxide synthase (NOS)-dependent generation of superoxide anion via uncoupling of endothelial NOS (eNOS),

iv. disruption of extracellular superoxide dismutase from endothelial surfaces, and

v. activation of NADPH oxidases.

vi. Interestingly, mutual tissue production of strong oxidant peroxynitrite stimulates tyrosine nitration, which leads to protein functional alterations and cellular dysfunction [26]. Auto-oxidation of Hcy metabolites results in H_2O_2 accumulation and as shown by [9] and later by [8] prolonged incubation of neurons with Hcy metabolites leads to necrotic cell death.

Homocysteine is also converted to the thioester forming the Hcy-thiolactone in an error-editing reaction in translation mechanism. Accidentally in proteosynthetic process, Hcy is erroneously selected in place of methionine by methionyl-tRNA-synthetase. As shown by animal and human experiments, the Hcy-thiolactone remarkably contributes to Hcy pathobiology. Its toxicity is based on reaction which leads to protein N-homocysteinylation through the formation of amine bonds with protein lysine residues [27], which impairs or alters the structural and functional properties of particular protein. Several clinical studies have reported that increased plasma homocysteine levels may provoke neurological seizures. Systemic administration of homocysteine at high doses is able to induce convulsions in mice and it can be suggested that similar detrimental effects might occur in patients affected by temporal lobe epilepsy [28].

A number of papers from our and also other laboratories [13, 29–31] documented that global ischemia/reperfusion injury (IRI) in rats follows with the time-dependent dysbalance of redox balance in cortex and hippocampus. The insult also activates different gene expression at both the mRNA and protein levels. In addition, experiments of [32] proved that the redox status and gene expression are influenced by preconditioned pre-ischemic treatment. In spite of high clinical relevance, the data from literature which deals with the mutual effect of IRI and endogenously produced homocysteine as verified risk factor to ischemic injury are very limited [2]. Observations of [6] which described the effect of chronic dietary supplementation of Hcy for 2 weeks (to initiate hyperhomocysteinemia-hHCy) documented remarkable elevation of lipoperoxidative and protein oxidative products in rat cortex and hippocampus. Experimental hyperhomocysteinemia was induced by the subcutaneous administration of homocysteine in saline solution (0.45 μmol/g body weight) twice a day at 8-h interval for 14 days [6, 30]. It has been proved that Hcy crosses the blood/brain barrier and exhibits a maximum level in the cerebrum and parietal cortex between 15 and 60 min after subcutaneous injection. Remarkably, plasma Hcy concentration in rats treated this way achieved levels similar to those found in homocystinuric patients (moderate hyperhomocysteinemia). Groups of rats were subdivided as described earlier [6, 30]:

1. sham-operated control (naive) animals,
2. sham-operated control (preconditioning) animals,
3. the animals that underwent 15-min ischemia (naive),
4. the animals with induced 5-min IPC following 15-min ischemia,
5. sham-operated hyperhomocysteinemic control animals,
6. the hyperhomocysteinemic animals that underwent 15-min ischemia,
7. the hyperhomocysteinemic animals with induced preconditioning animals following 15-min ischemia.

Experiments evidently document that hyperhomocysteinemia induces remarkable elevation of lipoperoxidative and protein-oxidative products, the results which are in a good correlation with previously published experiments [24]. Moreover, as documented by the number of Fluoro-Jade B-positive- and TUNEL-positive cells (as indicator of neuronal degeneration) [30, 33–37], the number and proportion of degenerated neurons over intact cells evidently exceeds in the hippocampus of hHCy animals and reached the level which almost competes with the levels documented after ischemic insult in nontreated, naive group. As was shown in earlier studies, an auto-oxidation of Hcy metabolites results in higher H_20_2 production, and prolonged incubation of neurons with Hcy metabolites elevates the number of necrotic cell death [8, 9]. Interestingly, as was documented by [38], single intracerebroventricular injection of homocystein was followed by the elevation of typical apoptotic features of cells of *substantia nigra,* which results to the typical Parkinson's disease-like behavior in rats. As was detected earlier, an increased Hcy level is potent to induce and accumulate hydroxyl radicals as the most potent, powerful-free oxygen species with the high efficiency to remove electrons from other cellular biomolecules such as lipids, proteins, carbohydrates, and DNA [39]. Remarkably, results of experiments from our laboratory and also previous results have documented that in hyperhomocysteinic model in rats [6, 30, 36, 37, 40], the elevation of homocysteine was followed by significant neurotoxic effect. As was proposed earlier, the effect is probably caused by the hHCy-induced oxidative dysbalance and cellular stress. Interestingly, as was detected in a human study on Alzheimer's patients and patients with the mild cognitive impairment, an increased level of plasma homocysteine positively correlated with alterations of hippocampal volume. This effect is not mediated by cerebral beta-amyloid deposition and vascular burden but likely due to the oxidative dysregulation induced by homocysteine as part of direct homocysteine adverse effect [2, 41].

Results from another study from this laboratory [42] have shown that hyperhomocysteinic differently express mRNA and protein of calcium pump in secretory pathways (SPCA1). SPCA has a remarkable role in the development of neural cells and their migration [43] and its loss can finalize to the stress of Golgi apparatus expressed by alterations of membrane structure and redox dysregulation in neuronal cells. The effect of Hcy on the expression profile of the Ca^{2+}-transport proteins in neuronal cells is not yet fully described. The transcription factors Sp1 and YY1 were identified in the gene expression regulation by the cis-enhancing elements in 5′-untranslated regions. Hyperhomocysteinemia is followed in intracellular Ca^{2+} elevation, release of calcium and endoplasmic reticulum (ER) stress [6, 44], leading to apoptotic events, endothelial dysfunction, and remodeling of the extracellular matrix also in the brain parenchyma. Moreover, homocysteine itself by metabolic interfering with the level of S-adenosylmethionine (donor of methyl group) has also been reported to induce the modulation of gene expression through the alteration of the gene methylation status [10].

Remarkably, the processes, such as modifications of protein structure, have been proved in the etiology eventually leading to homocysteine-induced neurotoxicity. Homocysteinylation can be subdivided into the two main types:

i. S-homocysteinylation and

ii. N-homocysteinylation,

both of which are typical examples of posttranslational protein modifications. The extent of the homocysteinylated modifications correlates with increased plasma Hcy level [39], and the chemical conversion of Hcy to Hcy-thiolactone followed by protein N-homocysteinylation is an etiological factor, which contributes to the expressed Hcy neuronal and tissue toxicity. As shown by [45], homocysteinylation follows functional protein modification and enhances protein degradation processes which can finalize to cell damage.

In this context, Petras et al. [6] in a recent study observed remarkable decrease of Mn^{2+}-activated superoxide dismutase (Mn-SOD) activity in cortical mitochondria in the 14-day hHCy model in rats. This catalytic activity is included in the first line of cellular defense against oxidative injury, and has been shown to be suppressed in the hHCy group compared to the control group. These results might be explained by putative increased posttranslational modifications of Mn-SOD due to the higher level of Hcy leading to the enzyme homocysteinylation and thiolation. As was shown recently by Li et al. [46], the imbalance among antioxidant enzymes caused by an increased Hcy level might alter ROS elimination, and thus lead to the increasing amount of free radicals and likely to homocysteine-induced stress of endoplasmic reticulum, which can result in the dysfunctional consequences in rat hippocampus.

4. Impact of hyperhomocysteinemia on ischemic/reperfusion injury and ischemic tolerance induced by ischemic preconditioning

Now, the clinical comorbid effect of hHCy to the stroke incidence and severity is clearly recognized. However, a bit surprisingly, the experimental results, which are focused on the mutual influence of the comorbid hyperhomocysteinemia to ischemic damage on the animal models of human stroke, are only limited [12, 32, 47]. Ischemic insult/reperfusion insult in the animal models is followed by the degeneration of majority (more than 64%) of hippocampal neurons [3, 33]. Experiments from this laboratory [33, 34, 42], which combine 14 days of hyperhomocysteinemia with 15-min forebrain ischemia/reperfusion, show that insult initiates manifestations of morphologically changed neurons and disturbances of glial cells of the hippocampal area. On the other hand, the combination of both approaches elevated the percentage of morphologically intact and probably nondegenerated cells in comparison to the naive ischemic/reperfusion insult. In this context, Sato et al. [47] in experiments on hippocampal CA1 neurons after ischemic insult in rats have proved concentration-dependent cell protection by S-adenosyl-L-methionine (SAMe). The effect was concealed by the concomitant administration of S-adenosyl-L-homocysteine, a potent inhibitor in transmethylation. From these results, the authors considered that the enhancement of intraparenchymal SAMe level followed by the activation of transmethylation using SAMe as a methyl donor in postischemic brain is inevitable for the tissue protection and prevention of delayed neuronal death.

The pre-ischemic treatment has been recognized to save the majority of hippocampal neurons which exceeds more than 75% of all neurons [1, 33]. If we combined 14 days of hyperhomocysteinemia with preconditioning [6, 33, 34, 36, 37, 40, 42], this particular treatment has finalized by the larger suppression of cell degeneration not crossing 5% of the total number of neurons. It is remarkable that in this particular hyperhomocysteinic model in rats, the protective effect of IPC maneuver is influenced by not-yet fully clarified mechanism. One appealing candidate that has been described is a novel regulatory epigenetic mechanism, which encompasses both the gene environment interactions and also tissue functionality. The recent evidence proves that several epigenetic mechanisms are also involved in the stroke pathogenesis and the tolerance etiology. Participation of several important enzymes regulating DNA methylation including DNA-N-methyltransferase has been proved, and the high level of Hcy may eventually finalize to the increase in the level of S-adenosyl methionine. As a result, its higher enzymatic activity might stimulate hypermethylation of the genomic DNAs and silencing of functional genes [44].

In the recent study [35], the authors have analyzed whether hyperhomocysteinemia (risk factor of brain ischemia) alone or in combination with the ischemic preconditioning (IPC) affects the ischemia-induced neurodegenerative changes and imbalance in the intracellular-signaling pathway including the MAPK/p-ERK1/2 and MAPK/p-p38 gene and protein expression in the rat brains. We have used the model of hyperhomocysteinemia induced by the subcutaneous administration of homocysteine as well as the preconditioning maneuvers followed by global ischemia as was described above. Here, we suggest that hHCy alone (as an example of metabolic stress) and/or in combination with IR injury affects mechanisms of the ischemic tolerance induced by IPC maneuver. The study reveals that hHCy alone significantly increased neurodegeneration by Fluoro-Jade C and terminal deoxynucleotidyl transferase (TdT)-mediated dUTP nick end labeling (TUNEL) positive cells in hippocampus as well as in the cortical brain area. Prominent features of those changes were detected by using markers of cell damage/degeneration and changes in MAPKs expression in the CA1 hippocampal region and M1 cortical sector. We have also found in these experiments an elevated level of MAPK/p-ERK and the decreased level of MAPK/p-p38 after pre-ischemic challenge by Western blot and fluorescent immunohistochemistry.

Experiments from this laboratory previously showed that IR insult leads to the neurodegeneration of neurons in the CA1 region of hippocampus as detected by Fluoro-Jade C and TUNEL analysis. As expected, IPC leads to the suppression of the number of positive cells and conferred neuroprotection [33, 34]. Interestingly, the effect of homocysteine on cellular degeneration and following morphological changes was observed in the rat hippocampal and cortical regions. The increased number of Fluoro-Jade C+ and TUNEL+ neuronal and glial elements supports this effect of hHCy. The thickened and collapsed processes that poorly extend to the area of pyramidal neurons in CA1 region and M1 cortex are presumably due to the morphological alterations of astrocytes and cytoskeletal remodeling. This might suggest for the ensuing development of hHCy-associated neuronal cell damage [23, 48, 49]. Astrocytes are highly plastic cells and their dynamic morphological changes could affect the intercellular communication with surrounding synapses that are important in the development of brain lesions [40]. Maler et al. [50] reported that Hcy doses of 2 mmol/l and above induced a dose-dependent cytotoxic effect on cortical astrocytes. Astrocytes regulate the expression of the N-methyl-D-aspartate (NMDA) receptor subtypes, which increase neuronal sensitivity to glutamate toxicity and thus accelerate the initial step in a program of reactive astrogliosis and dynamics of the astrocyte response to damage [51]. On the other hand, in response to the injury, astrocytes synthesize a number of factors that may play either neuroprotective or neurotoxic roles.

Recently, we have shown that IPC prior to lethal ischemia affects MAPK/ERK and MAPK/p38 pathways in the cerebral cortex [33] as well as in hippocampus [34]. There is only sparse literature data focusing on the effect of Hcy on the MAPKs protein expression in neuronal cells [48, 52]. Our results suggest that the combination of both stressors (ischemia + Hcy) affects considerably the MAPKs pathways expression. hHCy-IR induces the MAPK/p38 expression as detected by Western blot and immunoanalysis. Poddar and Paul [52] showed a biphasic response of MAPK/p38 activation in the Hcy-NMDA-induced neuronal damage *in vitro*, characterized by the initial rapid elevation followed by a delayed and more prolonged secondary increase, where the later peak was primarily involved in mediating the Hcy-induced cell death. They also showed that this secondary activation of MAPK/p38 correlates with the upstream MAPK/ERK activation, which plays a role in facilitating of the Hcy with the conclusions of this study. Interestingly, we found that the MAPK/p38 pathway was activated also in hHCy control group. We previously reported that IR injury induces only slight increase of MAPK/p38 expression [33, 34]. However, the combination of both stressors (ischemia + hHCy) leads to the massive activation of MAPK/p-p38 with maximum at 24 h after reperfusion. This dynamic MAPK/p38 activation could contribute to more extensive progression of tissue injury [52, 53]. Remarkably, the effect of the IPC maneuver on the decreasing of MAPK/p-p38 expression in ongoing reperfusion times indicates for proposed neuroprotective mechanism. The MAPK/p-p38 pathway was suppressed also by the combination of two stressors.

MAPK/ERKs are versatile protein kinases that are ubiquitously expressed in the CNS. We have already shown that in the hippocampus and cerebral cortex activated MAPK/ERK parallels neuroprotection induced by IPC [33, 34]. The robust expression changes in hippocampus and modest posttranslational changes in MAPK/ERK pathway in less sensitive vulnerable neurons of the cortical layers III and V corresponds with results of similar experimental models [53, 54]. Extensive studies have shown an interplay and tight integration of MAPK/ERK signaling in promoting neuronal cell death both in development and in neurodegenerative disorders [49, 52]. It has been proposed that transient activation of MAPK/ERK has different consequences as compared with sustained activation [49, 52]. Transient activation of MAPK/ERK plays a pivotal role in neuronal maturation, survival, and long-term potentiation. On the other hand, the sustained activation of MAPK/ERK may play a critical role in triggering proapoptotic signals and neuronal cell death. As documented in our study [35], the immunoreactivity of MAPK/p-ERK after IPC with induced hHCy was found in the early stages of reperfusion, with maximum level at 24 h, and its activation is probably associated with neuronal protection induced by IPC [54]. The slight activation of MAPK/ERK was detected also in the hHCy- control group. It is well known that hHCy mediates glutamate-mediated NMDA receptor stimulation, which eventually leads to the activation of both stimulatory and inhibitory pathways involved in the modulation of MAPK/ERK signaling [49]. In fact, the dual role of MAKP/ERK kinases in cell survival and death suggests that a unique profile of gene expression may be elicited depending on the duration and/or magnitude of MAPK/ERK kinase activation [52]. Thus, the duration of MAPK/ERK kinase activation following MAPK/p38 stimulation depends on the nature of the extracellular stimuli and may have different consequences on intracellular signaling pathways eventually leading to different cellular responses.

To summarize, results from our and other experiments show that hHCy is associated with a selective degeneration of cortical and limbic brain structure including hippocampal area. The degeneration involves the loss of neurons, glial growth, hypertrophy of astrocytes, and probably sprouting of new connections. The morphological findings indicate that the astrocytes are the first neural cells participating in the deleterious actions of Hcy on the CNS. Apparently, astrocytes are able to respond to mild hHCy by reorganizing their cytoskeleton, surviving and protecting neurons from the damage [55].

Moreover, our studies also suggest that there are at least two different ways in which the neuronal tissue responds to hHCy. The induction of hHCy alone leads to neuronal cell death and morphological changes in the hippocampus and cortex that corresponds with findings of previous reported studies [48, 55, 56]. Combination of hHCy with more intense stimuli (ischemia) causes more prominent changes in cortex than in hippocampus. Importantly, IPC maneuver, even if combined with hHCy, still preserves the neuronal tissue from lethal ischemic effect. The other important finding that arose from our studies is that MAPK/p38 promotes neuronal cell death, whereas MAPK/ERK activation opposes apoptosis. Finally, all the above-mentioned studies provide evidence for the interplay and tight integration between ERK and p38 MAPK-signaling mechanism in response to mild hHCy and also in association with IR insult/IPC challenge in rat brain. Conclusively, preconditioning even if combined with hHCy could still preserve the neuronal tissue from lethal ischemic effect.

The one carbon unit metabolic pathway, which is involved in the regulation of homocysteine metabolism, is also part of the process which methylates amino acids in functional proteins and histones as well as the bases within the RNA and DNA. As a result, demethylation of S-adenosyl methionine, which is converted to S-adenosyl-homocysteine, exclusively provides methyl groups for the cells. Derangement of this phase might cause wide implications on plenty of cellular processes including the modulation of the expression of functional genes as well as the epigenetic regulation [10, 44, 21].

Elimination of Hcy-thiolactone, a metabolite of HCy, is performed by the high-density lipoprotein (HDL)-associated enzyme, Hcy-thiolactonase/paraoxonase 1 (PON1). This enzyme hydrolyzes Hcy-thiolactone in human serum [57] and similarly in the brain, it has been proposed that PON1 protects mice against Hcy-thiolactone neurotoxicity by enzymatic hydrolysis [58].

In summary, the experiments proved that pre-ischemic challenge in 14 days of hyperhomocysteinemic model in rats initiates responses of neuronal cells, which probably coordinate several etiological/protective mechanisms such as antioxidant defense [58], Ca^{2+} transport, and epigenetic mechanisms, such as DNA methylation and chromatin remodeling in the manifestation of the phenomenon of ischemic damage and ischemic tolerance [1, 12, 20, 32, 33].

5. Conclusion, challenges, and future directions

Hyperhomocysteinemia manifested as an elevated plasma level of homocysteine is now a widely recognized risk factor of human ischemic stroke. Elevated plasma homocysteine level leads to an increase in cerebrovascular permeability and causes several biochemical alterations such as thiolation and homocysteinylation to plasma proteins and enzymes and remarkably also in the brain parenchyma. These hHCy induced posttranslational protein modifications can have a causative role to the altered function and activity of the functional enzymes involved in the free radical protection also in brain parenchyma. Homocysteine metabolism itself leads also to the redox imbalance and to increased oxidative stress and the production of free radicals with the consequence in the damaging neuronal lipoperoxidation and cellular protein oxidation. The paper also highlights protective effect of pre-ischemic challenge to the subsequent lethal ischemia in rats. The pre-ischemic maneuver itself and also combined with hyperhomocysteinemia diminished the extent of neuronal degeneration as well as the intracellular signaling. Recent studies also underscore an opposing effect of MAPK/ERK and MAPK/p38 on cell survival and cell death in hyperhomocysteinemic conditions in brain parenchyma also if combined with IPC challenge in rat model of global ischemic stroke. Interestingly, a novel protective paradigm, such as postconditioning and/or remote conditioning, has already been observed as an effective in reducing ischemic reperfusion injury. As was proved in the experimental studies and also in clinical trials, those paradigms affect all the cells of the neurovascular network (consisting of neurons, glial cells, vascular endothelial cells, pericytes, smooth muscle cells, and venule/veins) [59, 60]. In the context of clinical applications, it is strongly suggested that the identification of the effects of comorbid factors in the mechanisms of ischemic damage and if combined with the ischemic tolerance evolution can potentially lead to improved therapeutics, especially the brain tissue. Additional studies of these molecular pathways are strongly needed to validate the role of hHCy in the etiology of neurological disorders.

Acknowledgements

This project is financed by grants VEGA 1/0128/16, from the Ministry of Education of the Slovak Republic, and by the project "Identification of Novel Markers in Diagnostic Panel of

Neurological Diseases," code:26220220114, "Martin Biomedical Center (BioMed Martin)," ITMS code: 26220220187co-financed from EC sources and the European Regional Development Fund and project of MZ SR No. 2012/30-UKMA-7.

Author details

Ján Lehotský[1*], Maria Kovalská[1,2], Barbara Tothová[1], Anna Beňová[1], Dagmar Kalenská[1] and Peter Kaplán[1]

*Address all correspondence to: lehotsky@jfmed.uniba.sk

1 Comenius University in Bratislava, Jessenius Faculty of Medicine, Institute of Medical Biochemistry and BioMed, Martin, Bratislava, Slovakia

2 Comenius University in Bratislava, Jessenius Faculty of Medicine, Institute of Histology and Embryology, Martin, Bratislava, Slovakia

References

[1] Lehotsky J., Burda J., Danielisová V., Gottlieb M., Kaplán P., et al. (2009) Ischemic tolerance: the mechanisms of neuroprotective strategy. Anat Rec. 292: 2002–2012.

[2] Kwon H.M., Lee Y.S., Bae H.J., Kang D.W. (2014) Homocysteine as a predictor of early neurological deterioration in acute ischemic stroke. Stroke. 45: 871–873.

[3] Dirnagl U., Becker K., Meisel A. (2009) Preconditioning and tolerance against cerebral ischaemia: from experimental strategies to clinical use. Lancet Neurol. 8: 398–412.

[4] Schaller B., Graf R. (2004) Cerebral ischemia and reperfusion: the pathophysiologic concept as a basis for clinical therapy. J Cereb Blood Flow Metab. 24(4): 351–371.

[5] Refsum H., Ueland P.M., Nygard O., Vollset S.E. (1998) Homocysteine and cardiovascular disease. Annu Rev Med. 49: 31–62.

[6] Petras M., Tatarkova Z., Kovalska M., Mokra D., Dobrota D., Lehotsky J., Drgova A. (2014) Hyperhomocysteinemia as a risk factor for the neuronal system disorders. J Physiol Pharmacol. 65:15–23

[7] Williams S.R., Yang Q., Chen F., Liu X., Keene K.L., Jacques P., Chen W.M., Weinstein G., Hsu F.C., Beiser A., Wang L., Bookman E., Doheny K.F., Wolf P.A., Zilka M., Selhub J., Nelson S., Gogarten S.M., Worrall B.B., Seshadri S., Sale M.M. (2014) Genomics and Randomized Trials Network; Framingham Heart Study. Genome-wide meta-analysis of homocysteine and methionine metabolism identifies five one carbon metabolism loci and a novel association of ALDH1L1 with ischemic stroke. PLoS Genet. 10:e1004214.

[8] Boldyrev A., Bryushkova E., Mashkina A., Vladychenskaya E. (2013) Why is homocysteine toxic for the nervous and immune systems? Curr Aging Sci. 6: 29–36.

[9] Ziemińska E., Stafiej A., Łazarewicz, J.W. (2003) Role of group I metabotropic glutamate receptors and NMDA receptors in homocysteine-evoked acute neurodegeneration of cultured cerebellar granule neurons. Neurochem Int. 43: 481–492.

[10] Dionisio N., Jardin I., Salido G.M., Rosado J.A. (2010) Homocysteine, intracellular signaling and thrombotic disorders. Curr Med Chem. 17: 3109–3119.

[11] Schaller B. (2005) Ischemic preconditioning as induction of ischemic tolerance after transient ischemic attacks in human brain: its clinical relevance. Neurosci Lett. 377(3): 206–211.

[12] Thompson J.W., Dave K.R., Young J.I., Perez-Pinzon M.A. (2013) Ischemic preconditioning alters the epigenetic profile of the brain from ischemic intolerance to ischemic tolerance. Neurotherapeutics 10: 789–797.

[13] Danielisova V., Gottlieb M., Bonova P., Nemethova M., Burda J. (2014) Bradykinin postconditioning ameliorates focal cerebral ischemia in the rat. Neurochem Int. 72: 22–29.

[14] Schaller B., Graf R. (2003) Hypothermia and stroke: the pathophysiological background. Pathophysiology. 10(1): 7–35.

[15] Schaller B., Graf R., Jacobs A.H. (2003) Ischaemic tolerance: a window to endogenous neuroprotection? Lancet. 362(9389): 1007–1008.

[16] Cox-Limpens K.E., Gavilanes A.W., Zimmermann L.J., Vles J.S. (2014) Endogenous brain protection: what the cerebral transcriptome teaches us. Brain Res. 1564: 85–100.

[17] Medina M., Urdiales J.L., Amores-Sánchez M.I. (2001) Roles of homocysteine in cell metabolism. Eur J Biochem. 268: 3871–3882.

[18] Obeid R., Hermann W. (2006) Mechanisms of homocysteine neurotoxicity in neurodegenerative diseases with special reference to dementia. FEBS Lett. 580: 2994–3005.

[19] Herrmann W., Obeid R. (2011) Homocysteine: a biomarker in neurodegenerative diseases. Clin Chem Lab Med. 49: 435–441.

[20] Kalani A., Kamat P.K., Familtseva A., Chaturvedi P., Muradashvili N., Narayanan N., Tyagi S.C., Tyagi N. (2014) Role of microRNA29b in blood-brain barrier dysfunction during hyperhomocysteinemia: an epigenetic mechanism. J Cereb Blood Flow Metab. 34: 1212–1222.

[21] Smulders Y.M., Smith D.E., Kok R.M., Teerlink T., Swinkels D.W., Stehouwer C.D., Jakobs C. (2006) Cellular folate vitamer distribution during and after correction of vitamin B12 deficiency: a case for the methylfolate trap. Br J Haematol. 132: 623–629.

[22] Škovierová H., Mahmood S., Blahovcová E., Hatok J., Lehotský J., Murín R. (2015) Effect of homocysteine on survival of human glial cells. Physiol Res. 64: 747–754.

[23] Kim S.J., Lee B.H., Kim Y.M., Kim G.H., Yoo H.W. (2013) Congenital MTHFR deficiency causing early-onset cerebral stroke in a case homozygous for MTHFR thermolabile variant. Metab Brain Dis. 28: 519–522.

[24] da Cunha M.J., da Cunha A.A., Ferreira A.G., Machado F.R., Schmitz F., Lima D.D., Delwing D., Mussulini B.H., Wofchuk S., Netto C.A., Wyse A.T. (2012) Physical exercise reverses glutamate uptake and oxidative stress effects of chronic homocysteine administration in the rat. Int J Dev Neurosci. 30: 69–74.

[25] Dayal S., Arning E., Bottiglieri T., Boger R.H., Sigmund C.D., Faraci F.M., Lentz S.R. (2004) Cerebral vascular dysfunction mediated by superoxide in hyperhomocysteinemic mice. Stroke 35: 1957–1962.

[26] Postea O., Krotz F., Henger A., Keller C., Weiss N. (2006) Stereospecific and redox-sensitive increase in monocyte adhesion to endothelial cells by homocysteine. Arterioscler Thromb Vasc Biol. 26: 508–513.

[27] Jakubowski H. (2011) Quality control in tRNA charging—editing of homocysteine. Acta Biochim Pol. 58: 149–163.

[28] Baldelli E., Leo G., Andreoli N., Fuxe K., Biagini G., Agnati L.F. (2010) Homocysteine potentiates seizures and cell loss induced by pilocarpine treatment. Neuromol Med. 12: 248–259.

[29] Lehotský J., Urban P., Pavlíková M., Tatarková Z., Kaminska B., Kaplán P. (2009) Molecular mechanisms leading to neuroprotection/ ischemic tolerance: effect of preconditioning on the stress reaction of endoplasmic reticulum. Cell Mol Neurobiol. 29: 917–925.

[30] Pavlíková M., Tatarková Z., Sivoňová M., Kaplán P., Križanová O., Lehotský J. (2009) Alterations induced by ischemic preconditioning on secretory pathways Ca^{2+}-ATPase (SPCA) gene expression and oxidative damage after global cerebral ischemia/reperfusion in rats. Cell Mol Neurobiol. 29: 909–916.

[31] Urban P., Pavlíková M., Sivonová M., Kaplán P., Tatarková Z., Kaminska B., Lehotský J. (2009) Molecular analysis of endoplasmic reticulum stress response after global forebrain ischemia/reperfusion in rats: effect of neuroprotectant simvastatin. Cell Mol Neurobiol. 29: 181–192.

[32] Stetler R.A., Leak R.K., Gan Y., Li P., Zhang F., Hu X., Jing Z., Chen J., Zigmond M.J., Gao Y. (2014) Preconditioning provides neuroprotection in models of CNS disease: paradigms and clinical significance. Prog Neurobiol. 114: 58–83.

[33] Kovalska M., Kovalska L., Pavlikova M., Janickova M., Mikuskova K., Adamkov M., Kaplan P., Tatarkova Z., Lehotsky J. (2012) Intracellular signaling MAPK pathway after cerebral ischemia-reperfusion injury. Neurochem Res. 37: 1568–1577.

[34] Kovalska M., Kovalska L., Mikuskova K., Adamkov M., Tatarkova Z., Lehotsky J. (2014) p-ERK involvement in the neuroprotection exerted by ischemic preconditioning in rat hippocampus subjected to four vessel occlusion. J Physiol Pharmacol. 65: 767–776.

[35] Kovalska M., Kovalska L., Tothova B., Mahmood S., Adamkov M., Lehotsky J. (2015) Combination of hyperhomocysteinemia and ischemic tolerance in experimental model of global ischemia in rats. J Physiol Pharmacol. 66: 887–897.

[36] Lehotský J., Pavlíková M., Kovalska M., Kaplan P., Tatarková Z., Racay P. (2011) Hyperhomocysteinemia and ischemic preconditioning in rat brain: response of SPCA Ca^{2+} ATPase gene expression. J Neurochem. 118(Suppl. 1): 154.

[37] Lehotsky J., Kovalská M., Drgová A., Kaplán P., Tatarková Z., Petráš M. (2014) Protective mechanisms induced by ischemic preconditioning in hyperhomocysteinemic rats. 8th International Symposium on Neuroprotection Neurorepair 2014, Magdeburg, I, 1-1-15.

[38] Ataie A., Ataee R., Mansoury Z., Aghajanpour M. (2013) Homocysteine intracerebroventricular injection induces apoptosis in the substantia nigra cells and Parkinson's disease like behavior in rats. Int J Mol Cell Med. 2: 80–85.

[39] Kolling J., Scherer E.B., da Cunha A.A., da Cunha M.J., Wyse A.T. (2011) Homocysteine induces oxidative-nitrative stress in heart of rats: prevention by folic acid. Cardiovasc Toxicol. 11: 67–73.

[40] Murín R., Škovierová H., Mahmood S., Blahovcová E., Lehotský J. (2014) Homocysteine affects the survival of cultured human glial cells. 8th International Symposium on Neuroprotection Neurorepair 2014, Magdeburg II-2-15.

[41] Choe Y.M., Sohn B.K., Choi H.J., Byun M.S., Seo E.H., Han J.Y., Kim Y.K., Yoon E.J., Lee J.M., Park J., Woo J.I., Lee D.Y. (2014). Association of homocysteine with hippocampal volume independent of cerebral amyloid and vascular burden. Neurobiol Aging. 35: 1519–1525.

[42] Pavlikova M., Kovalska M., Tatarkova Z., Sivonova-Kmetova M., Kaplan P., Lehotsky J. (2011) Response of secretory pathways Ca2+ ATPase gene expression to hyperhomocysteinemia and/or ischemic preconditioning in rat cerebral cortex and hippocampus. Gen Physiol Biophys. 30: 61–69.

[43] Sepulveda M.R., Marcos D., Berrocal M., Raeymaekers L., Mata A.M., Wuytack F. (2008): Activity and localization of the secretory pathway Ca^{2+} ATPase isoform 1 (SPCA1) in different areas of the mouse brain during postnatal development. Mol Cell Neurosci. 38: 461–473.

[44] Kalani A., Kamat P.K., Tyagi S.C., Tyagi N. (2013) Synergy of homocysteine, microRNA, and epigenetics: a novel therapeutic approach for stroke. Mol Neurobiol. 48: 157–168.

[45] Jakubowski H. (2004) Molecular basis of homocysteine toxicity in humans. Cell Mol Life Sci. 61: 470–487.

[46] Li M.H., Tang J.P., Zhang P., Li X., Wang C.Y., Wei H.J., Yang X.F., Zou W., Tang X.Q. (2014) Disturbance of endogenous hydrogen sulfide generation and endoplasmic reticulum stress in hippocampus are involved in homocysteine-induced defect in learning and memory of rats. Behav Brain Res. 262: 35–41.

[47] Sato H., Hariyama H., Moriguchi K. (1998) S-adenosyl-l-methionine protects the hippocampal CA1 neurons from the ischemic neuronal death in rat. Biochem Biophys Res Commun. 150: 491–496.

[48] Matte C., Mussulini B.H., dos Santos T.M., et al. (2010). Hyperhomocysteinemia reduces 20 glutamate uptake in parietal cortex of rats. Int J Dev Neurosci. 28: 183–187.

[49] Poddar R., Paul S. (2009) Homocysteine-NMDA receptor-mediated activation of extracellular signal-regulated kinase leads to neuronal cell death. J Neurochem. 110: 1095–1042.

[50] Maler J.M., Seifert W., Huther G., et al. (2003) Homocysteine induces cell death of rat 40 astrocytes in vitro. Neurosci Lett. 347: 85–88.

[51] Buffo A., Rolando C., Ceruti S. (2010) Astrocytes in the damaged brain: molecular and cellular insights into their reactive response and healing potential. Biochem Pharmacol. 79: 77–89.

[52] Poddar R., Paul S. (2013) Novel crosstalk between ERK MAPK and p38 MAPK leads to homocysteine-NMDA receptor-mediated neuronal cell death. J Neurochem. 124: 558–570.

[53] Liu A.J., Hu Y.Y., Li W.B., Xu J., Zhang M. (2011) Cerebral ischemic pre-conditioning enhances the binding characteristics and glutamate uptake of glial glutamate transporter-1 in hippocampal CA1 subfield of rats. J Neurochem. 119: 202–209.

[54] Zhang Q.G., Wang R.M., Han D., Yang L.C., Li J., Brann D.W. (2009) Preconditioning neuroprotection in global cerebral ischemia involves NMDA receptor-mediated ERK-JNK3 crosstalk. Neurosci Res. 63: 205–212.

[55] Loureiro S.O., Romão L., Alves T., et al. (2010) Homocysteine induces cytoskeletal remodeling and production of reactive oxygen species in cultured cortical astrocytes. Brain Res. 1355: 151–64.

[56] Lehotsky J., Petras M., Kovalska M., Tothova B., Drgova H., Kaplan P. (2015) Mechanisms involved in the ischemic tolerance in brain: effect of the homocysteine. Cell Mol Neurobiol. 35: 7–15.

[57] Domagała T.B., Łacinski M., Trzeciak W.H., Mackness B., Mackness M.I., Jakubowski H. (2006) The correlation of homocysteine-thiolactonase activity of the paraoxonase (PON1) protein with coronary heart disease status. Cell Mol Biol. (Noisy-le-grand) 52: 4–10.

http://dx.doi.org/10.5772/64611

[58] Borowczyk K., Shih D.M., Jakubowski H. (2012). Metabolism and neurotoxicity of homocysteine thiolactone in mice: evidence for a protective role of paraoxonase. J Alzheimers Dis. 30: 225–231.

[59] Sandua N., Schaller B. (2010) Postconditioning: a new or old option after ischemic stroke? Expert Rev Cardiovasc Ther. 8(4): 479–482.

[60] Wang Y., Reis C., Applegate R. 2nd, Stier G., Martin R., Zhang J.H. (2015) Ischemic conditioning-induced endogenous brain protection: applications pre-,per- or post-stroke. Exp Neurol. 272: 26–40.

Chapter 6

Immune System Involvement in the Degeneration, Neuroprotection, and Restoration after Stroke

Yolanda Cruz, Karla A Cantú-Saldaña and
Antonio Ibarra

Additional information is available at the end of the chapter

http://dx.doi.org/10.5772/64318

Abstract

Cerebrovascular diseases are currently among the three primary causes of death worldwide and are the first cause of disability in adults. Nevertheless, there are no neuroprotective or neurorestorative therapies that have shown considerable beneficial effects, except for the FDA-approved recombinant tissue plasminogen activator (rtPA), which has been used for decades for the treatment of stroke and its effectiveness is still controversial. This is why it is very important to develop effective therapeutic options. In order to achieve this objective, it is essential to recognize the secondary mechanisms involved in the pathological development. The immunological system is one of these mechanisms that participate during the acute and chronic phases of disease, both in deleterious and beneficial manners. It is known that the immune system's duality contributes to the ischemic injury through proinflammatory cytokine (tumor necrosis factor-α (TNF-α), interleukin-1 (IL-1), interleukin-6 (IL-6)), and oxygen reactive species production, etc. Nevertheless, it also provides protection and even restoration through anti-inflammatory cytokine (interleukin-4 (IL-4), interleukin-10 (IL-10), transforming growth factor-β (TGF-β)), and growth factor (brain-derived neurotrophic factor (BDNF), insulin-like growth factor-1 (IGF-1), neurotrophin-3 (NT-3), neurotrophin-4 (NT-4)) production. This states that innovative therapeutic options must be proposed with the goal of protecting and restoring the tissue after the ischemic event. Such therapies are exposed in the present chapter.

Keywords: cerebral ischemia, neuroprotection, immunomodulation, inflammation protective autoimmunity, neurorestoration

1. Introduction

Cerebrovascular diseases (CVD) include hemorrhagic and ischemic brain injuries, the latter being the most common since 85% of cases arise from atherothrombotic (artery stretching) and atheroembolic etiologies. Both of these diseases are the first cause of permanent disabilities in adults, primarily in developed countries, where 30% of patients that have suffered from stroke become incapable of performing their daily routines [1]. Stroke is, in addition, among the first three causes of premature death worldwide; according to the World Health Organization (WHO), 6.7 million deaths were caused by cerebral ischemia in 2012, as well as 46% of deaths being caused by stroke and ischemic heart disease altogether, with mayor incidence in low-income countries, with 80% of cases [2]. As for the United States (which has the most available information), the American Heart Association (AHA) reported in an updated statistics report that the death rates associated with stroke have been dropping over the years, and from 2009 to 2012, the prevalence is estimated in 2.6% with an incidence of almost 800,000 cases a year, one every 40 s [3]. And according to the Center for Disease Control (CDC), there is one death out of every 20 stroke cases, or one every 4 min [4]. On the other hand, European countries experience dramatic differences in disease burden. The EuroHOPE study performed on data from 2007 observed higher incidence of ischemic stroke in Hungary, and Finland and less in Scotland and Sweden and different mortality rates among regions in different countries [5].

The incidence and prevalence of stroke and its recurrence continue to be high due to the low attention and awareness to symptoms which create delay in the seeking of medical attention, allowing damage to progress. People are not aware that time is critical for stroke treatment due to the short therapeutic window of available treatments. Disabilities and dependence among patients tend to get worse in the 6–12 months following stroke; mobility and functionality related to dressing and toileting are the most affected, and deterioration is related to prior-to-stroke comorbidities [6]. Depression is one of the major outcomes and is associated with stroke recurrence [7].

There are a vast array of risk factors associated with cerebrovascular diseases and specifically to cerebral ischemia. The most common are chronic diseases that could be modified through behavioral and lifestyle changes or pharmacological treatment such as diabetes, hypertension, obesity, and atherosclerosis; besides, alcoholism and tabaquism, high salt consumption, and sedentarism are behaviors that are associated with a greater risk of developing stroke [2]. On the other hand, there are a series of risk factors that cannot be controlled and predispose a person to cerebral ischemia: they are age, gender, and ethnicity. For instance, postmenopausal women have greater risk of developing stroke than men the same age, but premenopausal women are protected by estrogenic hormones [8, 9]. It has also been reported in 2010 by the Global Burden of Disease (GBD) that 31% of strokes are among young adults (20–64 years of age) and strokes are common in people below 45 years of age [10]. Non-Caucasians are also at greater risk of stroke than Caucasians [8].

2. Pathophysiology

Usually, when speaking about stroke, two stages of damage to the integrity of the neural tissue are considered. The first stage is the lesion *per se*, caused by the restriction of blood flow from an obstruction in a major vessel and presents the characteristic physiopathology that ends in neural death. This area of the lesion, which is almost immediately damaged at this stage is called the "infarct core." The second stage of damage is that of secondary degeneration that further injures tissue not originally damaged by the restricted blood flow, but that is adjacent to and surrounds the infarct core. This area of lesion is called "ischemic penumbra," it preserves some energy metabolism, and its degeneration is caused primarily by excitotoxicity and inflammation.

Nonetheless, inflammation previously contributes to the development of stroke, since people who suffer from chronic proinflammatory state diseases like hypertension, dyslipidemia, atherosclerosis, and type-two diabetes have endothelial alterations, as well as irregularities in rheology and hemodynamics [11]. Galectin-3 (GAL-3) concentration is increased in these patients; this protein favors atherosclerotic plaque formation and might participate in the development of cerebrovascular disease [12] GAL-3 is also a very important inflammatory and fibrogenic mediator [13, 14]. Interleukin-1β (IL-1β) is a proinflammatory cytokine that has been related to atherosclerotic plaque formation and vascular inflammation [15]; other factors have also been associated with it, such as Von Willebrand coagulation factor, selectin E, and others [16].

Atherosclerotic plaque is characterized by accumulation of molecules of cholesterol and low-density lipoproteins (LDL) in the vessel walls, after being oxidized they chemo-attract monocytes to the site, and they phagocytose these oxidized LDL, which in turn causes them to become foam cells. Foam cells loaded with high amounts of LDL stay trapped in the endothelium and suffer from apoptosis and necrosis. This situation generates a lipidic plaque covered by connective tissue and are infiltrated by activated T cells, macrophages and mastocytes that will chronically produce inflammatory mediators in the endothelial wall [17]. Oxidized cell and molecule accumulation generate endothelial wall activation, thus promoting adhesion molecule expression and easing immune cell aggregation.

Several investigators consider that the severity of endothelial inflammation can imply differences in atherosclerotic plaque rupture vulnerability, which will contribute to the development of ischemia in the surrounding tissue. For this reason, the use of imaging technology such as Computerized axial tomography Computerized axial tomography(CAT);Positron emission tomography (PET) scan, MRI, and Positron emission tomography (PET), has been considered in order to identify the degree of endothelial inflammation and to assess risk of developing an ischemic event [18].

Stroke originates from either a reduction in the arterial lumen, or the release of a thrombus that becomes trapped in a major artery, most commonly the middle cerebral artery (MCA). This occlusion causes diminished blood flow to the site irrigated specifically by that vessel and so glucose and oxygen supply will stop, triggering metabolic insufficiency. The incapacity for glucose to reach the cells causes a decrease in adenosine triphosphate (ATP) production which interferes with Na^+ and K^+ pump function; in light of this, intracellular K^+ decreases dramatically causing membrane depolarization [19], and thus, further voltage-dependent Ca^{2+} channel dysfunction and opening, unlocking of some CA^{2++} receptor-dependent channels, Na^+/Ca^{2+} channels from cellular and mitochondrial membrane, and CA^{2+} pump deterioration in cell membrane, and endoplasmic reticulum [20].

All of these events triggered by membrane depolarization drive a secretion of excitatory neurotransmitters, especially glutamate that upon binding to its receptors induces greater depolarization and glutamate release, giving rise to the excitotoxicity phenomenon [21]. The massive amounts of calcium will activate a series of enzymes (e.g., calpaines, phospholipases, and endonucleases), and free radicals that in turn lead to neuronal death.

On the other hand, the proinflammatory milieu that is present in the occluded vessel endothelium is lacking in oxygen and altogether with the changes in vascular pressure generate a major reactive oxygen species (ROS) production [22] that promotes higher expression of: Matrix metalloproteinases 2 and 9 (MMP 2 and 9) that digest the basal endothelial sheet [23] and cyclooxygenase 2 (COX-2) and subsequent prostanoid production [24]. Increased ROS production also cause complement and endothelial cell activation that promotes the secretion of proinflammatory mediators such as IL-1 and IL-6, and increased expression of intercellular adhesion molecule (ICAM), vascular adhesion molecule (VCAM), and leukocyte adhesion receptors such as selectins P, E, and L; all this promotes leukocyte adherence and extravasation [25].

When, or if the occlusion is not permanent, the vessel experiences reperfusion (spontaneously or after treatment). During this process blood flow is restored, thus once again providing glucose and oxygen to the already injured tissue. This situation worsens neural tissue damage as a result of an increase in substrate availability that causes an increment of free radical production, lipoperoxidation, and a rise in cell death protein activation, as well as adhesion molecules [26] and metabolic detriment [27].

As free radicals such as nitric oxide (NO) and ROS increase, they interact with their target molecules and activate mechanisms such as apoptosis, arachidonic acid metabolism, and respiratory chain inhibition that, as a consequence, increase inflammatory mediators [26, 27] that contribute to the secondary degeneration.

Although it is worth mentioning that the amount of neural damage depends on how long the vessel is occluded, since it has been observed in several studies that early reperfusion reduces infarct sizes [27].

3. Secondary degeneration due to inflammation

Microglia is specialized macrophages that live in the cerebral parenchyma, when at rest or quiescent, these normally exhibit a phenotype characterized by thin processes. These cells are also very sensitive to changes in the cerebral milieu since their primary functions are to eliminate cell debris from apoptosis [28], regulate neural synapses [29], neurogenesis [30], trophic factor production [30], inflammatory process [31], damaged cell phagocytosis, and the repair and remodeling processes of the central nervous system (CNS) [32].

During early stages of ischemia, when there is a progressive decrease in oxygen and ATP in the cerebral parenchyma, glial cells release molecules such as lipocalin 2 (LCN2) [33] and IL-4 [34] secreted by neurons as an immediate response to injury. These molecules are capable of activating microglia and induce a protective M2 phenotype characterized by the production of anti-inflammatory cytokines IL-10, IL-4, and increased phagocytosis [33]. This phenotype has been observed during the first 7 days post-ischemia; it reaches it max peak at 3–5 days, and decreases by day 14, suggesting that microglia promotes neuronal survival during this first stage by attempting to reduce inflammatory mediator release by synthesizing transforming growth factor-β (TGF-β), arg-1, and CD206 [35, 36], apart from producing growth factors such as insulin-like growth factor-1 (IGF-1) and ciliary neurotrophic factor (CNTF) that facilitate mechanisms of repair [34].

While the milieu changes from day 3 through day 14 post ischemia toward high concentrations of Ca^{2+}, free radicals, glutamate, and debris from neuronal necrosis, microglial phenotype gradually changes from M2 to M1, and begins to express genes such as nitric oxide synthase (INOS), CD16 and CD32 as well surface markers such as CD11b and MCHII [36]. M1 phenotype is distinguished by a decrease in phagocytosis activity and an increase in the production of proinflammatory mediators: IL-1β, IL-6, and tumor necrosis factor α (TNF-α) and an increase in NO, H_2O_2, ROS, MMPs, and chemokines such as CXCL10, CCL2, MCP-1, CXCL1, and CCL5 [35, 37]; through the Notch pathway signaling [38], all of which propitiate the support for a proinflammatory milieu.

This polarization of microglial activation gives rise to the opportunity to search for ways to modulate it in order to induce an M2 phenotype and through it, be able to get the beneficial effects of an anti-inflammatory milieu, accompanied by trophic factors that ease cellular repair.

On the other hand, macrophages and mast cells dwell around the cerebral parenchyma and the perivascular spaces, also called Virchow-Robin spaces, these cells activate in presence of inflammatory mediators secreted as a result of ischemia/reperfusion [39, 40]. These produce high concentrations of histamine, catepsines, matrix metalloproteinases that further contribute to endothelial damage, blood-brain barrier (BBB), hyperpermeability, and the vasogenic edema formation as well increased production of TNF-α and CXCR, CXCL1/2/3 chemokines that will promote massive leukocyte recruitment to the perivascular region [39, 41], specifically neutrophils monocytes and T lymphocytes.

Neutrophil arrival at the injured perivascular space depends on time and type of occlusion, Nina Vindegaard Groberg et al. published in 2013 that when the occlusion lasts 120 min, there is an important number of neutrophils that arrive 12 h post-ischemia, reaching a peak concentration at 24 h; when the occlusion lasts 60 min concentration peak is observed as far as 3 days post-ischemia [42]. Notwithstanding, Isabel Pérez de Puig et al. results published in 2015 point out neutrophil presence as early as 6 h post-ischemia in permanent MCA occlusion (MCAo), which opens to consideration the fact that neutrophil quantity and distribution are different among patients [43]. Nevertheless, postmortem tissue analysis from people who suffered from cerebral ischemia in various vessels yielded no difference in neutrophil amount in perivascular zones, leptomeninges, and cerebral parenchyma around the lesion site.

As neutrophils arrive to the injury site, they react almost immediately to damage-associated molecular patterns (DAMPS), TNF-α and Interferon gamma (INF-γ) which are found widely distributed around the perivascular zone and cerebral parenchyma. This promotes their activation, and thus, they acquire the ability to secrete cytokines, primarily IL-1β, IL-6, also lytic enzymes, free radicals, and angiogenic factors, as well as chemokines such as CXCL9 and CXCL10 which influence Th1 and Th17 lymphocyte migration [44, 45], triggering an increased amount of cells and a proinflammatory milieu.

In the clinical field, it has been observed that patients who suffered from cognitive deterioration after an ischemic event have high concentrations of neutrophils, showing a high correlation between the degree of tissue damage secondary to inflammation and functional recovery [46]. Even patients that have been treated with recombinant tissue plasminogen activator (rtPA) but that previously presented high neutrophil amount have had the worst results associated with neuroprotection exerted by rtPA [47].

Large efforts are being made to conduct scientific investigations oriented toward the decrease of secondary damage through the inhibition neutrophil recruitment, the adherence of these to endothelial cells through cannabinoid 2 (CB2) receptor activation [48], or through Neurogenin1 (NRG1) growth factor that reduces response to endothelial inflammation causing a decrease in ICAM-1, VCAM-1, and selectin E [49] or by the use of competitive antagonist CXR2/CXR3 [50] all of which have demonstrated to have beneficial effects in the decrease of infarct size in animals subjected to these treatments.

Nonetheless, in the clinical setting, the use of some molecules such as Enlimomab, which reduces leukocyte adhesion, have had negative effects in stroke patients because it made them more prone to suffer from secondary infections that increased complications during their recovery [47].

In response to CCL2, MCP-1, and CXCL1 chemokines, to mention a few, monocytes infiltrate into the perivascular and brain tissue, and as thought up to a few years ago, they differentiated in macrophages indistinguishable from activated microglia, stimulating and exacerbating brain injury [51]; nonetheless, thanks to the identification of different monocyte subtypes investigators have been able to identify some of their roles in the injured tissue.

Recently, two different monocyte population types that express different markers have been identified in mice. Classical or proinflammatory monocytes expressing Ly-6C^{high}, CCR2^{high}, and CX3CR1^{low} markers have short half-lives and are actively recruited into inflamed tissues, boosting inflammation. The other types, expressing Ly-6C^{low}, CCR2^{low}, and CX3CR1^{high} markers, have longer half-lives and are found inspecting vessel integrity, aiding its maintenance [52]. Trying to identify the precise roles of each type of monocyte subpopulation is an essential task, since in 2015, Ritzel and his team conducted an experiment in which they demonstrate that 90 min after ischemia; there is a large forfeiture of microglia and a very high rise in monocytes coming from the periphery and reach up to 90% of monocytes in the ischemic brain at 72 h post-ischemia, making evident their very important role in injured tissue [53].

Several studies conducted in mice have also demonstrated that the rise of monocytes in blood and cerebral tissue express pro inflammatory markers, from subpopulation Ly-6C^{high} during the acute phase of ischemia [52, 53]. The rise of this subpopulation is correlated with the infarct size and neurological deficit in mice subjected to ischemia/reperfusion [54]. Also, a rise in TNF-α and IL-1β production, characteristic of this subtype, is observed during the first 72 h post-ischemia [53]. Nonetheless, it has also been observed that there is a change of phenotype during monocyte differentiation into macrophages, acquiring anti-inflammatory characteristics along with the synthesis of TGF-β around the sixth day post-ischemia [55, 56]; but it is still not clear how such differentiation occurs, or what characteristics induce the process.

Experimentally, it has been observed that T lymphocytes reach the cerebral parenchyma later in time, between 24 and 96 h post-ischemia, reaching a max peak at 3–7 days post-ischemia [57, 58]. The increase of monocyte differentiation into macrophage infiltration, the expression of major histocompatibility complex II (MHCII), and costimulatory molecules in the activated microglia and the presence of CNS antigens such as myelin basic protein (MBP), NR2A/2B subtype of the N-methyl-D-aspartate receptor) and the human neuron-specific enolase (NSE) to mention a few, all products of necrosis and neural cell rupture found in systemic circulation and brain parenchyma [59, 60] stimulate antigen presentation. It is worth mentioning that at clinical level, concentration of these proteins has been related to the severity of neurological damage and extent of brain lesion in humans [61].

The characteristics of the immune response to these antigens that have modified their nature due to the degree of necrosis resulting from ischemia, differ depending on the presented epitope [62]. Different from other CNS pathologies, in ischemia, Th1-type immune response to antigens like MBP is infrequent, but exacerbated when exposed in combination to lipopolysaccharides (LPS), since secondary-to-stroke infections are very common [62]. Nonetheless, it has not been possible to clearly establish which mechanism of autoantigens is involved in damage exacerbation.

There are a series of experiments that show the harmful role of T lymphocytes, among which are those performed by Gokhan [26] and his team in 2006 where they observed that lymphocytes are the primary producers of INF-γ and other proinflammatory cytokines, that promotes an increment in infarct size [26]; and those performed by Liesz in 2011 [63], in which they observed that by eliminating lymphocytes, infarct size was reduced in animals subjected to cerebral ischemia, all of which matches with Xiong et al.'s results in 2013 [64], where they observed that T lymphocyte deficiency significantly reduces infarct volume in a transient cerebral ischemia model, but not in distal permanent occlusion, which highlights that the model and level of reperfusion used are essential and differential to evaluate damage.

Thanks to new arrangement of more specific cellular markers, some new functions and mechanisms have been identified during stroke for the different T cell subtypes. INF-γ production, primarily by T $CD4^+$ cells, is what fundamentally compromises injury exacerbation [63]. T $CD8^+$ cell activation conducts to neural cell death through perforin-granzyme pathway. Natural killer (NK) cells have a less noxious effect. T $\gamma\delta$ cells show an injurious effect at the experimental level through the production of IL-17, IL-23 [38, 63, 64] and IL-6 at the clinical level [65]. Treg lymphocytes have been implicated mostly in neural tissue protection, preventing autoimmunity and inflammation through IL-10 [66].

Immune tolerance to autoantigens is based on the regulation of autoreactive T lymphocytes through various mechanisms involving: elimination, anergy, or suppression via Treg cells, even though several studies have not found benefit from them, since after being eliminated, injured tissue did not present further damage [65].

Recent studies have observed that autoreactive T cells have the ability to promote neuroprotection. This physiological mechanism appears when the CNS suffers from damage and can be potentiated or modulated through active immunization with neural-derived peptides. Such has been demonstrated in several models, like: spinal cord injury [66], multiple sclerosis [67], partial injury to the optic nerve [68], among others. Using T lymphocytes for the bone morphogenic protein (BMP) autoantigen neuroprotection is observed, under morphological, anatomical and functional criteria. Through this immunomodulation mechanism, a major production of anti-inflammatory cytokines and trophic factors has been observed, which is a crucial event to look for in neuroprotection and even neurorestoration.

Each comprised mechanism of immune system participation in cerebral ischemia represents an opportunity to explore immunomodulation and contention that shall not be wasted, in order to look for tissue neuroprotection and neurorestoration.

4. Inhibition of immune response as a neuroprotective mechanism

The cytokine accumulation and cellular infiltration increase mentioned above drive an expansion in damage, even though molecules that try to limit it are released. This prejudicial effect increases in relation to passing time and ischemia intensity, which provides a relatively small therapeutic window to look for protection alternatives. Initially, because the immune system has always been considered as one of the responsible mechanisms for damage increase, most neuroprotective therapies are being investigated toward its inhibition, looking to eliminate proinflammatory cytokine production and cell recruitment.

For this reason, strategies to try and delay or stop the biochemical and molecular damaging process are being investigated since over four decades ago in preclinical phases [69, 70] using different compounds that exert neuroprotective mechanisms.

Neuroprotection is a term that refers to the use of different therapies, alone or in combination that protect the brain or the neural cells against damage from immune degeneration, apoptosis, and dysfunction [70, 71].

Neuroprotection is aimed at not only protecting neurons, but also other brain constituents, such as microglia and endothelial cells of the penumbra region [72], and can be achieved through different mechanisms such as: anti-excitotoxic agents, anti-inflammatory agents, antioxidants [71], but our main focus will be in those that are involved with the immune system.

Studies have been conducted in different settings and performed in animals in order to prove the existence neuroprotective characteristics of several molecules through all of these different mechanisms, focusing on those with immunomodulatory and immune inhibition activity [73].

Among those studied, the most recent substances that have demonstrated to have neuroprotective mechanisms through anti-inflammatory activity in the preclinical field, the following are included.

Lycium barbarum polysaccharides are derived from a traditional Chinese plant that when used in a stroke model in mice, the investigators observed a reduced number of apoptotic cells in the peri-infarct zone, as well as a reduction in neurological deficit. This extract has neuroprotective effects through the inhibition of the ERK and JRK pathways, it inhibits MMP-9 and thus protect the BBB integrity, and it also regulates aquaporin-4 in order to reduce brain edema [74].

Piperine (1-peperoylpiperidine) is an extract from pepper usually used in folk medicine to treat different ailments since it appears to be anti-inflammatory. A group led by F. Islam investigated its effect in ischemic brain injury. They pretreated Wistar rats and investigated its neuroprotective role in a period of 24 h after the MCAo and observed a down regulation of COX-2, nitric oxide synthase (NOS-2), and nuclear factor κβ (NF-κβ) in the penumbra region, thus reducing the secretion of proinflammatory cytokines. A decrease in infarct size and less neuronal loss was also observed in the pretreated group [75].

Simvastatin is a pharmacological agent used in the treatment of atherosclerosis and high blood cholesterol, it has shown neuroprotective effects in ischemic brain injury through the upregulation of Nitric Oxide synthase, decrease in ROS production, the fibrinolysis activation through the upregulation of tissue plasminogen activator (tPA), and downregulation of plasminogen activator inhibitor-1 (PAI-1), as well as the recruitment of inflammatory components of the ischemic cascade from monocytes, macrophages, and T lymphocytes [76].

Neuro-erythropoietin (EPO) has proven to be neuroprotective in ischemic models. It decreases susceptibility to glutamate toxicity and nitric oxide, thus being antioxidant, it also induces the production of ant apoptotic and neurotrophic factors and decreases inflammation. Another proposed mechanism for neuroprotection by EPO is the use of the released iron by the ischemic lesion for erythropoiesis, thus limiting its oxidative effects [77].

Levodopa/benserazide is a pharmacological agent that during an investigation was given to rats 2 days after experimental stroke, and at day 7, T cells and chemokines were analyzed. It was discovered that CD3 and CD8 T cell population was diminished in the treated group, as well as lower levels of ICAM-1 in the ischemic hemisphere [78].

Fingolimod modulates the activity of the membrane receptor (S1PR) responsible for the reduction in lymphocyte migration into the brain tissue and the microvasculature; this increases cerebral blood flow by attenuation of adhesion and thrombus formation and protects the brain indirectly [79].

Other molecules occurring naturally, such as fatty acids, have neuroprotective effects through immunomodulation and antioxidation. Omega-3 fatty acids are essential for human consumption since humans lack the ability to synthesize them. *In vivo* and *in vitro* experiments performed by Zhang et al. using fish oils and/or omega-3 fatty acids demonstrate the importance of their consumption since the animals treated and subjected to MCAo showed lesser infarct size and neurological deficit. The mechanisms proposed by these authors are antioxidation through the enhancement of the expression of hemeoxigenase-1 (HO-1) and nuclear translocation of Nrf 2 in the *in vitro* model. The *in vitro* experiment showed increased levels of HO-1 in microglia and astrocytes, and they later proved its involvement in neuroprotection after stroke. Other studies have also shown that they exhibit anti-inflammatory properties, reduce microglial activation, and inhibit neutrophil activation. Altogether, they found that fish oil and omega-3 enriched diets have neuroprotective effects since treated animals showed less infarct size and neurological deficit, and treated cultures showed increased cellular viability [80].

5. Modulation of immune response as a therapy for stroke

Immunomodulation refers to the therapeutic approach to alter or modify the immune response for the benefit of the patient. Cytokine production, e change in cellular phenotype, and the complement are manipulated to modify the milieu to which the immune system shall react [81]. Immunomodulation can also be achieved through induction of anti-inflammatory milieu (L-4, TGF-β, other cytokines) in which Tregs and microglia can be induced toward a beneficial response.

The immunomodulation area of study is being increasingly explored, having already found a great diversity in pharmacological proposals that induce this type of response, among which we can mention: *Ganoderma lucidum*, another traditional Chinese plant extract has been used too in ischemic models with neuroprotective effects. This extract has shown these beneficial effects through the decrease of TNF-α and IL-8 and IL-6, as well as MDA levels in the hippocampus, and increases levels of IL-2, IL-4, and IL-10, all of which reduces neuronal loss. On the other side, it has antioxidant effects through the increase of superoxide dismutase activity. Overall, it reduces neurological deficit and the infarct size [82].

Yang et al. demonstrate that by treating animals with minocycline previous to an ischemic event increases blood flow, increases tight junction protein concentration in the ischemic cortex, maintained levels of MMP 2, 9, and 3 needed for repair. It also decreased microglial/macrophage activation, compared to the non-treated group, and activation was alternate at 4 weeks, meaning that microglia/macrophage expressed phenotype M2. This supports the observed decrease in TNF-α and IL-1β and increase in TGF-β and IL-10. Animals treated with minocycline Chad lesser infarct sizes assessed by MRI and (2,3,5-Triphenyltetrazolium chloride) TTC staining [83].

IL-4 is a naturally occurring cytokine produced mainly by Th2 cells, mast cells, eosinophils, and basophils. It is thought to be essential for the promotion of macrophage phenotype differentiation toward an M2 response, rather than the classical M1. IL-4 production reduces over time, and this is associated with neurodegenerative diseases. Liu and his team proved the importance of IL-4 after acute ischemic stroke, since IL-4 Knockout (KO) mice exhibited greater tissue loss at day 5 and functional deficit including memory impairment and spatial learning decrease. Overall, they suggest that immunomodulation IL-4 plays a key role in recovery after stroke [84].

Another cytokine involved in immune modulation and anti-inflammation is INF-β. It has been already approved by the FDA for MS treatment and Kuo et al. studied it for experimental stroke, demonstrating a protective effect, since animals treated had less infarct volume and neurological scores. The authors suggest that this is mediated through the INF-β receptor, since animals lacking this receptor ($Ifnar1^{-/-}$ MCAO/R mice) showed no protective effect from the treatment. The mechanisms involved in INF-β neuroprotection are: decrease in inflammatory cytokine expression (IL-1β, IL?6, IL-23p19, and TNF-α), reduction in microglial activation and soma size (suggestive of resting state), decrease in macrophage/monocyte, $CD4^+$ and $\gamma\delta$ T cell and neutrophil infiltration, inhibits TNF-α induced ICAM-1 (but not VCAM-1) and E selectin upregulation and inhibition of MMP-9, CCL3 and CXCL3 [85].

Under the bases of the new concept conceived by Dr. Michal Schwartz "protective autoimmunity," various non-encephalitogenic peptides have been tested. These have shown to potentiate neuroprotective effects of the immune system itself, such as Cop-1 is a modified neural peptide used in the treatment of multiple sclerosis that has shown beneficial effects in previous stroke models. Cop-1 competes for binding to MHCII since it has a high, fast, and efficient binding to several MHC molecules in several murine and human antigen-presenting cells without the need of being processed. It is also a MBP epitope 82-100 antagonist, which present a high cross-reaction with this molecule, thus competing with it for the MHC binding site. This copolymer helps modify the milieu since immunization with COP-1 after stroke has shown to induce a Th2 response [86]. Overall, these changes provide an anti-inflammatory milieu (cytokine production: IL-4, IL-5, IL-10, and TGF-β). Under this background effect of Cop-1 in MCAo model where rats were immunized with this neuropeptide after being subjected to the occlusion. Results analyzed 7 days post-ischemia yielded a decreased infarct size and lesser neurological deficit in animals treated with Cop-1, results consisting with neuroprotective benefits [87].

Poly-YE is a high molecular weight copolymer that has proven to exert immunomodulatory effects through the downregulation of Treg, modulation of microglial and macrophage response in the thalamus and an increase in production of insulin-like growth factor-1 (IGF-1) by $Nestin^+$ cells. After subjecting rats to experimental stroke, those treated with poly-YE presented diminished infarct size and neurological deficit [88].

Myelin oligodendrocyte glycoprotein (MOG) administered nasally demonstrated reduction in infarct size through the induction of IL-10-secreting $CD4^+$ T regulatory cells and reduction of $CD11b^+$ cells which contribute to the NO synthesis. Overall, infarct size and neurological deficit were reduced by the nasal MOG administration in a MCAo stroke model [69].

A different mechanism that has also been explored is ischemic tolerance; such consists in bring about a pre-conditioning of the tissue, in order to promote neuroprotection [89]. Among the activated mechanisms are an increase in anti-inflammatory cytokines such as IL-4 and IL-13 that ease hippocampal pyramidal neuron survival after an ischemic event in gerbils [90]. Tu

XK and his team also demonstrated that neuroprotection can be originated by pre-conditioning through modulation of the phosphatidyl inositol 3-kinase (PI3K/Akt) and ERK1/2 pathway modulation [91] (**Table 1**).

Therapy	**Mechanism of neuroprotection** **↑Increase** **↓Decrease**	**Treatment outcome**	**Reference**
Lycium barbarum	• Inhibition of proinflammatory pathway • →׀MMP-9 • Regulation of aquaporin-4	Reduction in the number of apoptotic cells in the peri-infarct zone Reduction of edema Decreased neurological deficit	Yang et al. 2012
Piperine (1-peperoylpiperidine)	• Immunomodulation: ↓COX-2, NOS-2, and NF-kB	Decrease in infarct size and neuronal loss	Vaibhav et al. 2012
Simvastatin	• Immunomodulation: recruitment and modulation of macrophage, monocyte, and T lymphocyte activity Antioxidation: ↑NO synthase, ↓ROS • ↑Blood flow: ↑tPA →PAI-1	Reduce changes in BBB and protect brain against cell stress Reduced amounts of inflammatory proteins in the brain	Campos-Martorell et al. 2014
Neuro-EPO	• Neurotrophic effects • ↓Glutamate NO, use of released Iron • Anti-Inflammation	Higher survival in treated animals, reduced neurological deficit. Increased histological protection	Lagarto Parra et al. 2012
Levodopa/ Benserazide	• Immunomodulation: ↓CD3, CD8 T cells. • ↓ICAM-1.	Attenuation of inflammation, reduced number to T cells, reduced ICAM-1, and T cell-associated IL-5.	Kuric et al. 2014
Fingolimod (FYT720)	• Immunomodulation: ↓lymphocyte migration through ↓S1PR • ↑Blood flow: ↓adhesion molecules, ↓thrombi	Reduction of infarct size Reduction of lymphocytes in cerebral vasculature→increased blood flow	Kraft et al 2012

http://dx.doi.org/10.5772/64318

Therapy	Mechanism of neuroprotection ↑Increase ↓Decrease	Treatment outcome	Reference
Omega-3	• Anti-inflammation: proinflammatory cytokines • Antioxidation: ↑Hemeoxigenase-1, Nrf2 • ↓Neutrophil infiltration, microglial activation	→Reduction of infarct size Reduced neurological deficit Increased cell viability (*in vitro*)	Zhang et al. 2014
Ganoderma lucidum	• Immunomodulation: ↓TNF-α, IL-8, IL-6. ↑IL-2, IL-4, IL-10 • Antioxidation: ↑superoxide dismutase activity	Reduction of infarct size Reduced neurological deficit	Zhang et al. 2014
Minocycline	• ↑Blood flow • Immunomodulation: M2 phenotype, maintenance of MMP's, ↓TNF-α, IL-1β, ↑TGF-β, IL-10	Reduction of infarct size	Yang et al. 2015
IL-4	• Immunomodulation: ↑M2 phenotype ↓M1 phenotype	Decreased tissue loss Better spatial learning and memory	Zhao X, et al. (2015)
INF-β	• Immunomodulation: ↓MMP-9 • ↓Iba1 cells, ↓ TNF-α, IL-1b, IL-6 • ↓Adhesion molecules, selectin E • ↓Monocyte, macrophages	Reduction of infarct size Decreased neurological deficit	Kuo PC, et al. (2016)
Cop-1	• Immunomodulation: ↑Th2 reg response. ↑IL-4, IL-5, IL-10, ↑M2 microglial phenotype	Reduction of infarct size Decreased neurological deficit	A. Ibarra et al. 2007
Poly-YE	• Immunomodulation: ↓Treg, modulation of microglial and macrophage response • ↑IGF-1	Reduction of infarct size Decreased neurological deficit	Ziv et al. 2007

Therapy	Mechanism of neuroprotection ↑Increase ↓Decrease	Treatment outcome	Reference
MOG	• Immunomodulation: ↑IL-10-secreting $CD4^+$ Treg • ↓$CD11b^+$, ↓NO	Reduction of infarct size Decreased neurological deficit	Frenkel et al. 2004
IL-10	• ↑Stem cell proliferation	Neurogenesis	Wang et al 2015
Noggin	• Modify activated microglial phenotype from M1 to M2	Neurogenesis and angiogenesis	Shin et al, 2014
Antibodies	• Inhibit signaling pathways that limit axonal growth	Increased neuroplasticity and neurological recovery	Weissner et al, 2003.
ALA	• Anti-inflammaton: ↓: IL-1 β, TNF-α, MIP1, Iba-1 • ↑SOX2	Reduction of infarct size Increased neurological recovery	Choi et al, 2015
Tetrmetylpyrazine	• Anti-inflammatory • Antioxidant	Induce dendritic plasticity Greater neurological recovery	Lin et al, 2015
Ischemic pre-conditioning	• Anti-inflammation: ↑IL-4, IL-13 • Pathways: PI3K/Akt) and ERK1/2	Reduction of infarct size	Schaller et al. 2003
		Increased neurological recovery	Tu XK et al 2015
		Pyramidal neuron survival	Kim DW et al 2015

Table 1. Neuroprotective mechanisms exerted by diverse therapies.

6. Immune response as a neurorestorative mechanism

Even though neuroprotection is a targeted treatment that might be useful in a variety of ailments above mentioned, it does not restore tissue to its original anatomical state. In order to achieve "anatomical normality," alternative and promising therapies are being studied for achieving neurorestoration through different mechanisms [71] involving the immune system, given that these new strategies have shown that immune cells are able to secrete factors that intervene in neurorestoration processes like neurogenesis.

Different studies have demonstrated that autoreactive T lymphocytes support neurogenesis in young and old animals, and are essential for memory development and spatial learning [92]. This was observed before by studies where the circulating T lymphocyte depletion drives a cognitive deficit from neurogenesis decrease [93].

Active immunization with Cop-1 has demonstrated to be able to increase trophic factor production, such as: IGF-1 in retinal ganglion cells [94] experimental autoimmune encephalitis (EAE) [95], as well as in combination neurotrophin-3 and neurotrophin-4 (NT-3 and NT-4) in EAE [96].

Both brain-derived neurotrophic factor (BDNF) and NT-3/NT-4 have been implicated in neurogenesis regulation mechanisms, differentiation, and neuron survival through its receptors Trks or p75 [97], also, BDNF has been implicated in neuroblast migration processes through the rostral migratory stream [98]. In healthy conditions, neuroblasts are conducted to the olphactory bulb where they mature and contribute to site plasticity [99], or in pathological conditions such as ischemia, they can be conducted toward periphery of the damage zone where they incorporate.

IGF also promotes neural cell proliferation by interacting with its receptor IGF-IR in the sub-ventricular zone as well as the hippocampal dentate gyrus (neurogenic niches in adults) in adult rats [100]. Furthermore, it participates in oligodendrogenesis after being stimulated by Cop-1 in a multiple sclerosis model [95].

Immunization with Cop-1 has demonstrated to induce an increment in neurogenesis and neuron survival during acute and chronic phases of an ischemic event [101]. In the same way, Poli-Y immunomodulator has also shown an increment in cortical and hippocampal neurogenesis, as well as reduction of neural loss [88].

IL-10 use has also shown to have a positive effect on neurogenesis after cerebral ischemia, in 2015 Wang J and his work team observed that Treg cells are capable of increasing stem cell proliferation in the sub ventricular zone through IL-10 production [102].

Noggin is a bone morphogenic protein (BMP) antagonist that has also been tested in a MCAo model and has had neuroprotective as well as neurorestorative results through its ability to modify activated microglial response from M1 to M2 phenotype and induce an increase in several molecule production such as: vascular endothelial growth factor IL-10, Growth Associated Protein-43 (GAP-43), and vascular endothelial growth factor (VEGF) which intervene in neurogenesis and angiogenesis [103].

Antibodies have also been used successfully to inhibit signaling pathways that limit axonal and neurite growth and remodeling, thus allowing an increment neuronal plasticity and neurological recovery in ischemic rats [104].

On the other hand, the use of cell-based therapies is being studied for their neurorestorative properties; for instance, it has been demonstrated that microglia participates in neuronal precursor cell (NPC) migration and differentiation [105], as well as in neurogenesis, synaptogenesis, and tissue remodeling increase through the release of IGF-1 and neurotrophic growth factor (NGF), among others, in animals subjected to experimental stroke [106].

Other animal models, such as traumatic brain injury (TBI), have had success in the use of combined therapies composed of stem cell co-transplants and pharmacological a or immunomodulatory agents that modify neural tissue milieu in order to favor recovery and restoration. For example, the use of granulocyte-colony stimulating factor (GCSF) and human umbilical cord blood cell (hUCB) transplantation has demonstrated to reduce proinflammatory cytokine expression, increases trophic factor production, and promotes synaptic circuit reestablishment. For this reasons, it has been proposed as a therapy for stroke models [107].

Another mechanism through which brain tissue restoration is pursued is neuroplasticity or synapse plasticity, which is an inherent neurophysiological adaptive trait in which preexisting connections between two neurons can gain or lose strength during neural activity [108], as well as change in structure, function and organization [109]. It responds to different experiences and emphaticism and has been observed in different sections of the CNS [109].

Treatment with tetramethylpyrazine, which has anti-inflammatory and antioxidant effects, has shown to be able to induce dendritic plasticity, observing maintenance of neuroarchitecture through microtubule-associated protein 2 (MAP-2), which has been observed in greater density in peri-infarct zone found dendrites, causing a greater neurological recovery in rats with cerebral ischemia [110].

Alpha-lipoic acid (aLA) has yielded very good results in preclinical investigation since it has shown that its anti-inflammatory capacity through a decrease in proinflammatory cytokine expression such as: IL-1β, TNF-α, MIP1, Iba-1, and the increase in expression of transcription factor SOX2, which is essential for maintenance of auto regeneration properties, as well as an increase in neuron precursor cell proliferation accompanied by a significant reduction in infarct volume and better functional recovery. For all these reasons, aLA is a great candidate to start clinical trials as neurorestorative of brain tissue [111].

7. Advances in the clinical field

Even though preclinical trials have yielded promising results, translation into clinical human stroke trials has been unsuccessful. Clinical trials have been conducted very scarcely and have shown very little results [72, 112]. Some agents have been used in the clinical setting after having been observed beneficial in animal models. By 2008, Ginsberg had reported the existence of 160 clinical trials for neuroprotection after stroke and one-third of the by-then-finished 120 trials included more than 200 subjects; nonetheless, most of them failed to prove any benefit [70]. As of March 2016, a search in "www.strokecenter.org" for clinical trials involving neuroprotection yields 25 results of which 12 involve neuroprotection for acute ischemic stroke and only one of them is already in already phase 4. A different search in involving the word "immune" yielded another 25 matches, of which only two are related to immunomodulation in stroke.

One of them, Nasal Selectin E administration is being studied by Hellenbeck, M.D. at the National Institute of Neurological Disorders and Stroke (NINDS) in patients that have suffered from stroke, seeking induction of mucosal tolerance to this adhesion molecule through low-dose nasal administration, in order to promote a response shift from Th1 toward Th2 or Th reg at inflammation sites. This trial is currently at phase I and has not yet published results [113].

Fingolimod, which has been mentioned earlier, is also being used in an ongoing clinical trial with the goal of analyzing neurofunctional effects in stroke patients at different time points after being orally administered. The secondary purpose is to identify if there are any cellular and structural brain modifications through the use of flow cytometry and MRI [114].

In accordance, a pilot trial was conducted combining the use of rtPA and Fingolimod in a randomized multicenter pilot trial that included 47 patients in China. Treatment was provided within 3 and 3.1 h from symptom onset. Whole blood was used to assess lymphocyte and mononuclear cells at day 1, 7, and 90. After day 1, $CD4^+$ T cells, $CD8^+$ T cells, $CD19B^+$ cells, and NK cells had significant decreases in the fingolimod + alteplase group, as opposed to the alteplase only group. At day 7, this trend continued and normalized by day 90th. Other results included lesser infarct volume expansion, smaller hemorrhage, and greater functional recovery in the short and long term in the combined treatment group. Safety was assured during this trial, and further investigation needs to be considered [115].

On the other hand, stem cell therapies are also under clinical scrutiny, their use has proven to be feasible, but not necessarily practical, and it is safe. Most clinical trials have proven that stem cell therapy improves functional recovery but other factors have to be taken into account too, such as cost-effectiveness, comparison to other stroke treatments, time, and type of stroke. According to Young, there are currently nine ongoing stem cell clinical trials for stroke, testing safety, and efficacy as well as most accurate patient selection [116].

Knowledge about the molecular dynamics of cerebral ischemia pathophysiology and the study of neuroprotective mechanisms has promoted the use of combined therapies [89].

The use of combined therapies has also been tried in the clinical field in different diseases. For example, two quadriplegic patients were transplanted with differentiated neural stem cells (NSC) and autoreactive autologous T lymphocytes. These patients regained motor and sensitive functions without adverse effects [117], all the more reason to try these therapies in stroke.

Some stem cell trials have shown to have some beneficial effects on stroke patients, such as the use of human placenta derived adherent (PDA001) cells, isolated from *postpartum* placenta, and were studied for their neurorestorative effects after stroke. Animals were injected with these cells 4 h after being subjected to stroke. Results show an increase in functional recovery 7- and 14 days post-ischemia, as well as an increase level of BDNF, vascular endothelial growth factor (VEGF) which is an angiogenic factor, increases axonal outgrowth, stop apoptosis and increases neurogenesis, and hepatocyte growth factor (HGF) which is also angiogenic, and decreased TUNEL and cleaved caspase 3, showing a decreased infarct volume. Although not many cells survived until day 14, beneficial effects were still observed [118] (**Table 2**).

Treatment	Outcome	Reference
Nasal selectin E	Promote a response shift from Th1→Th2 or Th reg Ongoing	[113]
Fingolimod	No outcome, still ongoing	[114]
rtPA + Fingolimod	Reduced infarct volume Greater neurological recovery	[115]
NSC + Autoreactive Autologous T cells	Recovery of motor and sensory functions No adverse effects	[117]
PDA001	Increased functional recovery	[118]

Table 2. Results of some clinical trials.

Most preclinical investigations focus on delivering treatment in the first hour after reperfusion and happen in strictly controlled environments, which is why they have shown beneficial effects. Lack of results in clinical trials is attributed to uncontrolled real life settings, different populations, comorbidity existence, different ischemic territories, duration of occlusion before reperfusion, and a single target for treatment, leaving behind other neural components that might aid recovery. Also, patients are selected after arrival to hospitals and thus, other environmental variables and time window are not accounted for in results [72, 112].

The study and application of new therapies that will aid the ischemic patient recover more effectively needs to continue to be worked on in the basic and preclinical fields, specially through the exploration of immune system characteristics that might be beneficial for stroke therapy and thus achieve a decrease in mortality and an increase in functional recovery after hemiplegia (one-sided paralysis) hemi-hypoesthesia (one-sided decrease in sensory perception) hemianopsia (one eyed decreased vision), paresia (partial paralysis), aphasia (inability to comprehend language), and memory alterations; favorably increases stroke patients quality of life.

Author details

Yolanda Cruz, Karla A Cantú-Saldaña and Antonio Ibarra*

*Address all correspondence to: iantonio65@yahoo.com.mx

Health Sciences Center for Investigation (CICSA), Health Sciences Faculty, Anáhuac México Norte University, Huixquilucan, Mexico

References

[1] Prieto-Arribas R, Moreno-Gutierrez A, Simal-Hernández P, Pascual-Garvi JM, Matías-Guiu J, Roda JM, et al. Experimental models of cerebral ischemia. Revista de neurología. 2008;47(8):414-26.

[2] WHO. Global Status Report on Noncommunicable Diseases World Health Organization; 2014. Report No.: Contract No.

[3] Mozaffarian D, Benjamin EJ, Go AS, Arnett DK, Blaha MJ, Cushman M, et al. Heart disease and stroke statistics—2016 update: a report from the American Heart Association. American Heart Association; 2016. Report No.: Contract No.

[4] CDC. STROKE FACT SHEET <+http://www.cdc.gov/stroke/facts.htm

[5] Malmivaara A, Meretoja A, Peltola M, Numerato D, Heijink R, Engelfreit P, et al. Comparing ischemic stroke in six European countries. The EuroHOPE register study. European Journal of Neurology. 2015;22(2):284–91.

[6] Ullberg T, Zia E, Petersson J, Norrving B. Changes in functional outcome over the first year after stroke. Stroke. 2015;46:389–94.

[7] Guiraud V, Gallarda T, Calvet D, Turc G, Oppenheim C, Rouillon F, et al. Depression predictors within six months of ischemic stroke: the DEPRESS Study. Int J Stroke. 2016;11(5):519–25.

[8] Haast AMR, Gustafson RD, Kiliaan A. Sex differences in stroke. Journal of Cerebral Blood Flow and Metabolism. 2012;32:2100–7.

[9] Durukan A, Tatlisumak T. Acute ischemic stroke: overview of major experimental rodent models, pathophysiology, and therapy of focal cerebral ischemia. Pharmacology Biochemistry and Behavior. 2007; 87;(1):179–197.

[10] Krishnamurthi RV, Moran AE, Feigin VL, Barker-Collo S, Norrving B, Mensah GA, et al. Stroke prevalence, mortality and disability-adjusted life years in adults aged 20–64 years in 1990–2013: data from the Global Burden of Disease 2013 Study. Neuroepidemiology. 2015;45(3):190–202.

[11] Diaw M, Pialoux X, Martin C, Samb A, Diop S, Faes C, et al. Sickle cell trait worsens oxidative stress, abnormal blood rheology and vascular dysfunction in type 2 diabateres. Diabetes Care. 2015;38(11):2120-7.

[12] Edsfeldt A, Bengtsson E, Asciutto G, Dunér P, Björkbacka H, Fredrikson GN, et al. High plasma levels of Galectin-3 are associated with increased risk for stroke after carotid endarterectomy. Cerebrovascular Diseases. 2016;41:199–203.

[13] Wan L, Liu FT. Galectin-3 and inflammation. Glycobiology Insights. 2016;6:1–9.

[14] Jin QH, Lou YF, Li TL, Chen HH, Liu Q, He XJ. Serum galectin-3: a risk facor for vascular complication in type 2 diabetes mellitus. Chinese Medical Journal (Engl). 2013;126(11): 2109–15.

[15] Sheedy FJ, Moore KJ. IL-1 signaling in atherosclerosis: sibling rivalry. Nat Immunol. 2013;14;(10):1030–2.

[16] Nadar SK, Lip GYH, Lee KW, Blann AD. Circulating endothelial cells in acute ischemic stroke. Thrombosis and Haemostasis. 2005;94:707–12.

[17] Hansson GK, Hermansson A. The immune system in atherosclerosis. Nat Immunol. 2011;12(3):204–12.

[18] Goel S, Miller A, Agarwal C, Zakin E, Acholonu M, Gidwani U, et al. Imaging modalities to identity inflammation in an atherosclerotic plaque. Radiology Research and Practice. 2015;2015:13.

[19] Castillo J, Álvarez-Sabin J, Dávalos E, Díez-Tejedor E, Lizasoain I, Martínez-Villa E, et al. Consensus Revision. Pharmacological Neuroprotection in cerebral ischemia: Is it still a therapeutic option? Neurología. 2003;18(7):368–84.

[20] Cross JL, Meloni BP, Bakker AJ, Lee S, Knuckey NW. Modes of Neuronal Calcium Entry and Homeostasis following Cerebral Ischemia. Stroke Research and Treatment. 2010;2010:316862:1–9.

[21] Marambaud P, Dreses-Werringloer U, Vingtdeux V. Calcium signaling in neurodegeneration. Molecular Neurodegeneration. 2009;4(20).

[22] Al Ahmad A, Gassmann M, Ogunshola OO. Involvement of oxidative stress in hypoxia-induced blood-brain barrier breakdown. Microvascular Research. 2012;84(2):222–5.

[23] Cavdar Z, Egrilmez MY, Altun ZS, Arslan N, Yener N, Sayin O, et al. Resveratrol reduces matrix metalloproteinase-2 activity induced by oxygen-glucose deprivation and reoxygenation in human cerebral microvascular endothelial cells. International Journal of Vitamin and Nutrition Research. 2012;82(4):267–74.

[24] Frankowski JC, DeMars KM, Ahmad A, Hwkins KE, Yang C, Leclerc JL, et al. Detrimental role of the EP1 prostanoid receptor in bloodbrain barrier damage following experimental ischemic stroke. Scientific Reports. 2015;5:17956.

[25] Huang J, Upadhyay UM, Tamargo RJ. Inflammation in stroke and focal cerebral ischemia. Surgical Neurology. 2006;66(3):232–45.

[26] Gokhan Y, Arumugam TV, Stokes KY, Granger N. Role of T lymphocytes and interferon-y in ischemic stroke. Circulation. 2006;113:2015–112.

[27] Schaller B, Graf R. Cerebral ischemia and reperfusion: the pathophysiologic concept as a basis for clinical therapy. Journal of Cerebral Blood Flow and Metabolism. 2004;24:351–71.

[28] Shastri A, Bonifati DM, Kishore U. Innate immunity and neuroinflammation. Mediators Inflamm. 2013;2013:342931:1–19.

[29] Besis A, Bechade C, Bernard D, Roumier A. Microglial control of neuronal death and synaptic properties. Glia. 2007;55:233–8.

[30] Butovsky O, Ziv Y, Schwartz A, Landa G, Talpalar A, Pluchino S, et al. Microglia activated by IL-4 or IFN-γ differentially induce neurogenesis and oligodendrogenesis from adult stem/progenitor cells. Neuroscience. 2006;31(1):149–60.

[31] Kofler J, Wiley C. Microglia: key innate immune cells of the brain. Toxicologic Pathology. 2011;39:103–14.

[32] Goldmann T, Prize M. Role of microglia in CNS autoimmunity. Clin Dev Immunol. 2013; 2013:208093. doi: 10.1155/2013/208093.

[33] Xing C, Wang X, Cheng C, Montaner J, Mandeville E, Leung W, et al. Neuronal production of lipocalin-2 as a help-me signal for glial activation. Stroke. 2014;45(7): 2085–92.

[34] Zhao X, Wang H, Sun G, Zhang J, Edwards NJ, Aronowski J. Neuronal interleukin-4 as a modulator of microglial pathways and ischemic brain damage. Journal of Neuroscience. 2015;35(32):11281–91.

[35] Patel A, Ritzel R, McCullough LD, Liu F. Microglia and ischemic stroke: a double-edged sword. International of Journal of Physiology, Pathophysiology and Pharmacology. 2013;5(2):73–90.

[36] Hu X, Li P, Guo Y, Wang H, Leak R, Chen S, et al. Microglia/macrophage polarization dynamics revea novel mechanism of injury expansion after focal cerebral ischemia. Stroke. 2012;43:3060–70.

[37] Lambertsen KL, Biber K, Finsen B. Inflammatory cytokines in experimental and human stroke. Journal of Cerebral Blood Flow and Metabolism. 2012;32:1677–1698.

[38] Wei Z, Chigurupati S, Arumugam TV, Jo DG, Li H, Chan SL. Notch activation enhances the microglia-mediated inflammatory response associated with focal cerebral ischemia. Stroke. 2011;42(25):2589–94.

[39] Lindsberg PJ, Strbian D, Karjalainen-Lindsberg ML. Mast cells as early responders in the regulation of acute blood-brain barrier changes after cerebral ischemia and hemorrhage. Journal of Cerebral Blood Flow and Metabolism. 2010;30:689–702.

[40] Mattila OS, Strbian D, Saksi J, Pikkarainen TO, Rantanen V, Tatlisumak T, et al. Cerebral mast cells mediate blood-brain barrier disruption in acute experimental ischemic stroke through perivascular gelatinase activation. Stroke. 2011;42:3600–5.

[41] Fang W, Sha L, Kodithuwakku ND, Wei J, Zhang R, Han D, et al. Attenuated blood-brain barrier dysfunction by XQ-1H following ischemic stroke in hyperlipidemic rats. Molecular Neurobiology. 2015;52:162–175.

[42] Grønberg NV, Johansen FF, Kristiansen U, Hasseldam H. Leukocyte infiltration in experimental stroke. J Neuroinflammation. 2013;10;(115):1–9.

[43] Perez-de-Puig I, Miró-Mur F, Ferrer-Ferrer M, Gelpi E, Pedragosa J, Justicia C, et al. Neutrophil recruitment to the brain in mouse and human ischemic stroke. Acta Neuropathologica. 2015;129(2):239–57.

[44] Ransohoff R, Brown M. Innate immunity in the central nervous system. Journal of Clinical Investigation. 2012;122(4):1164–71.

[45] Kolaczkowska E, Kubes P.: Neutrophil recruitment and function in health and inflammation. *Nat Rev Immunol*. 2013;13(3):159 ◎?75.

[46] Kumar AD, Boehme AK, Siegler JE, Gillette M, Albright KC, Martin-Schild S. Leukocytosis in patients with neurologic deterioration after acute ischemic stroke is associated with poor outcomes. J Stroke Cerebrovasc Dis. 2013;22(7):e1117.

[47] Maestrini I, Strbian D, Gautier S, Haapaniemi E, Moulin S, Sairanen T, et al. Higher neutrophil counts before thrombolysis for cerebral ischemia predict worse outcomes. Neurology. 2015;85(16):1408–16.

[48] Murikinati S, Jüttler E, Keinert T, Ridder DA, Muhammad S, Waibler Z, et al. Activation of cannabinoid 2 receptors protects against cerebral ischemia by inhibiting neutrophil recruitment. FASEB Journal. 2010;24:788–98.

[49] Wu L, Walas S, Leung W, Sykes DB, Wu J, Lo EH, et al. Neuroregulin 1-β decreases IL-1β-induced neutrophil adhesion to human brain microvascular endothelial cells. Translational Stroke Research. 2015;6(2):116–24.

[50] Connell BJ, Gordon JR, Saleh TM. ELR-CXC chemokine antagonism is neuroprotective in a rat model of ischemic stroke. Neuroscience Letters. 2015;606:117–22.

[51] OB D, Stamatovic SM, Keep RF, Andjelkovic AV. Absence of the chemokine receptor CCR2 protects against cerebral ischemia/reperfusion injury in mice. Stroke. 2007;38(4): 1345–53.

[52] ElAli A, Jean LeBlanc N. The Role of Monocytes in Ischemic Stroke Pathobiology: New Avenues to Explore. Front Aging Neurosci. 2016;8;(29):1–7.

[53] Ritzel RM, Patel AR, Grenier JM, et al. Functional differences between microglia and monocytes after ischemic stroke. J Neuroinflammation. 2015;12;(106):1–12.

[54] Zhang X, Li H, Li Y, Ma Y, Luo Y, Zhou X, et al. Increased circulating Ly6C(high); monocyte subsets are correlated with cerebral infarct size in cerebral ischemia/reperfusion mouse models. Xi Bao Yu Fen Yi Xue Mian Zhi. 2016;32(3):294–8.

[55] Miró-Mur F, Pérez-de-Piug I, Ferrer-Ferrer M, Urra X, Justicia C, Chamorro A, et al. Immature monocyte recruited to the ischemic mouse brain differentiate into macrophages with features of alternative activation. Brain, Behaviour and Immunity. 2016;53:18–33.

[56] Chu HX, Kim HA, Lee S, Broughton BRS, Drummond GR, Sobey C. Evidence of CCR2-independent transmigration of Ly6 Chi monocytes into the brain after permanent cerebral ischemia in mice. Brain Research. 2015;16(37):118–27.

[57] Stevens SL, Bao J, Hollis J, Lessov NS, Clark WM, Stenzel-Poore MP. The use of flow cytometry to evaluate temporal changes in inflammatory cell following focal cerebral ischemia in mice. Brain Research. 2002;932(1–2):110–9.

[58] Kim HA, Whittle SC, Lee S, et al. Brain immune cell composition and functional outcome after cerebral ischemia: comparison of two mouse strains. Front Cell Neurosci. 2014;8;(365):1–12.

[59] Becker K, Kalil AJ, Tanzi P, Zierath D, Savos A, Gee JM, et al. Autoimmune responses to the brain after stroke are associated with worse outcome. Stroke. 2011;42:2763–9.

[60] Planas AM, Gómez-Choco M, Urra X, Gorina R, Caballero M, Chamorrow Á. Brain-derived antigens in lymphoid tissue of patients with acute stroke. Journal of Immunology. 2012;188:2156–63.

[61] Urra X, Miró F, Chamorro A, Planas AM. Antigen-specific immune reactions to ischemic stroke. Front Cell Neurosci. 2014;8; (278): 1–15.

[62] Zierath D, Kunze A, Fecteau L, Becker K. Promiscuity of autoimmune responses to MBP after stroke. Journal of Neuroimmunology. 2015;285:101–5.

[63] Liesz A, Zhou W, Mracskó E, Karcher S, Bauer H, Schwarting S, et al. Inhibition of lymphocyte traffiking shields the brain against deleterious neuroinflammation after stroke. Brain. 2011;134(Pt.3):704–20.

[64] Xiong X, Gu L, Zhang H, Xu B, Zhu S, Zhao H. The protective effects of T cell deficiency against brain injury are ischemic model-depentent in rats. Neurochemistry International. 2013;62(3):265–170.

[65] Stubbe T, Ebner F, Richter D, Engel O, Klehmet J, Royl G, et al. Regulatory T cells accumulate and proliferate in the ischemic hemisphere for up to 30 days after MCAO. Journal of Cereberal Blood Flow and Metabolism. 2013;33(1):37–47.

[66] Ibarra A, Hauben E, Butovsky O, Schwartz M. The therapeutic window after spinal cord injury can accommodate T cell-based vaccination and methylprednisolone in rats. European Journal of Neuroscience. 2004;19:2984–90.

[67] Revesz T, Kidd D, Thompson A, Barnard R, McDonald W. A comparison of the pathology of primary and secondary progressive multiple sclerosis. Brain. 1994;117:759–65.

[68] Schwartz M, Kipnis J. Protective autoimmunity and neuroprotection in inflammatory and noninflammatory neurodegenerative diseases. Journal of Neurological Sciences. 2005;233:163–6.

[69] Frenkel D, Huang Z, Maron R, Koldzic DN, Hancock WW, Moskowitz MA, et al. Nasal vaccination with myelin oligodendrocyte glycoprotein reduces stroke size by inducing IL-10-producing $CD4^+$ T cells. The Journal of Immunology. 2004;172:6549–55.

[70] Ginsberg MD. Neuroprotection for ischemic stroke: past, present and future. Neuropharmacology. 2008;55(3):363–89.

[71] Zarros A. In which cases is neuroprotection useful? Advances & Alternative Thinking in Neuroscience. 2009;1(s1):3–5.

[72] Tymianski M. Novel approaches to neuroprotection trials in acute ischemic stroke. Stroke. 2013;44:2942–50.

[73] Liesz A, Hagmann S, Zschoche C, Adamek J, Zhou W, Sun L, et al. The Spectrum of systemic immune alteration after murine focal ischemia: immunodepression vs immunomodulation. Stroke. 2009;40:2849–58.

[74] Yang D, Li S-Y, Yeung C-M, et al. Lycium barbarum Extracts Protect the Brain from Blood-Brain Barrier Disruption and Cerebral Edema in Experimental Stroke. PLoS ONE. 2012;7(3):e33596:1–10. doi:10.1371/journal.pone.0033596.

[75] Vaibhav K, Shrivastava P, Javed H, Khan A, Ahmed E, Tabassum R, et al. Piperine suppresses cerebral ischemia-reperfusion-induced inflammation through the repression of COX-2, NOZ-2 and NF-κB in middle cerebral artery occlusion rat model. Molecular and Cellular Biochemistry. 2012;367(1):73–84.

[76] Campos-Martorell M, Salvador N, Mongge M, Canals F, García-Bonilla L, Hernández-Guillamon M, et al. Brain proteomics identifies potential simvastatin targets in acute phase of stroke in a rat embolic model. Journal of Neurochemistry. 2014;130:301–12.

[77] Lagarto Parra A, García Rodrígez JC. Nasal Neuro EPO Could be a reliable choice for neuroprotective stroke treatment. Central Nervous System Agents in Medicinal Chemistry. 2012;12:60–8.

[78] Kuric E, Ruscher K. Reduction of rat brain $CD8^+$ T-cells by levodopa/benserazide treatment after experimental stroke. European Journal of Neuroscience. 2014;40(2): 2463–70.

[79] Kraft P, Göb E, Schuhmann MK, Göbel K, Deppermann C, Thielmann I, et al. FTY720 Ameliorates acute ischemic stroke in mice by reducing thrombo-inflammation but not by direct neuroprotection. Stroke. 2013;44:3202–10.

[80] Zhang M, Wang S, Mao L, Leak R, Shi Y, Zhang W, et al. Omega-3 Fatty acids protect the brain against ischemic injury by activating Nrf2 and upregulating heme oxygenase 1. The Journal of Neuroscience. 2014;34(5):1903–15.

[81] Immunology WoMa. Immunomodulation http://www.encyclopedia.com/doc/1G2-3409800310.html2003.

[82] Zhang WX, Zhang QL, Deng W, Li YL, Xing GQ, Shi XJ, et al. Neuroprotective effect of pretreatment with ganoderma lucidum in cerebral ischemia/reperfusion injury in rat hippocampus. Neural Regeneration Research. 2014;9(15):1446–52.

[83] Yang Y, Salayandia VM, Thompson JF, Yang LY, Estrada EY, Yang Y. Attenuation of acute stroke injury in rat brain by minocycline promotes blood–brain barrier remodeling and alternative microglia/macrophage activation during recovery. J Neuroinflammation. 2015;12: 26.

[84] Liu X, Liu J, Zhao S, Zhang H, Cai W, Cai M, et al. Interleukin-4 is essential for microlia/macrophage M2 polarization and long-term recovery after cerebral ischemia. Stroke. 2016;47:498–504.

[85] Kuo PC, Scofield BA, Yu I-C, Chang F-L, Ganea D, Yen J-H. Interferon-β modulates inflammatory response in cerebral ischemia. J Am Heart Assoc.2016; 5: e002610.

[86] Aharoni R, Kayhan B, Eilam R, Sela M, Arnon R. Glatiramer acetate-specific T cells in the brain express T helper 2/3 cytokines and brain-derived neurotrophic factor *in situ*. Proceedings of the National Academy of Sciences of the United States of America. 2003;100(24):14157–62.

[87] Ibarra A, Avendaño H, Cruz Y. Copolymer-1 (Cop-1) improves neurological recovery-after middle cerebral artery occlusion in rats. Neuroscience Letters. 2007;425:110–3.

[88] Ziv Y, Finkelstein A, Geffen Y, Kipnis J, Smirnov I, Shpilman S, et al. A novel immune-based therapy for stroke induces neuroprotection and supports neurogenesis. Stroke. 2007;38:774–82.

[89] Schaller B, Graf R, Jacobs AH. Ischaemic tolerance: a window to endogenous neuroprotection? The Lancet. 2003;362:1007–8.

[90] Kim DW, Lee JC, Cho JH, Park JH, Ahn JH, Chen BH, et al. Neuroprotection of ischemic preconditioning is mediated by anti-inflammatory, not pro-inflammatory, cytokines in the gerbil hippocampus induced by a subsequent lethal transient cerebral ischemia. Neurochem Res. 2015;40(9):1984–95.

[91] Tu XK, Yang WZ, Chen JP, Chen Y, Chen Q, Chen PP, et al. Repetitive ischemic preconditioning attenuates inflammatory reaction and brain damage after focal cerebral ischemia in rats: involvement of P13K/Akt and ERK 1/2 signaling pathway. Journal of Molecular Neuroscience. 2015;55(4):912–22.

[92] Ziv Y, Avidan H, Pluchino S, Martino G, Schwartz M. Synergy between immune cells and adult neural stem/progenitor cells promotes functional recovery from spinal cord injury. Proceedings of the National Academy of Sciences of the United States of America. 2006;103(35):13174–9.

[93] Kipnis J, Cohen H, Cardon M, Ziv Y, Schwartz M. T cell deficiency leads to cognitive dysfunction: implications for therapeutic vaccination for schizophrenia and other

psychiatric conditions. Proceedings of the National Academy of Sciences of the United States of America. 2004;101(21):8180–5.

[94] Qian S, Tang Y, Cheng L, Sun X, Tian J, Buzoianu DA. Interaction of copolymer-1-activated T cells and microglia in retinal ganglion cell protection. Clinical and Experimental Ophthalmology. 2013;41(9):881–90.

[95] Skihar V, Silva C, Chojnacki A, et al. Promoting oligodendrogenesis and myelin repair using the multiple sclerosis medication glatiramer acetate. Proceedings of the National Academy of Sciences of the United States of America. 2009;106(42):17992–17997. doi: 10.1073/pnas.0909607106.

[96] Aharoni R, Eilam R, Domev H, Labunskay G, Sela M, Arnon R. The immunomodulator glatiramer acetate augments the expression of neurtrophic factors in brains of experimental autoimmune encephalomyelitis mice. Proceedings of the National Academy of Sciences of the United States of America. 2005;102(52):19045–50.

[97] Vilar M, Mira H. Regulation of Neurogenesis by Neurotrophins during Adulthood: Expected and Unexpected Roles. Front Neurosci. 2016;10; (26):1–9 doi:10.3389/fnins.2016.00026.

[98] Snapyan M, Lemasson M, Brill M, Blais M, Massouh M, Ninkovic J, et al. Vasculature guides migrating neuronal precursos in the adult mammalian forebrain via brain-derived neurotrophic factor signaling. Journal of Neuroscience. 2009;29:4172–88.

[99] Lledo PM, Merkle FT, Álvarez-Buylla A. Origin and function of olfactory bulb interneuron diversity. Trends in Neurosciences. 2008;31:392–400.

[100] Nieto-Estévez V, Defterali Ç, Vicario-Abejón C. IGF-I: A Key Growth Factor that Regulates Neurogenesis and Synaptogenesis from Embryonic to Adult Stages of the Brain. Front Neurosci. 2016;10;(5):1-9 doi:10.3389/fnins.2016.00052.

[101] Cruz Y, Loera J, Mestre H, Kim-Lee J, Herrera J, Mellado R, et al. Copolymer-1 promotes neurogenesis and improves functional recovery after acute ischemic stroke in rats. PLoS ONE 2015; 10(3): e0121854.

[102] Wang J, Xie L, Yang C, et al. Activated regulatory T cell regulates neural stem cell proliferation in the subventricular zone of normal and ischemic mouse brain through interleukin 10. Front Cell Neurosci. 2015;9;(361):1–11 doi:10.3389/fncel.2015.00361.

[103] Shin JA, Lim SM, Jeong SI, Kang JL, Park EM. Noggin improves ischemic brain tissue repair and promotes alternative activation of microglia in mice. Brain, Behaviour, and Immunity. 2014;40:143–54.

[104] Wiessner C, Bareyre F, Allegrini P, Mir A, Frentzel S, Zurini M, et al. Anti-Nogo-A antibody infusion after experimental stroke improved behavioral outcome and corticospinal plasticity in normotensive and spontaneously hypertensive rats. Journal of Cerebral Blood Flow Metabolism. 2003;23(2):154–65.

[105] Sierra A, Encinas J, Deudero J, Chancey J, Enikolopov G, Overstreet-Wadiche L, et al. Microglia shape adult hippocampal neurogenesis throush apoptosis-coupled phagocytosis. Cell Stem Cell. 2010;7(4):483–95.

[106] Liu Z, Xin H, Chopp M. Reactive astrocytes promote azonal remodeling and neurological recovery after stroke. Neural Regeneration. 2014;9(21):1874–5.

[107] Peña I, Borlongan CV. Translating G-CSF as an Adjunct Therapy to Stem Cell Transplantation for Stroke. Transl Stroke Res. 2015;6(6):421–9.

[108] De Pittá M, Brunel N, Volterra A. Astrocytes: Orchestrating synaptic plasticity? Neuroscience. 2015; 323: 43–61.

[109] Pelletier R, Higgins J, Bourbonnais D. Is neuroplasticity in the central nervous system the missing link to our understanding of chronic musculoskeletal disorders? BMC Musculoskeletal Disorders. 2015;16(1):1471–2474.

[110] Lin JB, Zheng CJ, Zhang X, Chan J, Liao WJ, Wan Q. Effects of Tetramethylpyrazine on function recovery and neuronal dendritic plasticity after experimental stroke. Evidence-Based Complementary and Alternative Medicine. 2015;2015:1–10 ID394926.

[111] Choi KH, Park MS, Kim HS, Kim KT, Kim HS, Kim JT, et al. Alpha-Lipoic acid treatment is neurorestorative and promotes functional recovery after stroke in rats. Mol Brain. 2015;8:9. doi: 10.1186/s13041-015-0101-6.

[112] Grotta J. Neuroprotection is unlikely to be effective in humans using current trial designs. Stroke.2002;33(1):306–307.

[113] Hellenbeck J. E-Selectin Nasal Instillation to Prevent Secondary Stroke. Clinical trials 2016. ClinicalTrials.gov Identifier: NCT00069069 https://clinicaltrials.gov/ct2/show/NCT00069069.

[114] Shi FD. Efficacy and Safety of FTY720 for Acute Stroke. 2014. ClinicalTrials.gov Identifier: NCT02002390 https://clinicaltrials.gov/show/NCT02002390.

[115] Zhu Z, Fu Y, Tian D, Sun N, Han W, Chang G, et al. Combination of an immune modulator fingolimod with alteplase in acute ischemic stroke: a pilot trial. Circulation. 2015; 132 (12):1104–12.

[116] Bang OY, Lee JS, Lee PH, Lee G. Autologous mesenchymal stem cell transplantation in stroke patients. Annals of Neurology. 2005;57(6):874–82.

[117] Moviglia G, Fernandez Viña R, Barizuela J, Saslavsky J, Vrsalovic F, Varela G, et al. Combined protocol of cell therapy for chronic spinal cord injury. Report on the electrical and functional recovery of two patients. Cytotherapy. 2006;8(3):202–9.

[118] Chen J, Shehadah A, Pal A, Zacharek A, Cui X, Cui Y, et al. Neuroprotective effect of human placenta-derived cell treatment of stroke in rats. Cell Transplantation. 2013;22(5):871–9.

Section 4

Clinical Science

Chapter 7

Cerebrovascular Anatomy, Neuropathology, Clinics of Stroke: Endovascular Treatment, Decompressive Craniectomy

Erion Musabelliu , Masahiro Oomura and Yoko Kato

Additional information is available at the end of the chapter

http://dx.doi.org/10.5772/64610

Abstract

Stroke, a disease of millions, and a financial burden for many more is still challenging health sciences, as we greatly increase our efforts to better understand stroke pathogenesis, early diagnose, prevent and treat high risk and major risk factors we still need to update our clinical and surgical skills in treating stroke event and its aftermath. Use of applied anatomical and physiological knowledge should apply the same everywhere, and based on these standard principles we should be able to predict the early course of stroke neuropathology and its potential consequences. Updated new guidelines of recombinant tissue plasminogen activator (r-tPA) indications should help in early intervention when correct diagnosis is promptly made, but as the list of contraindications as well has changed staff neuroscientists should consider all possible medical and or surgical options for treatment. With prompt actions to try to reinstate perfusion we should always try to do so within the first 4 h, and having a maximal additional 2 h in reserve to consider surgical therapeutic options (should the clinic/unit's infrastructure allow it). Treatment modalities, therapeutic/endovascular and or surgical (embolectomy, bypass, decompression) are the alternatives among which we should wisely chose to treat our patients based on the best medical practice not in the skills of the individuals performing each or either procedure. It is of critical importance to know when surgery should be performed, how to calculate craniotomy size, what are the intra-, extra-cranial surgical landmarks and when should we put the bone back in cases of decompression. We should be able to correctly predict at what extent volume and intracranial pressure values will change by the size of decompressive craniectomy and its effect on the patient's prognosis. Clinic is the best indicator for timing of surgical decompression as it is the sole determinant of any other treatment option, and what high risk and major risk factors are present (if any) at the time of diagnosis will predict the clinical outcome of the patient, but not the age (which should not be the limit).

Keywords: Cerebrovascular Anatomy, Neuropathology, Clinics of Stroke, Embolectomy, Vascular Bypass, Decompression Techniques

1. Stroke syndrome, preamble

In this chapter, we try to explain through principles of anatomy, physiology, and hemodynamics of fluids how does it happen and why these are the series of pathological events following a cerebrovascular occlusion. What can we do differently to treat stroke syndrome? The main focus is on the invasive modalities of the treatment of stroke syndrome, specifically endovascular and surgical techniques.

Is it the best possible way to treat stroke syndrome itself by preventing and treating all the disease processes that risk and cause stroke syndrome?

2. Epidemiology, facts, stroke

Some of the facts of stroke syndrome are as follows:

1. Major neurological disease of our times
2. Second leading cause of death worldwide
3. Second largest contributor to hospital care cost among cardiovascular diseases
4. The leading cause of serious long-term disability
5. Its risk varies by race, ethnicity, and age and geography.

According to World Health Organization (WHO), 15 million people suffer stroke worldwide annually, and of these

1. 5 million die, 5 million are permanently disabled;
2. Stroke can and do occur at any age;
3. Hypertension contributes to more than 12.7 million strokes worldwide;
4. Atrial fibrillation is an independent risk factor for stroke, increasing risk by fivefold;
5. Incidence is 1.5/1000/year and rising rapidly with age to 10/1000/year at 75 years;
6. Male/female ratio of >1:1 (male>female);
7. Life-threatening complete middle cerebral artery (MCA) infarction—up to 10%, with mortality from malignant infarction—up to 80%;

Early action is important, the chances of survival are greater when treatment begins quickly (within 3 h cutoff), and these patients tend to have less disability 3 months after stroke [1].

http://dx.doi.org/10.5772/64610

3. Brain anatomy, physiology, facts

At any moment in normal conditions *(Monro-Kellie equation)*:

$$Volume_{Intracranial\ space} = Vol_{Brain} + Vol_{Blood} + Vol_{CSF} \tag{1}$$

Average human brain of an adult, weight	1300–1400 g [2] – Comprising 80% of brain weight
Hemisphere of an adult, weight	400 g – 55% of blood supplied by MCA – 25% supplied by ACA – 15% supplied by PCA – 5% supplied by anastomotic branches
Average weight of an adult cerebellum	150 g
Inside skull volume	≈1600 ml – 80% made by brain tissue – 20% – 55% CSF – 45% blood – <5% (60–80 ml) virtual space between cranial bone, meningeal layers, and brain
Cerebral blood flow (CBF)	750 ml/min (≈20% cardiac output) 50 ml/100 g/min
Changes in intracranial volume before: – Clinical signs appear – Imagery signs appear	– ≥60 ml – ≥80 ml
Volume of adult human brain	1200 cm^3 – 1100 cm^3 female – 1200 cm^3 male
Cerebrospinal fluid (CSF) volume, adult	150–270 ml – 25 ml, volume of ventricles
CSF production rate	0.2–0.7 ml/min 600–700 ml/day
Cerebral metabolic rate of O_2 consumption ($CMRO_2$)	3–4 ml/100 g tissue/min

Average human brain of an adult, weight	1300–1400 g [2] – Comprising 80% of brain weight
Normal intracranial pressure (ICP)	5–15 mmHg – 1–5 mmHg, infants – 5–10 mmHg, children – 5–15 mmHg, adolescents, adults
Critically raised ICP	≥20 mmHg

Table 1. Brain anatomy, physiology, facts.

$$CBF = \frac{CPP}{CVR} = \frac{MAP - ICP}{CVR}$$

The only parameters in which we have some medical and or surgical control (however, with extreme limitations).

	Constantly changing variables
CBF, cerebral blood flow	Yes
CPP, cerebral perfusion pressure	Yes
CVR, cerebrovascular resistance	Yes
MAP, mean arterial pressure	No, within a wide normal range
ICP, intracranial pressure	Yes, but has a very narrow range

Main factors influencing cerebral blood flow circulation are as follows:

- Systemic blood pressure (BP)
- The arterial blood gas levels

In the range of 60–140 mmHg, systemic BP has minimal effect on the CBF, due to autoregulation (via cerebral blood vessel dilation and contraction). MAP has the widest range of autoregulation.

$\uparrow$ in BP $\geq$ 150 mmHg $\Rightarrow \uparrow$ CBF, $\uparrow$ ICP

$\downarrow$ in BP $\leq$ 50 mmHg $\Rightarrow \downarrow$ CBF, and can potentially cause cerebral ischemia.

Hypercapnic vasodilation:

$PaCO_2$, the most important regulator.

Control—central chemoreceptors, medulla, brain stem.

Except in patients with medullary damage, or long-standing COPD (chronic obstructive pulmonary disease), when PaO_2 levels become a significant contributor to the respiratory drive.

Hypoxic vasodilation:

PaO_2 has a less profound effect, only when

$PaO_2 \downarrow \leq$ 50 mmHg $\Rightarrow \uparrow$cerebral perfusion.

Control—peripheral chemoreceptors, carotid and aortic bodies.

Table 2. Determinants of cerebral blood flow.

http://dx.doi.org/10.5772/64610

All three variables, components in this equation, are inversely related in normal autoregulation. Changes in the increase of at least one of the variables that are not accompanied with inverse relations of the other variables will results in ↑ intracranial volume and pressure (↑ ICP) eventually.

For these mathematical reasons that any increase in the intracranial volume up to 60 ml can be accommodated first by spinal movements of cerebrospinal fluid (CSF) before clinical (>60 ml ↑ in volume) and radiological (>80 ml ↑ in volume) signs of herniation occur (**Table 1**).

In their review, Schaller et al. revoked the classical equation of Kellie-Monro and suggested a more differentiated description for the dynamic of ICP, and its relation to cerebral blood flow (CBF). Several experimental and clinical studies have given evidence that this equation and the consideration of the intracranial volume to be a closed system are not entirely true from the physiological and pathophysiological point of view; even so the understanding of this phenomenon is incomplete [3].

CBF and blood pressure have a direct relation, and the main determinants of CBF are mean arterial pressure (MAP) and cerebrovascular resistance (CVR) (**Table 2**) (**Graphic 1**).

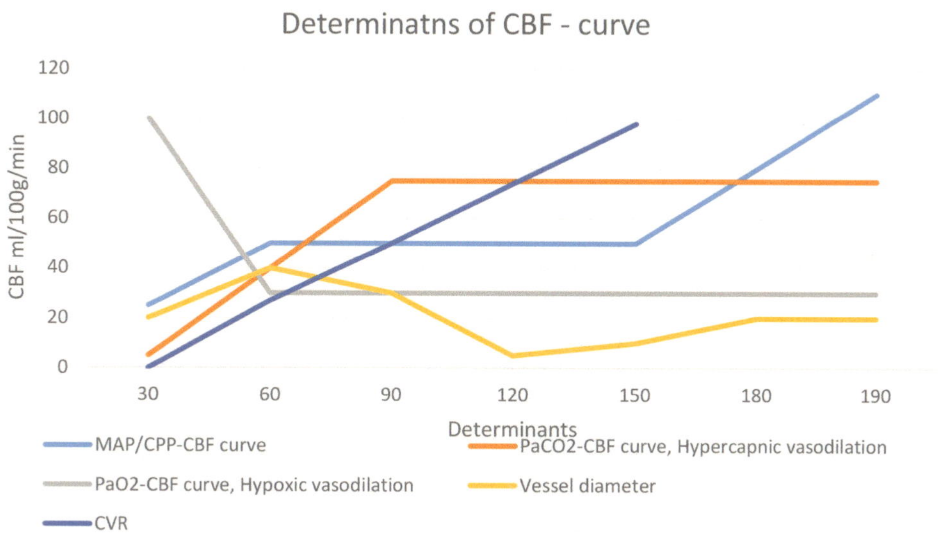

Graphic 1. Determinants of cerebral blood flow, correlation.

The arterial blood gases have a more powerful effect on the CBF. The medullary respiratory center controls the depth and the rate of respiration based on input from

- Chemoreceptors, located at
- Centrally, brain stem;
- Peripherally.

– Airway mechanoreceptors, regulate the duration of inspiration (Hering-Breuer reflex).

Cerebrovascular resistance (CVR) is affected by changes in

– $PaCO_2$;

– CPP (cerebral perfusion pressure).

The ratio, $\frac{CBF}{CMRO_2}$, is 14–18 (coupling ratio), when the brain is at the point of lowest O_2 consumption/g tissue.

For every region of cortex activated, the required ↑ of CBF by ≈ 30% will require a minimum ↑ of cerebral metabolic rate of oxygen consumption ($CMRO_2$) by ≈ 5% [4] (**Graphic 2**).

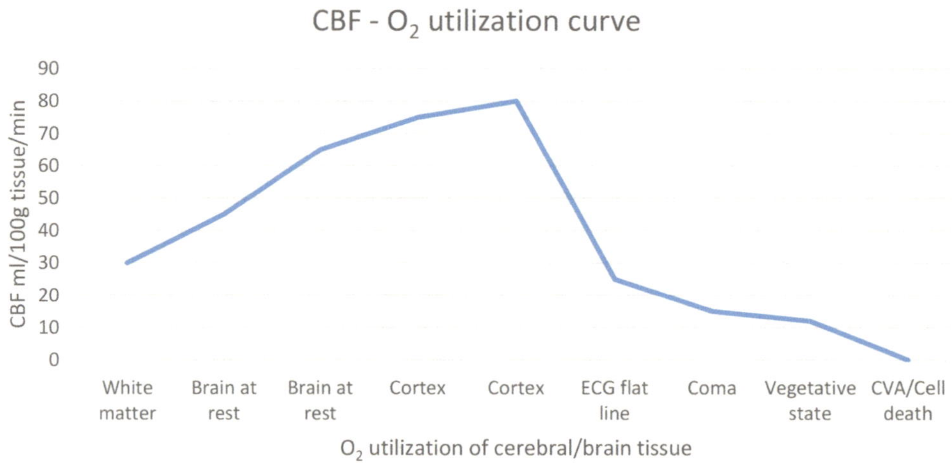

Graphic 2. Cerebral blood flow-O_2 utilization correlation.

Brain-tissue oxygen extraction exceeds that of any other tissue/organ (except for myocardial tissue); therefore, ↑ in the brain O_2 demand are met by a nearly proportional ↑ in vascular blood flow.

We can assume that by reducing the metabolic rate of the brain tissue, we may try and reach lower levels of oxygen consumptions during disease processes. The steps that can be taken to manipulate to some degree and reduce the $CMRO_2$ are by

1. Reducing the electrical activity of neurons (e.g., the use of barbiturates, general anesthesia);

2. Reducing the maintenance energy of neurons (e.g., hypothermia);

- Deep hypothermia (≈20°C) permits the brain to tolerate up to 1 h of circulatory arrest (more data required).

http://dx.doi.org/10.5772/64610

4. Cerebrovascular anatomy

We will use stroke imagery, and demonstrate simultaneously patent and occluded vessel as they mirror in the Circle of Willis, labeling the vessels most often affected (of particular interest for this chapter) in the stroke syndrome (**Figure 1**). A computerized tomography (CT) scan without contrast is the first diagnostic imagery, followed when possible by angio/angio-CT/ magnetic resonance imaging (MRI) scan. Angiography has its superiority in stroke syndrome as the diagnostic standard following the CT scan when possible; it can lead the way to endovascular procedures, should the infrastructure of the clinics support it [5, 6]. Successful endovascular treatment of the occluded vessel can save life. **Limitations** in the use of endovascular treatment exist in many clinics; they rely mostly on medical treatment options and surgical bypass and or decompression modalities for their patients.

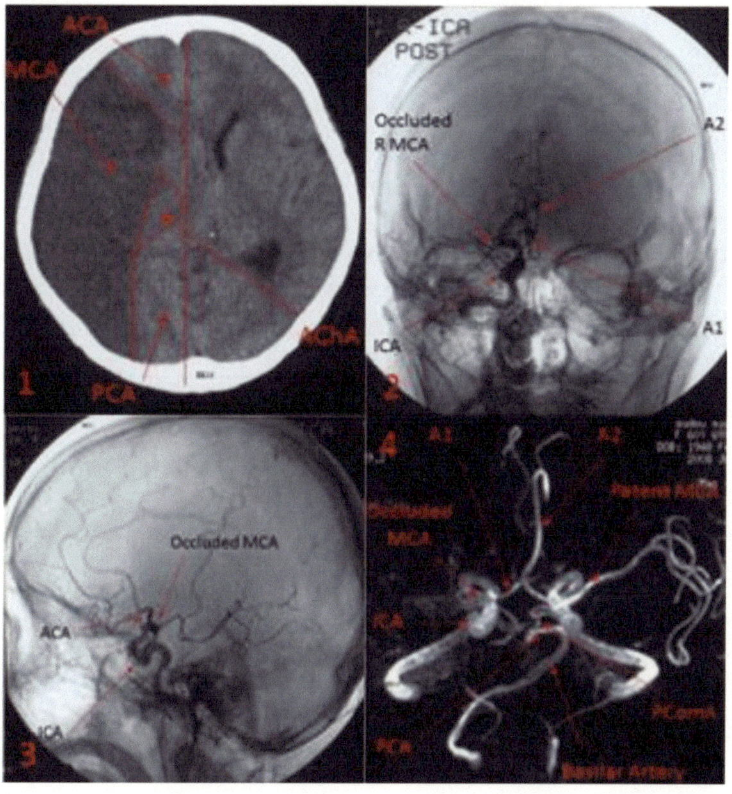

Figure 1. Imagery findings during stroke event, anatomical correlations. 1. A CT scan without contrast, illustrating main hemispheric cerebrovascular territories and ischemic zone under pathological progression in the MCA territory. 2. Anteroposterior view. 3. Lateral view, early diagnostic angiography images, demonstrating patent and occluded vessels. 4. Angio-MRI of Circle of Willis, mirroring the patent and occluded vessel after an acute ischemic accident.

Following internal carotid artery (ICA), MCA is the largest vessel in the anterior circulation. It supplies the largest brain-tissue territory, and it is for this anatomical reason that its occlusion is "malignant." Of its two branches (superior and inferior), occlusion of the superior has a devastating clinical course, if not the main MCA, and it supplies almost 60% of the main territory of the MCA main:

- There is considerable variability of the major arteries, and the central distribution [7];
- A balanced configuration of the Circle of Willis is present in only 18% of the population;
- Hypoplasia of one or both posterior communicating (P-comm) occurs in 22–32%;
- Absent or hypoplastic A1 segments occurs in 25%;
- 15–35% of patients supply their posterior cerebral artery on one or both sides from the carotid (via P-comm) instead of via the vertebrobasilar system *(fetal circulation)*;
- Large arteries are the primary conduit for blood delivery to the tissues, and contain a large amount of smooth muscle in their walls to regulate blood pressure and withstand high pressure/stress;
- Small arteries and arterioles are the primary site of hormonal regulation of systemic blood pressure and the primary vascular site of vasoactive anti-HTN (hypertension) drugs such as Ca^{2+} channel blockers or alpha-adrenergic blockers.

5. Biophysics of fluids and flow hemodynamics in normal vasculature

Cerebral blood flow is supplied by vessels connected in series and in parallel (**Figure 4**).

For each individual vessel, the law of the conservation of mass applied to the steady state of an incompressible fluid through a system of cylinders of varying cross-sectional areas tells us that

$$\textit{Total flow} = \textit{flow velocity}(V) \times \textit{cross sectional area}(A) = \text{constant} \tag{2}$$

This principle may be applied to blood flow in the cerebrovascular system. The law of conservation of mass as applied to fluid dynamics tells us that the total flow of mass into a contained system (before any vessel is damaged) must be equal to the total outflow of mass from the system steady state (**Figure 3**).

Applying this principle:

Flow/Q_{in} = grams of fluid material in/unit time = volume in × density (in)/time;

Flow/Q_{out} = grams of fluid material out/unit time = volume out × density (out)/time.

For a relatively incompressible fluid (e.g., blood), density may be considered constant; therefore, in a steady state,

Volume in (Vol in) = Volume out (Vol out)

$$\text{Vol in} = A1 \times V1 = \text{Vol out} = A2 \times V2$$

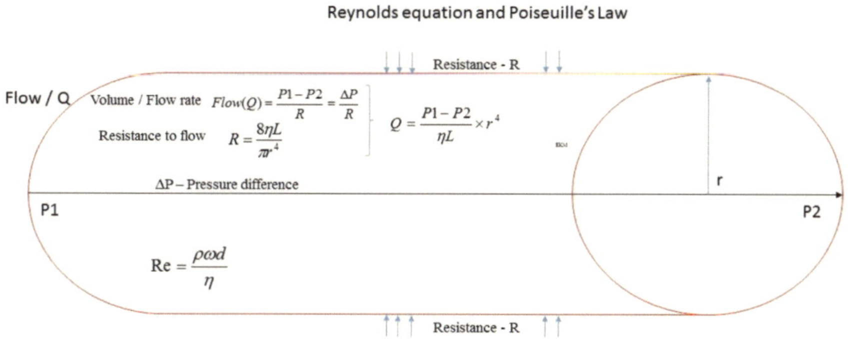

Figure 2. Biophysics of fluids and hemodynamic in normal vasculature.

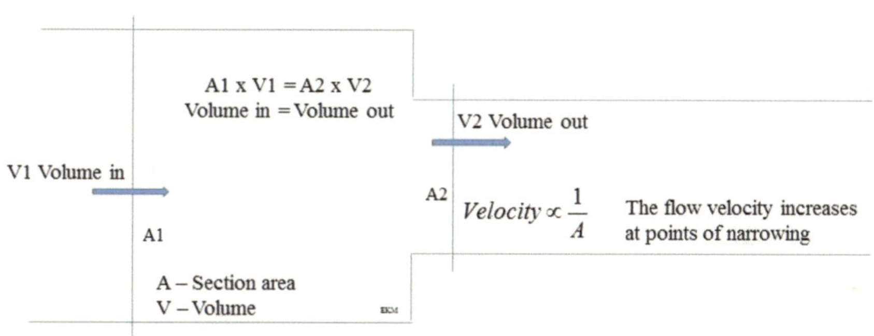

Figure 3. Relation of section area with flow velocity, in a steady state.

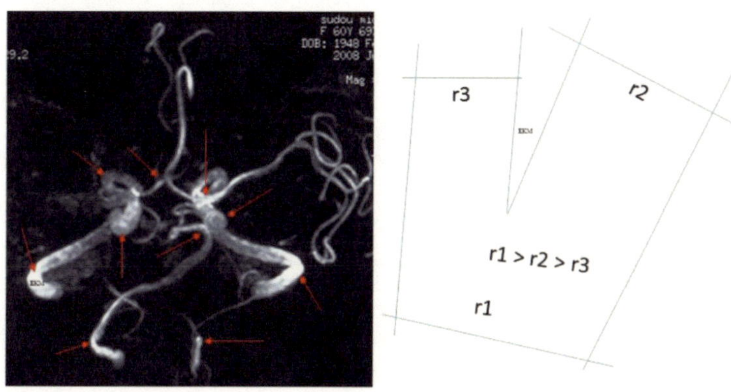

Figure 4. The most common sites of atherosclerotic events in the Circle of Willis. r1—vessel radius proximal to bifurcation. r2, r3—vessel radius distal to bifurcation.

In a steady state, the flow at a given point is directly proportional/related to the cross-sectional (A) area at that point (**Figure 2**) (**Table 3**). This explains why immediate distal to bifurcation, wall tension is higher/greater than proximal. This principle of hemodynamics of fluids in cylinders explains the reason of increased frequency of vascular-wall changes (atherosclerosis) at points of narrowing and or curvatures (red arrows), in the Circle of Willis (**Figure 4**). The same principles are used in Doppler echographic measurements.

$Re = \frac{\rho \omega d}{\eta} Q = \frac{P1 - P2}{\eta L} \times r^4$	**Constantly changing variables**
Re, Reynolds number	No
ρ, density of the liquid	No, it has a very narrow range
ω, flow velocity of the liquid	Yes
d, orifice/vessel diameter	Yes
r, radius of the vessel	Yes
η, viscosity	Yes, but to a narrow range
L, length of the blood vessel	No
ΔP, pressure gradient between two points in the vessel	Yes
R, resistance to flow in the vessel	Yes

A small change in blood vessel radius can have a profound effect on the flow through a vessel; it is based on these simple principles of hemodynamics that we can explain the changes in the flow and pressure when larger vessels bifurcate to smaller ones (**Figures 3** and **4**).

Table 3. Variables in the Reynolds equation and Poiseuille's law/equation.

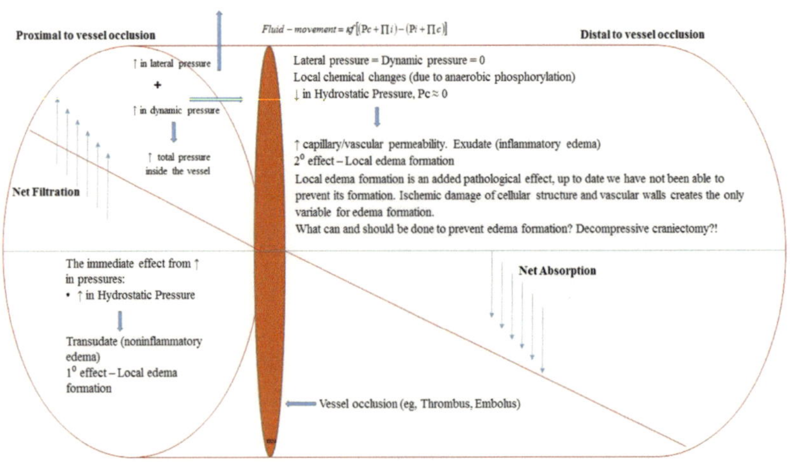

Figure 5. Biophysics of occlusive cerebrovascular disease pathology.

Note: although individual capillaries have a small cross-sectional area, the flow velocity through these vessels is slow. This is because numerous capillaries *arranged in parallel* receive flow from a given feeder vessel; thus, the functional cross-sectional area combined is actually

http://dx.doi.org/10.5772/64610

much larger than that of the feeder vessel from which they receive their flow. Applying this principle, we can explain why:

Blocking of one of the vessels in parallel in this system (e.g., thrombus) ⇒ ↑ pressure and flow in the rest of the system

This is due to the fact that the resistance to flow in a blood vessel is inversely proportional to the radius raised to the fourth power (**Figure 2**).

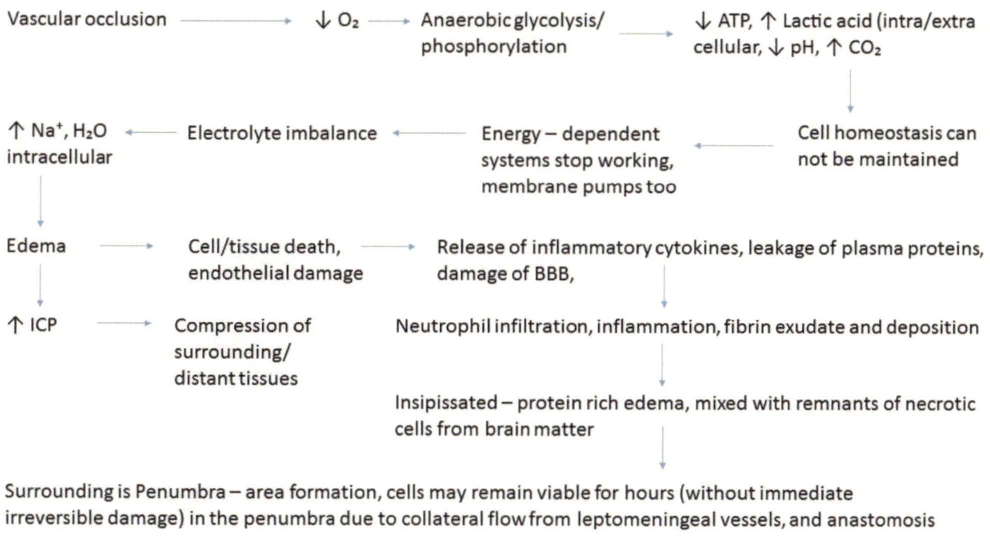

Diagram 1. Stroke-event progression.

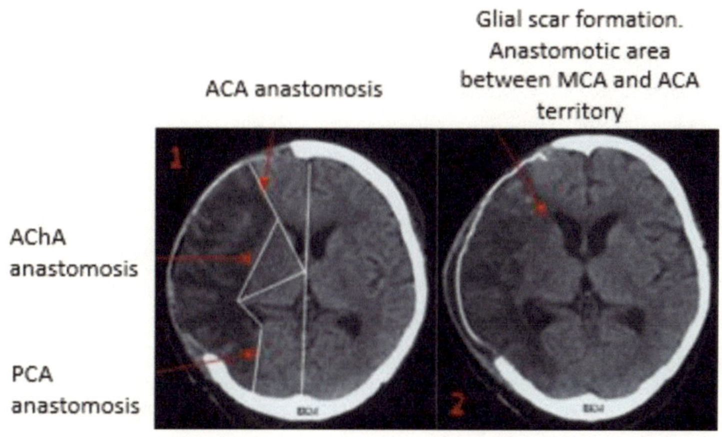

Figure 6. Reactive gliosis and glial scar formation. Cleaning of debris starts from the periphery (where possible anastomoses supply the area with blood and metabolites first, this is the route for neutrophils and macrophages to arrive and signal for more astrocytes stimulation/activation) to the center. 1. Non-contrast CT scan, second week of stroke event.

Reactive gliosis and vascular proliferation around the necrotic area are indicated. 2. Non-contrast CT scan, third week of stroke event.

The cerebral metabolic rate of oxygen consumption arises from neurons utilizing energy for two functions:

1. Maintenance of cell integrity, cell homeostasis, which normally accounts for ≈40% of energy consumption;

2. Conduction of electrical impulses (neuronal work, ≈ 60%).

Oxidative phosphorylation produces ≈99.99% of energy/adenosine triphosphate (ATP). Anaerobic phosphorylation produces only ≈0.01% of energy required for utilization by neurons. In an event of stroke, it is the 0.01% time-energy during which we depend to try and reverse hypoxia and/or treat stroke and its consequences (**Figure 5**) (**Diagram 1**).

6. Neuropathology of occlusive cerebrovascular disease

- Probably/regardless of proper treatment, the transudate of edema proximal to vascular occlusion tends to resolve (**Figure 5**). But our patient's progressive clinical and pathological deterioration suggests a less reversible exudation process (**Table 4**).

Time from injury/event	Microscopic changes	Macroscopic changes (Figure 7)
12–24 h	"Red neurons" eosinophilic cytoplasm, pyknotic nuclei, loss of Nissl substance. ***Sings of irreversible damage, from this moment onward.***	First changes appear that can be seen macroscopically as well. At any time, the patient is at risk for extracranial complication and superimposed conditions.
24–72 h	Neutrophils infiltrate the area after the interruption of blood supply; they do not phagocytize myelin remnants.	
3–7 days	Macrophage/microglia infiltration and phagocytosis begin. Neutrophils continue moving into the area, followed by microglia.	
1–2 weeks	Reactive gliosis and vascular proliferation around the necrotic area. Repair is performed by astrocytes that migrate to the area during this time [8].	Liquefactive necrosis (1–4 weeks) **(Figure 6)**
>2 weeks	Glial scar formation. As necrotic tissue is resorbed, a cystic space forms, which is then surrounded by astrocyte and newly formed capillaries. The enlargement and proliferation of astrocytes peripherally around the area of necrosis forms the glial scar.	Cystic area surrounded by dense glial fibers (>4 weeks) **(Figure 6)**

Table 4. Stroke phenomenon—event, neuropathological time line.

http://dx.doi.org/10.5772/64610

7. Cerebrovascular Accidents (CVAs)

7.1. Clinical signs

Sudden onset, or a step-wise progression over hours (even days), is typical presentation. In theory, focal signs relate to the distribution of the artery and or arteriole affected, but when collateral supplies have the capacity to supply their territory it will cloud the issue of a pure clinical presentation depending on the vascular territory of the vessel involved as we know its anatomy.

Clinical presentation includes the following:

- 1° signs of vascular territory affected;
- 2° signs due to mass effect from edema formation and or brain herniation, and clinical signs of increased ICP (Cushing syndrome), bradycardia, hypertension, and bradypnea.

7.2. Neurological and/or psychiatric new focal deficits

From all emergencies, abrupt onset of a new focal neurological deficit [9] occurs

- 95% are vascular pathologies:
  - 85% ischemic infarcts;
  - 15% hemorrhagic.
- 5% are nonvascular pathologies:
  - seizure, tumors, psychogenic.

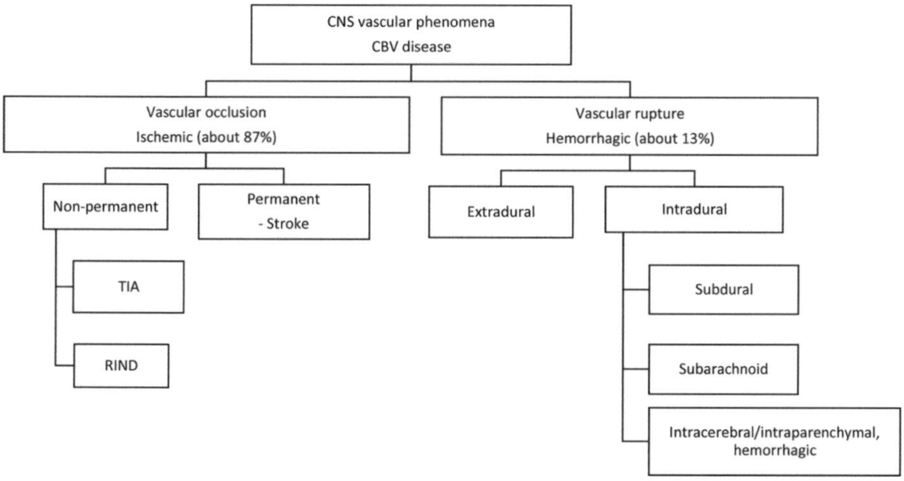

Diagram 2. Cerebrovascular accidents.

7.3. Stroke syndrome

This is caused by inadequate perfusion of a region of CNS. Many causes but same clinic/end results (**Diagram 3**) can occur.

7.4. Occlusive cerebrovascular disease

TIA (transient ischemic attack): a focal neurologic deficit that lasts ≤24 h (by definition), but in up to 70% of cases lasts only ≤10 min [10] (**Diagram 2**) (**Tables 5** and **6**). Of patients with a deficit persisting >60 min, only 14% will resolve with 24 h [11]. Ninety percent of patients with TIAs will have had reversal within 4 h of onset. An ischemic deficit resolves rapidly.

Infarct types/classification	**Major causes of stroke (Diagram 3):**	
– Lacunar – Territorial (e.g., MCA,– ACA) – End-zone infarcts – Border-zone/watershed infarcts – Global cerebral hypoxia/ischemia	– Thrombosis in situ/local – Atherothromboembolism distant/nonlocal – Heart emboli • Atrial fibrillation • Infective endocarditis • MI – CNS bleed • ↑ in BP • Trauma • Aneurysms/AVMs	
	Arteries with a diameter ≥ of MCA, superior branch of MCA included	**Arteries with a diameter < of MCA**
The most important risk factors are	Atrial fibrillation	– HTN (associate long-standing HTN with time and severity. Hence the age effect) – Diabetes – Smoking
Treatment, options	– r-tPA – Mechanical thrombectomy – Embolectomy, surgically – Vascular bypass – Decompression	Therapeutic, preventive.

Table 5. Infarct types, major causes of stroke, and treatment options.

The major clinical types of cerebrovascular diseases:	Vascular distribution:
– Thrombosis (atherothrombotic)-carotid (most common site of origin)	– ≈50% cerebral hemisphere infarcts
– Embolism-MCA (most commonly occluded vessel)	– ≈25% brainstem infarcts
– Hemorrhage	– ≈25% lacunar infarcts

Table 6. Major clinical types of cerebrovascular diseases and vascular distribution.

RIND (reversible ischemic neurologic deficit): a focal deficit lasting ≥24 h but less than 1 week. It comprises only 2.5% of patients admitted with TIA, RIND, or CVA [11].

Cerebrovascular accidents: also known as stroke. A permanent (irreversible) neurologic deficit caused by inadequate perfusion of a region of the brain or brain stem.

7.5. Common clinical problems in cerebrovascular disease

- The patient with a history of an ischemic attack or small stroke in the past;
- The patient with atrial fibrillation;
- The patient with a recent stroke that may not be complete;
- The non-evident or misconstrued syndromes of cerebrovascular disease;
- The comatose-stroke patient:
- The most common cause (MCC) of vascular coma is intracranial hemorrhage
    - Usually deep in the hemisphere
    - Less often in the
        - Cerebellum/brainstem
        - Extensive subarachnoid hemorrhage
        - Basilar artery occlusion.
- Seizure following stroke

7.6. "Malignant" middle cerebral artery territory infarction

- Occurs in up to 10% of stroke patients [12];
- Mortality of up to 80% (mostly due to severe postischemic cerebral edema) [13].

7.7. Cerebellar infarction

Relatively rare, seen on up to 1% of all CTs obtained for any reason [14].

7.8. Cardiogenic brain emboli

About one stroke in six is cardioemb [15]

- Fibrin-rich thrombi (mural thrombi);
- Platelets (nonbacterial thrombotic endocarditis);
- Calcified material (aortic stenosis);
- Tumor particles (atrial myxoma).

7.9. Following acute myocardial infarction (MI)

- 2.5% of patients will have a CVA within 1–2 weeks, higher risk with anterior wall MI (≈6%) versus inferior wall MI (≈1% risk).

7.10. Atrial fibrillation (A-fib)

Nonrheumatic patients with A-fib have a three- to five fold increased risk of stroke [16]:

- With a 4.5% rate of stroke/year without treatment [17];
- About 75% of CVAs in patients with A-fib are due to left atrial thrombi [18].

Independent risk factors for CVA in patients with A-fib are as follows:

- Advanced age;
- Prior embolism (CVA or TIA);
- HTN;
- Diabetes mellitus (DM);
- Echocardiographic evidence of left atrial enlargement or left ventricular dysfunction.

Prosthetic heart valves: patients with mechanical prosthetic heart valves on long-term anticoagulation have an embolism rate of

- 3%/year for mitral valve, and −1.5%/year for aortic valve;
- with bioprosthetic heart valves and no anticoagulation, the risk is 2–4%/year.

Paradoxical embolism can occur with a patent foramen ovale, which is present in 10–18% of the general population, but in up to 56% of young adults with unexplained CVA [19]; for this process to occur,

- The defect must be old enough to create a reverse of shunt (Eisenmenger syndrome);
- Or there should be moments where differences in pressure from the right side of the heart are greater than those on the left.

A cerebrovascular event in the setting of a known venous thromboembolic disease is suspicious for paradoxical embolism, and they can occur in patients with

http://dx.doi.org/10.5772/64610

- patent foramen ovale, atrial septal defects, ventricular septal defects;
- large pulmonary arteriovenous malformations (AVMs) [20].

Lacunar strokes: They are small infarcts resulting from the occlusion of penetrating branches. The size of infarcts ranges from 3 to 20 mm. Although their clinic might be devastating, they are the object of prevention and/or medical treatment alone.

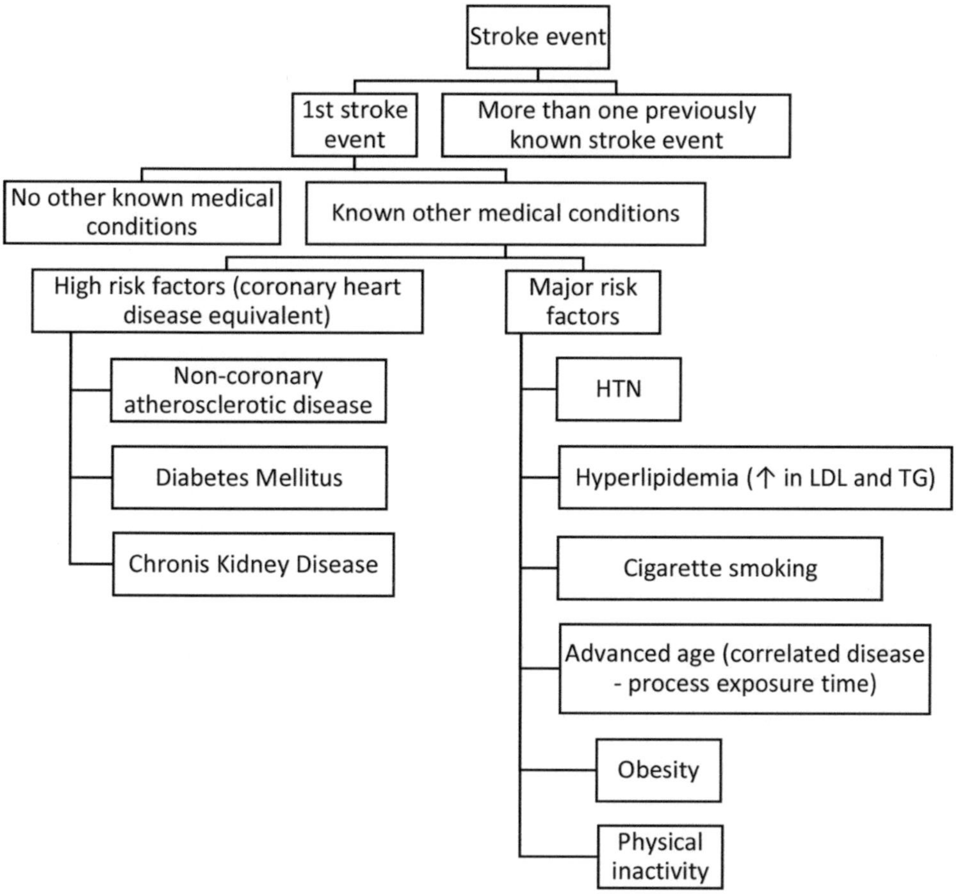

Diagram 3. Stroke event.

8. Diagnosis

Many centers now have strict protocols for the diagnosis and treatment of any stroke event, and such steps should be seriously considered even when a patient presents with minimal clinical signs because the next event might be fatal (**Table 7**).

Steps to the right path:	**Prompt investigation to confirm the diagnosis and avoid further stroke events, but consider whether results will affect management.** **Must Search for**

– Epidemiological data
– Clinical event
– Medical history
– Medical examination
  – Physical
  – Instrumental
    – Blood work
    – Imagery
      – CT scan/angio
      – Angio/ angio-MRI/MRI
      – Doppler
– Use NIH Stroke Scale
	• HTN
	• Cardiac sources of emboli
	• Noncardiac sources of emboli
	• Carotid artery stenosis (carotid causes of stroke are the source in >30% of patients affected, they may recur)
	• Hypoglycemia, hyperglycemia
	• Lipid metabolism disorders
	• Vasculitis
	• Infectious sources of emboli
	• Coagulopathies
	• Hematological diseases (most commonly)
	  ◦ Polycythemia vera
	  ◦ Sickle cell disease
	  ◦ Multiple myeloma

Table 7. Diagnosis of stroke and tests used.

8.1. Imaging

1. Emergency imaging of the brain is recommended before initiating any specific treatment for acute stroke [21]. In most instances, nonenhanced CT will provide the necessary information to make decisions about emergency management.

2. If endovascular therapy is contemplated, a noninvasive intracranial vascular study is strongly recommended during the initial imaging evaluation of the acute stroke patient but should not delay intravenous (IV) recombinant tissue plasminogen activator (r-tPA) if indicated. For patients who qualify for intravenous r-tPA according to guidelines from professional medical societies, initiating intravenous r-tPA before noninvasive vascular imaging is recommended for patients who have not had noninvasive vascular imaging as part of their initial imaging assessment for stroke. Noninvasive intracranial vascular imaging should then be obtained as quickly as possible.

3. The benefits of additional imaging beyond CT and CTA or MR and MRA, such as CT perfusion or diffusion- and perfusion-weighted imaging, for selecting patients for endovascular therapy are unknown. Further randomized, controlled trials may be helpful to determine whether advanced-imaging paradigms employing CT perfusion, CTA, and MRI perfusion and diffusion imaging, including measures of infarct core, collateral flow status, and penumbra, are beneficial for selecting patients for acute reperfusion therapy

http://dx.doi.org/10.5772/64610

who are within 6 h of symptom onset and have an ASPECTS (Alberta Stroke Program Early CT score).

8.1.1. CT scan

It is the emergency procedure, and we should always try to perform a non-contrast brain CT scan within 6 h of clinic occurrence, to help us rule out the following (**Figure 7**):

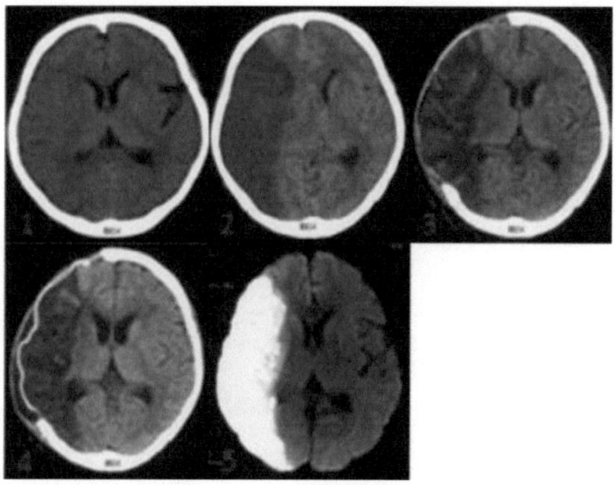

Figure 7. Stroke evolution followed with imagery, CT, and MRI. Non-contrast CT scan images at hour 2 (image 1), day 2 (image 2), week 2 (image 3), and week 3 (image 4) of stroke event. Non-contrast MRI at hour 12 of stroke event (image 5). CT scan findings in ischemic CVAs: *Note: These principles do not apply to small lacunar infarcts, or hemorrhagic CVAs.*

- Hemorrhage (intraparenchymal or SAH);
- Hematoma;
- Lesions (tumors, vascular).

CT scan, indicated in almost all situations of emergency, is strongly suggested in cases when

- Anticoagulation or thrombolytic therapy is indicated (first, we must rule out hemorrhage);
- ICH is suspected;
- Surgical lesions are suspected (vascular, tumoral).

First 12–24-h normal scan can be seen in between 10 and 70% of patients with MCA-CVAs. Early findings of imagery include the following:

1. Hyperdense artery sign (of the vessel involved, indicative of intra-arterial (IA) clot), 12% of patients, within 24 h of CVA, and in 23% of scans done within the first 6 h [22].
2. Focal low attenuation within the gray matter.
3. Mass effect (seen commonly from day 1 to week 4) as
    a. Effacement of cerebral sulci (often this change is subtle);

b. Midline shift (maximal effect: end of the first week, with a range between 2 and 5 days).

4. Loss of gray-white interface.

5. Attenuation/reduction in the strength of the signal of the lentiform nucleus.

6. Hypodensity involving the insular region.

7. Enhancement, 33% of the patients. CVA becomes isodense (masking effect) or hyperdense with normal brain, which rarely may be the only indication of the infarction.

At 48 h, most of CVAs can be seen as areas of low density.

In 1–2 weeks, we see a sharp demarcation of the CVA area.

In up to 10% of CVAs, there may be a short window, between the first and second weeks where the CVA becomes isodense (called fogging effect). An IV contrast scan and/or an MRI will demonstrate these.

Atrophy is usually seen by the end of the second week to the fifth.

At 3 weeks, the density of the CVA will approach that of the CSF.

Hyperdense artery sign on CT scan: This test has a low sensitivity, but a high specificity when the most common differential diagnosis of carotid dissection, calcified atherosclerosis of vessels (usually bilateral), or high hematocrit has been ruled out first. However, this test does not have independent prognostic significance [23].

8.1.1.1. CT enhancement with IV contrast in CVA:

- Many will enhance by day 6;
- Most will enhance by day 10;
- Some will enhance up to 5 months;
- Enhancement of gyri is common, seen by 1 week usually, predominantly in the gray matter. Differentiate with inflammatory infiltrating lesions due to the breakdown of blood-brain barrier (BBB).
- *Note: there should not be enhancement at the same time as there is mass effect.*

8.1.2. Magnetic resonance imaging

- More sensitive than CT scan, especially between hours 8 and 24, specifically for brain stem and cerebellar CVAs.

MRI enhancement patterns [24]:

1. Intravascular enhancement, 75% of patients, may indicate areas of the brain at risk of infarction.

http://dx.doi.org/10.5772/64610

2. Meningeal enhancement, especially with dural involvement, in 35% of cortical CVAs between days 1 and 3.

3. Transitional enhancement, two types coexist with early evidence of BBB breakdown, usually seen on days 3–6.

4. Parenchymal enhancement classically appears as a cortical/subcortical gyral enhancement. May not be apparent for the first 1–2 days, and gradually approaches 100% by 1 week. Enhancement may eliminate "fogging effect" (as on CT scan), which may obscure some CVAs at about 2 weeks on unenhanced T2WI.

8.1.3. Emergency cerebral angiography is used in the diagnosis of:

- Pathologies with early CVA in carotid distribution;
- If diagnosis is still questionable (e.g., aneurysms, vasculitis);
- Pathologies with rapid recovery, suggesting carotid TIA in the face of increasing stenosis.

Note: **Avoid** angio if the patient is

- Unstable or with severe disabling neurological deficit.

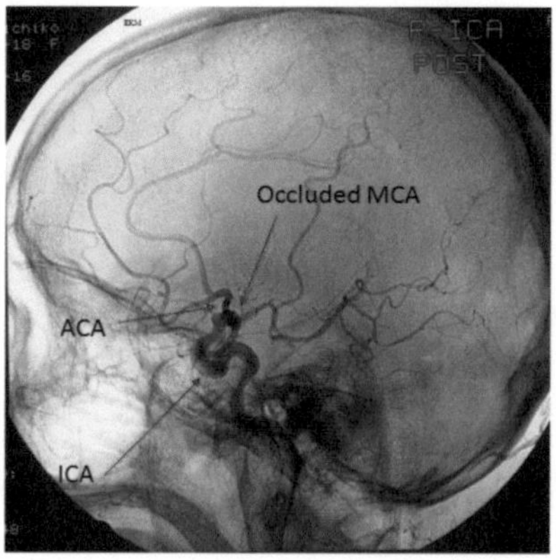

Figure 8. Emergency cerebral angiography. Cutoff sign: vessel ending abruptly at the point of the MCA occlusion.

Findings include the following:

1. Cutoff sign: vessel ends abruptly at the point of obstruction (**Figure 8**).

2. String sign: narrow strand of contrast in a vessel with high-grade stenosis.

3. **"Luxury perfusion"**: reactive hyperemia is a recognized response of cerebral tissue to injury (trauma, infarction, epileptogenic focus/foci). It is blood flow in excess of demand due to the abolition of CBF autoregulation due to acidosis [25]. It shows as accelerated circulation adjacent to the infarct with a stain or blush and early venous drainage.

9. Stroke prevention

As a general principle to prevent primary and or secondary stroke or TIA events, we must identify and control all modifiable risk factors and treat all comorbid diseases (**Table 8**).

Preventing stroke = Risk factor prevention
Preventing and treating:
– Diabetes
– HTN
– Lipid disorders
– Chronic kidney disease
– Atherosclerotic plaque formation
– Smoking

Table 8. How to prevent stroke

Patients with highest/strongest risk factors (coronary heart disease equivalent) (**Diagram 3**) are at the same risk of CV events (e.g., MI, stroke) as patients with known coronary heart disease.

Cardiovascular mortality in patients with type 2 DM increases by two to four times, of which

– 40% of patients die 2° to coronary heart disease;

– Coronary heart disease, not stroke, is the MCC of death.

In patients with type 2 DM,

– 40% die from coronary heart disease;

– 10% die from cerebrovascular accidents;

– 85% from stroke.

It will be of great pharmacological importance to study the chemical structure of thrombi, from autopsy studies. The study of chemical structure of the local-occluding thrombus and the possible site of its release and their comparison as well will help

- determine their nature (chemically) and how we can treat these elements (anticlot-drug development or thrombolytic/clot-lytic strategies);
- make a comparison between the locally found thrombus on the occluded vessel with the location of its release/formation and how different they are and local tissue changes from the site of origin with time.

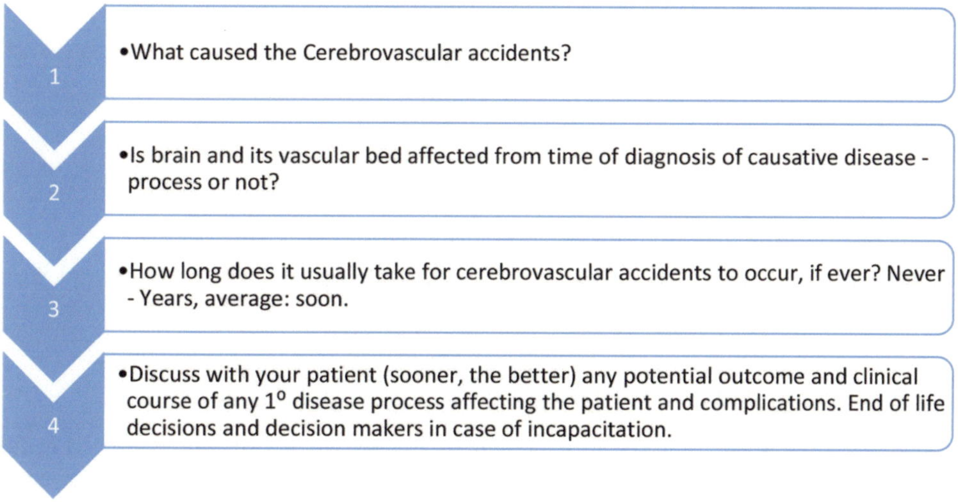

Diagram 4. Questioner of the first clinical encounter with the patient.

In a recent trial involving patients without diabetes who had insulin resistance along with a recent history of ischemic stroke or TIA, the risk of stroke or myocardial infarction was lower among patients who received pioglitazone than among those who received placebo. Pioglitazone was also associated with a lower risk of diabetes but with higher risks of weight gain, edema, and fracture [26]. Every clinic must have a systemic approach in preventive diseases, steps that answer important questions for future preventive measurements (**Diagram 4**).

10. Treatment

Start treatment after the first event and define vascular risks—do not wait for another one, it could be a stroke. Control risk factors for stroke and myocardial infarction, the commonest mode of death after TIA.

Protocols, treatment modalities (**Diagrams 5** and **6**) are designed in their simplicity to be applicable everywhere, although some limitations apply [5, 6]. We have to consider all standards and suggest applications accordingly, in simple steps that can be implemented anywhere. This is what in science we would call "Ideal."

Treatment of atherothrombotic infarction and TIAs includes the following:

- Preventive measures
- Management of the acute phase
- Measures to restore the circulation and arrest the pathological process
- Thrombolytic agents

- Acute surgical revascularization
- Treatment of cerebral-infarction edema, and raised intracranial pressure
- Anticoagulation drugs
- Antiplatelet drugs
- Other forms of medical treatment
- Surgery and angioplasty for symptomatic carotid stenosis
- Asymptomatic carotid stenosis evaluation
- Physical therapy and rehabilitation.

Of these modalities, surgical and endovascular treatment are technically indicated for stroke events caused by vascular accidents in arteries with diameter as or greater than MCA, of anterior and or posterior circulation. Smaller-size arteries have technical limitations in performing any of these modalities, except for r-tPA and in selected cases of bypass surgery when it can help restore flow in smaller-size arteries that are occluded (should the size allow the technique to be performed).

We know now that thrombus formation can occur in the absence of fibrin/fibrinogen and or vWF (von Willebrand Factor) or both, and either or both are target/s of pharmacological treatments. This might be one of the reasons why drug/medical thrombolysis and or prophylaxis were not successful for all the patients within the same risk group, giving us new trajectories to look in and think of new and better strategies in the medical treatment of stroke [27–31].

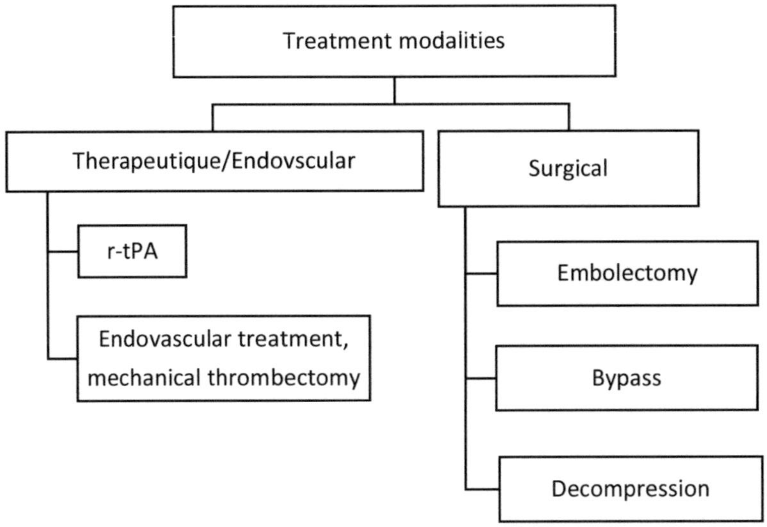

Diagram 5. Treatment modalities of stroke.

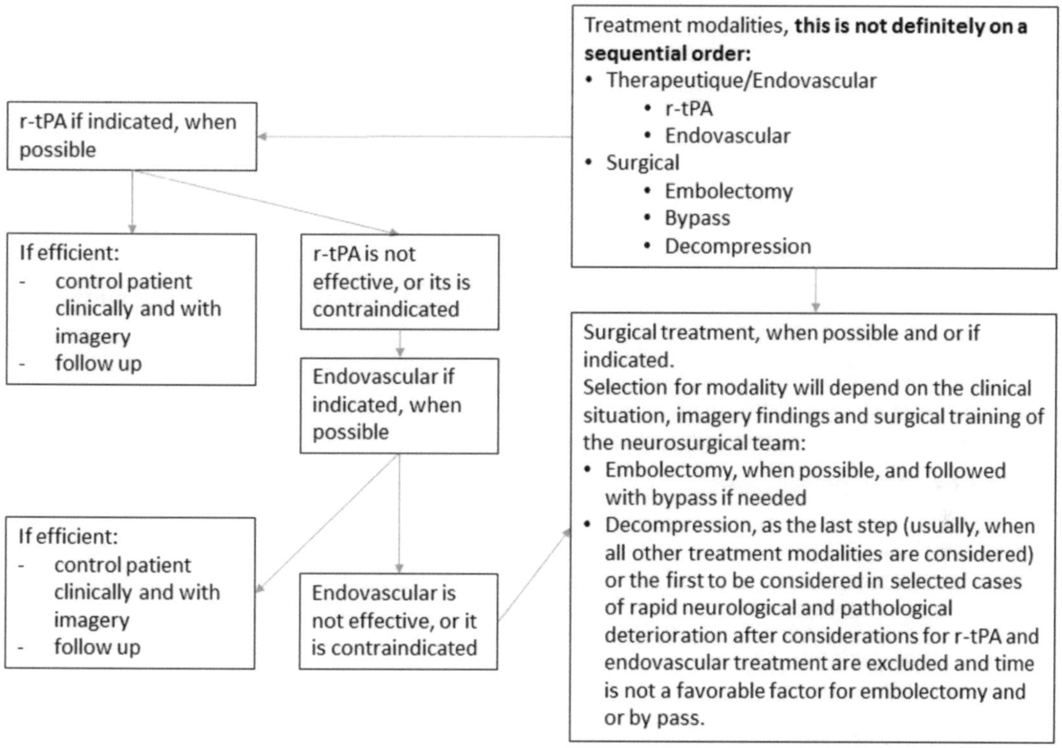

Diagram 6. Treatment modality steps followed during a (stroke) vascular accident.

10.1. Therapeutic/endovascular treatment for acute ischemic stroke – current concepts:

10.1.1. Ischemic penumbra

In 1981, Astrup et al. reported a reversible non-functioning brain tissue due to ischemia which is known as "ischemic penumbra" [32]. This ischemic but non-infarcted tissue is potentially salvageable. Without rapid reperfusion, however, the penumbral tissue goes to cell death, that is, infarction. As the purpose of ischemic stroke is to regain the lost neurological deficits, the salvage of penumbral tissue is a goal of acute stroke treatment.

How is penumbra identified?

Penumbral tissue can be inferred by showing both of underperfused brain tissue within a threshold of functional impairment and of infarction (ischemic core) [33]. The hypoperfused brain tissue without infarction can be considered as penumbra [33].

Cerebral blood flow is measurable by a single-photon emission CT (SPECT); however, performing SPECT is quite difficult in an emergent clinical setting. Perfusion CT and/or MRI is rather feasible compared to SPECT, and they can provide perfusion image of the brain. MR diffusion-weighted image (DWI) can visualize cytotoxic edema and are useful to detect hyperacute ischemic brain tissue. As a rule of thumb, significant underperfusioned brain tissue with symptoms without showing abnormalities in MR diffusion-weighted image is considered as "ischemic penumbra" [33, 34].

10.1.2. Approval of IV r-tPA

In 1995, the efficacy of intravenous (IV) thrombolysis in patients with acute ischemic stroke (AIS) was first reported (the National Institute of Neurological Disorders and Stroke (NINDS) study) [35] (**Table 9**). In the study, patients with AIS who were treated with IV recombinant tissue plasminogen activator (r-tPA) had a better prognosis compared to those without IV r-tPA [35]. In 1996, the next year, the US Food and Drug Administration approved the intravenous administration of rt-PA in patients with AIS within 3 h after the onset. After that, ECASS III reported an efficacy of IV r-tPA within 4.5 h in 2008 [46]; IV r-tPA is eligible for AIS patients within 4.5 h at the present time.

Indications	Contraindications
– Acute ischemic stroke age, 18–85 [21, 38–40]	**Absolute:**
– Onset of symptoms 3–4.5 h before r-tPA administration	– Acute or history of intracranial hemorrhage (intraparenchymal, subarachnoid (even if CT scan was normal), intraventricular hemorrhage, epidural, subdural hematoma, hemorrhagic conversion of infarction)
– Stroke symptoms present for at least 30 min with no significant improvement before treatment	– Severe uncontrolled hypertension (systolic pressure >185 mmHg or diastolic pressure >110 mmHg, or aggressive treatment (IV medication) necessary to reduce blood pressure to these limits)
– IV r-tPA should not be withheld from patients because of microbleeds seen on MRI [41]	– Serious head trauma or stroke in the previous 3 months
5. Severe hypertension does not need to preclude treatment with IV r-tPA for patients with acute stroke, provided it can be safely controlled with antihypertensive medications [38, 42, 43]	– Thrombocytopenia (platelet count <100,000/ml^3) and coagulopathy
	– Current use of anticoagulant with international normalization ratio (INR) >1.7 or partial thromboplastin (PT) >15 s
	– Administration of heparin within the 48 h preceding the onset of stroke, with an activated partial thromboplastin time at presentation exceeding the upper limit of the normal range
	– Low-molecular-weight heparin (LMWHs) within 24 h [43]
	– Oral anticoagulant treatment, direct thrombin inhibitors, and factor Xa inhibitors
	– Severe hypo- or hyperglycemia (blood glucose <50 mg/dl or >400 mg/dl)
	– Early radiographic ischemic changes

Indications	Contraindications
	Relative
	– Advanced age (older than 80 years [21, 43])
	– Mild or improving stroke symptoms (symptoms rapidly improving or only minor before start of infusion)
	– Severe stroke as assessed clinically (NIHSS score of >25) or by appropriate imaging techniques, or coma [44, 45]
	– Major surgery or severe trauma within the previous 3 months [44]
	– Arterial puncture of noncompressible vessel
	– Recent gastrointestinal or genitourinary hemorrhage
	– Seizure at the onset of stroke
	– Recent myocardial infarction
	– CNS structural lesions
	– Time of symptoms onset unknown
	– Combination of previous stroke and diabetes mellitus
	– Other major disorders associated within and increased risk of bleeding

Table 9. Indications and contraindications for treatment with r-tPA [36–38].

10.1.3. Drawbacks of IV r-tPA

One of the major drawbacks of IV r-tPA is systemic hemorrhagic complication. The clinicians should be cautious when using IV r-tPA in patients with AIS presenting with laterality in blood pressure of arms. Although it is very occasionally, some patients with acute aortic dissection presents with symptoms of AIS [47]. As the clinical feature of AIS can outweigh those of aortic dissection in an emergent clinical setting, IV r-tPA can be administered before a diagnosis of aortic dissection is established [47]. The number of reported cases is small; however, more than half of AIS associated with aortic dissection are reported to be fatal [47]. As intravenously infused r-tPA will be delivered to anywhere in a body, hemorrhage of any organs can develop. We experienced a case of AIS which developed fatal intraperitoneal hemorrhage following IV r-tPA [48]. The bleeding point was considered to be biopsied liver [48].

10.1.4. Limitation of r-tPA

After IV r-tPA was approved, findings of recanalization rate by occlusion site have been obtained. Recanalization rate just after IV r-tPA varies depending on reports; however, roughly it is reported as 10% in the internal carotid artery, 30% in the middle cerebral artery, M1, and 70% in the middle cerebral artery, M2 [49]. It is really less surprising when we consider a volume of a thrombus. Assuming that the diameter of the internal carotid artery is 4 mm and those of the distal middle cerebral artery is 2 mm and a thrombus is a sphere, a ratio of the volume of a thrombus lodging to the internal carotid artery to a thrombus lodging to the distal middle cerebral artery becomes 8. However, a dose of IV r-tPA is determined not by a size of thrombus but by a patient's body weight.

To overcome the drawbacks of IV r-tPA, a concept of additional neurointervention for patients who are refractory or not eligible to IV r-tPA has emerged. In 2004, the Interventional Management of Stroke (IMS) study investigators reported the feasibility and safety of a combination therapy (IV r-tPA alone vs. IV r-tPA plus intra-arterial (IA) administration of r-tPA) [50]. IMS-3, a final version of bridging study conducted by IMS study investigators, failed to show any benefits of additional neurointervention following IV r-tPA [51]. However, in 2015, another five randomized controlled trials succeeded in showing the effectiveness of the additional neurointervention [52–56].

10.1.5. Illustrative case

A 75-year-old man suddenly developed right hemiplegia and total aphasia. On examination, his National Institutes of Health Stroke Scale (NIHSS) score was 20. About 4.5 h had already past when he arrived at our hospital, and IV r-tPA was not eligible. Diffusion-weighted MR image showed a moderate ischemic change of the left middle cerebral artery (**Figure 9**); however, it was difficult to explain all of his neurological symptoms by the ischemic change. Neurointervention was performed, and a complete recanalization was obtained by a stent retriever (**Figure 10**). Improvement of his neurological deficits was obtained. The complete recovery of the right hemiplegia was obtained, and he was discharged with mRS2.

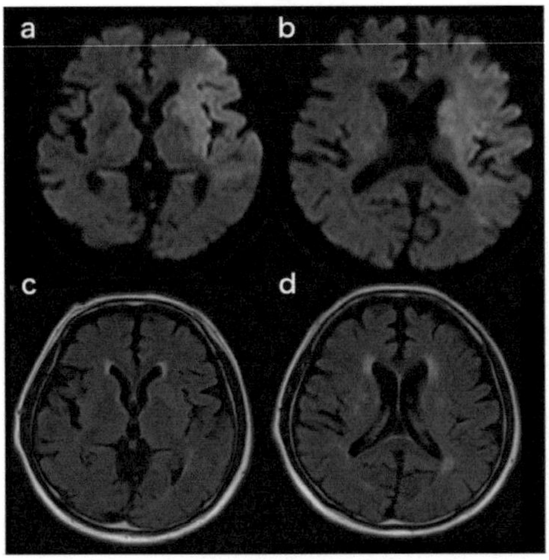

Figure 9. Diffusion-weighted MR image (a, b) and FLAIR image (c, d) on admission. Acute ischemia was noted in the left middle cerebral artery on diffusion-weighted MR image (a, b); however, no lesions were detected on FLAIR image (c, d), suggesting hyperacute ischemia.

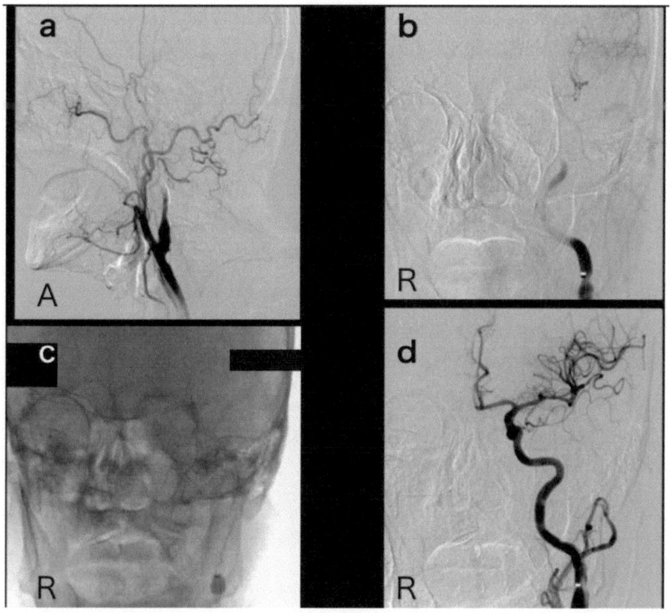

Figure 10. Lateral view of the left carotid angiogram before the neuroendovascular procedure (a). Microcatheter injection confirmed that a tip of the microcatheter was in distal to a thrombus (b). Solitaire FR 6 × 30 mm was deployed, and the Solitaire was pulled with a proximal flow control (c). After one passage of the Solitaire FR, a complete recanalization was obtained (d).

10.1.6. Future issues

Twenty years has been passed since the publication of NINDS study. It is quite evident that r-tPA is effective in patients with AIS within 4.5 h. It is and will be impossible to conduct randomized controlled trial comparing neurointervention and medical management without r-tPA in patients with AIS within 4.5 h. Thus, further issues to be addressed should be the methodology of how to recanalize occluded vessels in conjunction with IV r-tPA. Should we puncture a femoral artery during IV r-tPA? Which devices are most suitable to recanalize? Are there any necessary to choose devices depending on an occlusion site or nature? The next decade will answer these questions, we believe.

A recent trial involving predominantly an Asian patient with acute ischemic stroke did not show the noninferiority of low-dose alteplase to standard-dose alteplase with respect to death and disability at 90 days. There were significantly fewer symptomatic intracerebral hemorrhages with low-dose alteplase [57].

Although the INR and pTT are not adequately reliable indicators of the anticoagulation effect of direct thrombin inhibitors (dabigatran), the thrombin time (TT) is sensitive to the presence of dabigatran activity. Based on the current understanding of pharmacokinetics, IV r-tPA may be considered reasonable in some cases if patients have normal TT, aPTT, and PT, but this should be a subject of future research [38, 58].

10.1.7. The guidelines for the Early Management of Patients with Acute Ischemic Stroke Regarding Endovascular Treatment, Endovascular Interventions:

1. Patients eligible for intravenous r-tPA should receive intravenous r-tPA even if endovascular treatments are being considered (Class I; Level of Evidence A) [21, 59].

2. Patients should receive endovascular therapy with a stent retriever if they meet all the following criteria (Class I; Level of Evidence A):

    a. prestroke mRS scores 0–1,

    b. acute ischemic stroke receiving intravenous r-tPA within 4.5 h of onset according to guidelines from professional medical societies,

    c. causative occlusion of the internal carotid artery or proximal MCA (M1),

    d. age ≥18 years,

    e. NIHSS score of ≥6,

    f. ASPECTS of ≥6, and

    g. treatment can be initiated (groin puncture) within 6 h of symptom onset.

3. As with intravenous r-tPA, reduced time from symptom onset to reperfusion with endovascular therapies is highly associated with better clinical outcomes. To ensure benefit, reperfusion to TICI grade 2b/3 should be achieved as early as possible and within 6 h of stroke onset (Class I; Level of Evidence B-R).

4. When treatment is initiated beyond 6 h from symptom onset, the effectiveness of endovascular therapy is uncertain for patients with acute ischemic stroke who have causative occlusion of the internal carotid artery or proximal MCA (M1) (Class IIb; Level of Evidence C).

5. In carefully selected patients with anterior circulation occlusion who have contraindications to intravenous r-tPA, endovascular therapy with stent retrievers completed within 6 h of stroke onset is reasonable (Class IIa; Level of Evidence C). There are inadequate data available at this time to determine the clinical efficacy of endovascular therapy with stent retrievers for those patients whose contraindications are time-based or nontime-based (e.g., prior stroke, serious head trauma, hemorrhagic coagulopathy, or receiving anticoagulant medications).

6. Although the benefits are uncertain, the use of endovascular therapy with stent retrievers may be reasonable for carefully selected patients with acute ischemic stroke in whom treatment can be initiated (groin puncture) within 6 h of symptom onset and who have causative occlusion of the M2 or M3 portion of the MCAs, anterior cerebral arteries, vertebral arteries, basilar artery, or posterior cerebral arteries (Class IIb; Level of Evidence C).

7. Endovascular therapy with stent retrievers may be reasonable for some patients <18 years of age with acute ischemic stroke who have demonstrated large vessel occlusion in whom

http://dx.doi.org/10.5772/64610

treatment can be initiated (groin puncture) within 6 h of symptom onset, but the benefits are not established in this age group (Class IIb; Level of Evidence C).

8. Although the benefits are uncertain, the use of endovascular therapy with stent retrievers may be reasonable for patients with acute ischemic stroke in whom treatment can be initiated (groin puncture) within 6 h of symptom onset and who have prestroke mRS score of >1, ASPECTS.

9. Observing patients after intravenous r-tPA to assess for clinical response before pursuing endovascular therapy is not required to achieve beneficial outcomes and is not recommended (Class III; Level of Evidence B-R).

10. The use of stent retrievers is indicated in preference to the MERCI device (Class I; Level of Evidence A). The use of mechanical thrombectomy devices other than stent retrievers may be reasonable in some circumstances (Class IIb, Level B-NR).

11. The use of proximal balloon-guide catheter or a large bore distal access catheter rather than a cervical guide catheter alone in conjunction with stent retrievers may be beneficial (Class IIa; Level of Evidence C). Future studies should examine which systems provide the highest recanalization rates with the lowest risk for nontarget embolization.

12. The technical goal of the thrombectomy procedure should be a TICI 2b/3 angiographic result to maximize the probability of a good functional clinical outcome (Class I; Level of Evidence A). The use of salvage technical adjuncts including intra-arterial fibrinolysis may be reasonable to achieve these angiographic results, if completed within 6 h of symptom onset (Class IIb; Level of Evidence B-R).

13. Angioplasty and stenting of proximal cervical atherosclerotic stenosis or complete occlusion at the time of thrombectomy may be considered but the usefulness is unknown (Class IIb; Level of Evidence C). Future randomized studies are needed.

14. Initial treatment with intra-arterial fibrinolysis is beneficial for carefully selected patients with major ischemic strokes of <6-h duration caused by occlusions of the MCA (Class I; Level of Evidence B-R). However, these data derive from clinical trials that no longer reflect current practice, including the use of fibrinolytic drugs that are not available. A clinically beneficial dose of intra-arterial r-tPA is not established, and r-tPA does not have FDA approval for intra-arterial use. As a consequence, endovascular therapy with stent retrievers is recommended over intra-arterial fibrinolysis as first-line therapy (Class I; Level of Evidence E).

15. Intra-arterial fibrinolysis initiated within 6 h of stroke onset in carefully selected patients who have contraindications to the use of intravenous r-tPA might be considered, but the consequences are unknown (Class IIb; Level of Evidence C).

16. It might be reasonable to favor conscious sedation over general anesthesia during endovascular therapy for acute ischemic stroke. However, the ultimate selection of anesthetic technique during endovascular therapy for acute ischemic stroke should be individualized based on patient risk factors, tolerance of the procedure, and other clinical characteristics. Randomized trial data are needed (Class IIb; Level of Evidence C).

General anesthesia with intubation and conscious sedation are the two most frequently used anesthetic approaches for patients with an acute ischemic stroke receiving endovascular therapy.

An expert consensus statement of the Society of Neurointerventional Surgery and the Neurocritical Care Society recommends the use of general anesthesia for patients with severe agitation, low level of consciousness (the Glasgow Coma Scale (GCS) of <8), loss of airway protective reflexes, respiratory compromise, and in selected posterior circulation stroke presenting with these features [60].

10.1.8. Patient selection

- Intracranial vessel occlusion must be diagnosed with noninvasive imaging whenever possible before considering treatment with mechanical thrombectomy (Grade A, Level 1a, KSU Grade A) [59].
- If vessel imaging is not available at baseline, an NIHSS score of ≥9 within 3 h, and ≥7 points within 6 h may indicate the presence of large vessel occlusion (Grade B, Level 2a, KSU Grade B).
- Patients with radiological signs of large infarcts (e.g., using the ASPECTS score) may be unsuitable for thrombectomy (Grade B, Level 2a, KSU Grade B).
- Imaging techniques for determining infarct and penumbra sizes can be used for patient selection and correlate with functional outcome after mechanical thrombectomy (Grade B, Level 1b, KSU Grade B).
- High age alone is not a reason to withhold mechanical thrombectomy as an adjunctive treatment (Grade A, Level 1a, KSU Grade A).

10.2. Surgical treatment

10.2.1. Embolectomy and extracranial – intracranial (EC/IC) bypass; STA – MCA bypass is this the solution or a treatment – procedure?

Surgical embolectomy in conjunction with ligation of the cervical ICA followed by STA-MCA bypass might be a safe alternative method to endovascular recanalization, when the cervical dissection of ICA is extensive and when huge secondary emboli are present along the MCA when it is clinically indicated and or in centers that do not have a 24-h endovascular service [61]. In these centers, microsurgery is recommended as a first-line treatment, after exclusion of malignant profile based on MRI findings (i.e., minimal DWI lesion less than one-third of the entire MCA region despite large ICA/MCA occlusion on MRA) [5, 6, 62–64]. Spontaneous dissection of the internal carotid artery (ICA) is one of the main causes of ischemic stroke in young- to middle-aged patients. It can cause malignant brain infarction [65], and in addition tandem ICA and MCA occlusion independently predict poor outcomes in response to intravenous r-tPA [66–68]. We know that theoretically stent deployment for cervical ICA dissection could cause distal migration of secondary emboli, vessel laceration, and in-stent thrombosis [64, 69]. When other criteria are not meet, surgical embolectomy is recommended.

CBF increases significantly after bypass, and flow reservation improves significantly. Patients with TIA experience less or no recurrence of such episodes after bypass and the neurologic deficit remains unchanged in patients with complete stroke after bypass, with a very high satisfaction rate after surgery as assessed by the patients themselves, in comparison to the conservative treatment [70].

10.2.2. Bypass may be indicated and may be helpful in restoring CBF and reducing the risk of stroke in:

- Atherosclerotic plaque non treatable by endovascular or other means;
- Failure of medications to control TIA symptoms or stroke;
- Imagery (angio, CTA, and MRA) showing intra- and or extracranial arterial stenosis/ occlusion;
- CBF studies (CT perfusion, positron emission tomography (PET), and SPECT) show insufficient blood flow due to arterial stenosis [5, 64, 68-70]..

Bypass surgery might improve CBF, but it does not cure (with some exceptions) the underlying disease.

Outside	Inside
Frontal sinus, 1-cm superior	Superior sagittal sinus
Sagittal suture, 1-cm lateral	Transverse sinus
Lambda and lambdoid suture 1-cm superior	
Asterion and pterion	

With an extensive craniectomy, we can remove an area of bone≈60 cm^2.

At this range, the volume calculated to protrude through the opening will be a minimum of 60 ml.

This technique has a greater decompression effect on frontal, precentral, superior cerebral, and parietal veins, with the greatest effects expected on the superior sagittal sinus and the confluence of sinuses.

Sixty milliliter is the maximal volume of compensation before clinical signs of herniation appear during stroke event.

Table 10. Craniectomy landmarks to consider.

10.3. Decompressive craniectomy (DC)

10.3.1. Age is not the limit! DC is nor the solution, nor the cure! Hemicraniectomy for malignant MCA territory infarction

Treatment modalities for stroke has progressed and substantially changed from what we knew two decades ago; we have now the possibility to use noninvasive treatment options and/or a combination with surgical techniques as well. Although none of the surgical techniques is the first to be considered, they are absolutely the last options we can use to treat stroke event and complications (**Table 11**) (**Diagram 6**).

Indications	Contraindications
Failure of r-tPA and or endovascular treatment	Prestroke mRS score of ≥2
Failure of bypass	Prestroke score Barthel Index of <95
Refractory increase in ICP despite treatment (**Graphic 3**)	GCS of <8
	Brain stem involvement and or signs of herniation
Brain stem not involved and before signs of herniation	Hemorrhagic transformation of the infarct
Disease affecting ICA, and or MCA, M1, M2, or either of the last in	Related disease/conditions affecting outcome.
combination with ACA or PCA (rare occurrence) ipsilateral	Coagulopathy/systemic-blooding disorders.

Table 11. Hemicraniectomy indications and contraindications in brain malignant infarction.

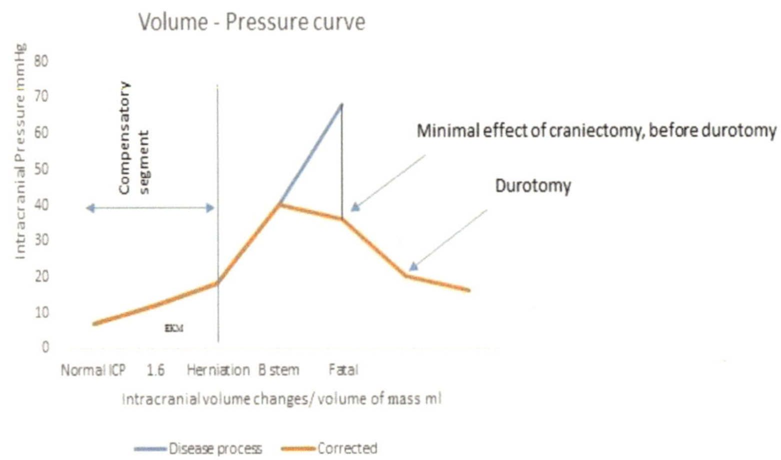

Graphic 3. Volume-pressure changes, graphic.

It may reduce mortality to as low as 32% in nondominant hemisphere CVAs [71], and it can reduce mortality up to 37% in all corners, with surprising clinical results. Better results occur with early surgery, before any changes associated with herniation occur [72], but it does not

http://dx.doi.org/10.5772/64610

treat the underlying cause/s of the edema formation (being it transudate or exudate). It is a very important treatment procedure that must be considered. As decompression has never been the first treatment modality, it has mostly been considered the last and in many clinical situations the first as well.

10.3.2. Surgical techniques and notes

Preferred skin incisions for a large decompressive craniectomy (**Table 8**, **Figure 11**) are as follows:

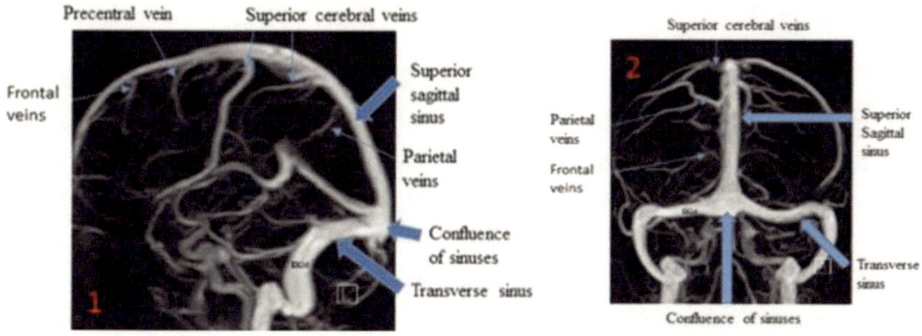

Figure 11. Images 1 and 2 identify the major intracranial surgical landmarks to be considered.

– Question mark extended;

– U shape extended.

Both incisions expose the scalp greatly, with its borders along the anastomotic segments. U-shape incision traumatizes the vascular supply to a lesser degree [73]. However, due to the extensive vascular collateral circulation in the scalp area, scalp necrosis is uncommon.

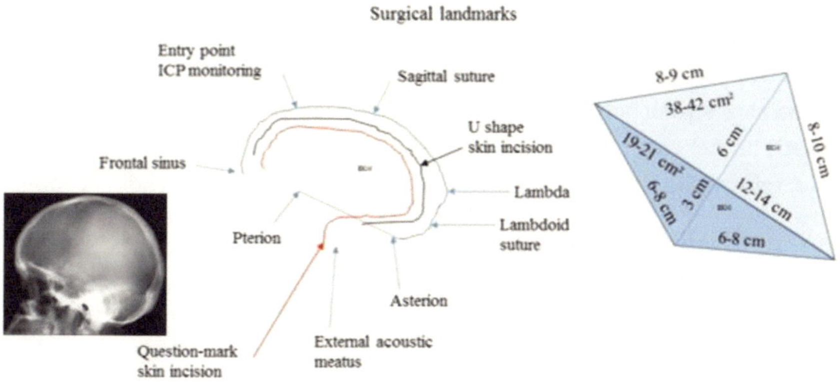

Figure 12. Surgical landmarks and area measurements [74, 75].

Craniectomy landmarks and indications are listed in **Tables 10** and **11** (**Figure 12**).

A larger craniectomy does not always mean better; however, a smaller craniectomy (the lower threshold of 12 cm for hemicraniectomy and decompression to the temporal base) is effective in relieving ICP. The size should always consider the risk of complications, including the parenchymal shear stress and hemorrhage [74, 75] (**Figure 12**).

Age should not be the limit (each disease categories), for medical and or surgical modality treatment decisions, but the existing and past medical conditions of the patient. By contrast, we should push the limit and provide support for longer life expectancy with a better quality for stroke-related diseases [76] (**Table 11**).

Hemicraniectomy is increasingly used as treatment option in stroke and in head trauma, but little is known on the physiological regional effects of hemicraniectomy in the normal brain. In their work, Schaller et al. [77] measured in consecutive hours regional CBF, CMR of O_2, and glucose from the brain tissue underneath the craniectomy (hemicraniectomy) of the animals used in the study. They demonstrated for the first time that decompressive hemicraniectomy decreases CBF, and to a lesser extent CMR of O_2 and glucose 2 h after hemicraniectomy in the normal brain tissues that last for at least 1 day. The underlying basis of these phenomena is not fully understood; however, their findings implied that persisting pathophysiological processes are induced by hemicraniectomy and should be taken into consideration for surgical indications [77].

We can use clinical findings and imagery, and analyze volumetric changes before neuronal injury and predict which patients may benefit from hemicraniectomy. It is a life-saving surgery when performed correctly; it can reduce disability and mortality and improve functional outcome as proved in several controlled trials [75, 78].

10.3.3. Dural incisions and duraplasty

- Cross, extended (**Figure 13 f**) or standard (**Figure 13 d, e**) [73, 79]. These incisions create two smaller triangles superiorly (one and two) (**Figure 13 d, e**), thus creating the possibility for a better supply from the anastomotic vessels opposite. If the axial plane of the dural incision creates equal half's 1–2 and 3–4), the area requiring blood supply from the anastomotic branches (one and two) will be greater than what the vasculature can supply, and this might create the risk of necrosis at the distal margins of each incision.

- "Maple leaf" (**Figure 13 a–c**): the incisions in this technique follow parallel with the vasculature of the major branches of the middle meningeal artery supplying the dura, and respect their segments of anastomosis. At the same time, the wide opening of the dural leafs exposes the brain-herniating tissue to a lesser pressure.

Standard duraplasty can be performed at the end of the decompression procedure, with a loose graft.

10.3.4. When should we put the bone back?

With the patient in stable clinical conditions, we should prepare to put the bone back any time after gliosis starts forming (≥4 weeks). Although ICP helps to set a baseline of when we should decide to put the bone back (**Graphic 3**), it is pathologically correct to do so during gliosis and scar formation (**Table 4**), usually >2 weeks when glial scar starts to form, and best after the fourth week when cystic area is surrounded by dense glial fibers.

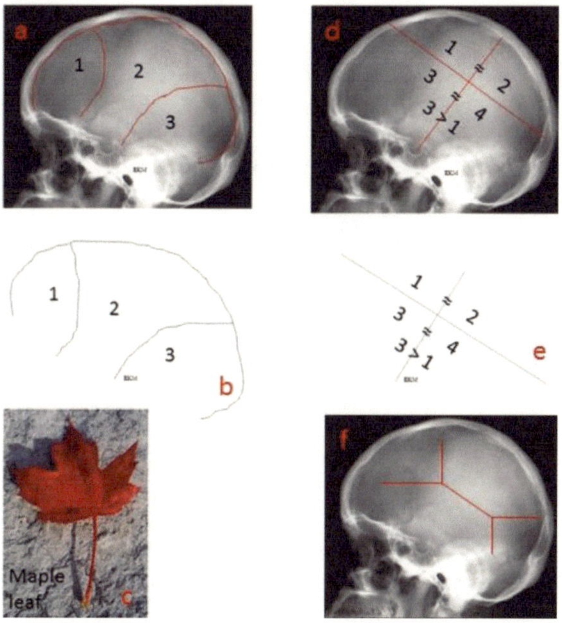

Figure 13. Dural incision's techniques.

10.3.5. Suturing of the skin (at the end of the surgery/craniectomy)

The most productive results are with a continuous suture, if a second surgical procedure will be required; this technique allows you to remove the suture with only two cuts, and pull.

10.4. Possible modality treatments of the future

In the last couple of years, the use of transcranial ultrasound has been modified for therapeutic use as well [80]. Its promising results will open doors for application in thrombus destruction during the ischemic event. Its use in trans-BBB (Blood Brain Barrier) delivery of medical therapy has been published now, as well as its use in functional neurosurgery. This is a novel technique, noninvasive that is starting to take shape beyond its initial plan of application and is promising.

We recommend the use of **Diagram 6** that indicates in a step-wise manner all possible treatment modalities we can chose based on clinical and imagery indications.

Acknowledgements

We thank our medical illustrators for their work and support.

Conflict of interest: The authors declare no conflict of interest.

Author details

Erion Musabelliu[1*], Masahiro Oomura[2] and Yoko Kato[1]

*Address all correspondence to: erionmusabelliu@gmail.com

1 Department of Neurosurgery, Fujita Health University, Toyoake, Aichi, Japan

2 Department of Neurology and Neuroscience, Nagoya City University Graduate School of Medical Sciences, Mizuho-cho, Mizuho-ku, Nagoya, Japan

References

[1] The ATLANTIS, ECASS, and NINDS rt-PA Study Group Investigators. Association of outcome with early stroke treatment: pooled analysis of ATLANTIS, ECASS, and NINDS rt-PA stroke trials. Lancet 363: 768–74, 2004.

[2] Hartmann P, Ramseier A, Gudat F, Mihatsch MJ, Polasek W. Normal weight of the brain in adults in relation to age, sex, body height and weight [article in German]. Pathologe 15(3): 165–70, 1994.

[3] Schaller B, Graf R. Different compartments of intracranial pressure and its relationship to cerebral blood flow. J Trauma 59(6): 1521–31, 2005.

[4] Raichle ME, Grubb RL, Gado MH, et al. Correlation between regional cerebral blood flow and oxidative metabolism. In vivo studies in man. Arch Neurol 33: 523–6, 1976. (Reference Henegar MM, Sillbergeld DL: Pharmacology for Neurosurgeons, Part II: Anesthetic Agents, ICP Management, Corticosteroids, Cerebral Protectants. Contemp Neurosurg 18 (10): 1–6, 1996.)

[5] Inoue T, Saito I, Tamura A. Emergent surgical embolectomy in conjunction with cervical internal carotid ligation and superficial temporal artery-middle cerebral artery bypass to treat acute tandem internal carotid and middle cerebral artery occlusion due to cervical internal carotid artery dissection. Surg Neurol Int 6: 191, 2015. DOI: 10.4103/2152-7806.

[6] Inoue T, Tamura A, Tsutsumi K, Saito I, Saito N. Surgical embolectomy for internal carotid artery terminus occlusion. Neurosurg Rev 38: 661, 2015. doi: 10.1007/s10143-015-0640-4.

[7] van der Zwan A, Hillen B, Tulleken CAF, et al. Variability of the territories of the major cerebral arteries. J Neurosurg 77: 927–40, 1992.

[8] Evans RJ, Wyllie FS, Wynford-Thomas D, Kipling D, Jones CJ. A P53-dependent, telomere-independent proliferative life span barrier in human astrocytes consistent with the molecular genetics of glioma development. Cancer Res 63(16): 4854–61, 2003.

[9] del Zoppo GJ, Poeck K, Pessin MS, et al. Recombinant tissue plasminogen activator in acute thrombotic and embolic stroke. Ann Neurol 32: 78–86, 1992.

[10] Werdelin L, Juhler M. The course of transient ischemic attacks. Neurology 38: 677–80, 1988.

[11] Levy DE. How transient are transient ischemic attacks? Neurology 38: 674–7, 1998.

[12] Moulin DE, Lo R, Chiang J, et al. Prognosis in middle cerebral artery occlusion. Stroke 16: 282–4, 1985.

[13] Hacke W, Schawb S, Horn M, et al. Malignant middle cerebral artery territory infarction: clinical course and prognostic signs. Arch Neurol 53: 309–15, 1996.

[14] Tomaszek DE, Rosner MJ. Cerebellar infarction: analysis of twenty-one cases. Surg Neurol 24: 223–6, 1985.

[15] Cerebral Embolism Task Force. Cardiogenic brain embolism. Arch Neurol 43: 71084, 1986.

[16] Blackshear JL, Kopecky SL, Litin SC, et al. Management of atrial fibrillation in adults: prevention of thromboembolism and symptomatic treatment. Mayo Clin Proc 71: 150–60, 1996.

[17] Atrial Fibrillation Investigators. Risk factors for stroke and efficacy of antithrombotic therapy in atrial fibrillation: analysis of pooled data from five randomized controlled trials. Arch Intern Med 154: 1449–57, 1994.

[18] Hart RG, Helperin JL. Atrial fibrillation and stroke: revisiting the dilemmas. Stroke 25: 1337–41, 1994.

[19] Lechat P, Mas JL, Lascault G, et al. Prevalence of patent foramen ovale in patients with stroke. N Engl J Med 318: 1148–52, 1988.

[20] Windecker S, Stortecky S, Meier B. Paradoxical embolism. J Am Coll Cardiol 29;64(4): 403–15, 2014. doi: 10.1016/j.jacc.2014.04.063.

[21] Powers WJ, Derdeyn CP, Biller J, Coffey CS, Hoh BL, Jauch EC, Johnston KC, Johnston SC, Khalessi AA, Kidwell CS, Meschia JF, Ovbiagele B, Yavagal DR; American Heart Association Stroke Council. 2015 American Heart Association/

American Stroke Association Focused Update of the 2013 Guidelines for the early management of patients with acute ischemic stroke regarding endovascular treatment: a guideline for health professionals from the American Heart Association/American Stroke Association. Stroke 46(10): 3020–35, 2015. doi: 10.1161/STR.0000000000000074.

[22] Tomsick TA, Brott TG, Olinger CP, et al. Hyperdense middle cerebral artery: incidence and quantitative significance. Neuroradiology 31: 312–5, 1989.

[23] Manelfe C, Larrue V, von Kummer R, et al. Association of hyperdense middle cerebral artery sign with clinical outcome in patients treated with plasminogen activator. Stroke 30: 760–72, 1999.

[24] Elster AD, Moody DM. Early cerebral infarction: gadopentetate dimeglumine enhancement. Radiology 177: 627–32, 1990.

[25] Lassen NA. Control of cerebral circulation in health and disease. Circ Res 34: 749–60, 1974.

[26] Kernan WN, Viscoli CM, Furie KL, Young LH, et al, for the IRIS Trial Investigators. Pioglitazone after ischemic stroke or transient ischemic attack. N Engl J Med 374: 1321–1331, 2016. doi: 10.1056/NEJMoa1506930.

[27] Hou Y, Carrim N, Wang Y, Gallant RC, Marshall AH, Ni H. Platelets in hemostasis and thrombosis: novel mechanisms of fibrinogen-independent platelet aggregation and fibronectin-mediated protein wave of hemostasis. J Biomed Res 2015. doi: 10.7555/JBR.29.20150121.

[28] Reheman A, Xu X, Reddy E, Ni H. Targeting activated platelets and fibrinolysis: hitting two birds with one stone. Circ Res 114: 1070–3, 2014. doi:10.1161/CIRCRESAHA.114.303600.

[29] Wang Y, Reheman A, Spring CM, Kalantari J, Marshall AH, Wolberg AS, Gross PL, Weitz JI, Rand ML, Mosher DF, Freedman J, Ni H. Plasma fibronectin supports hemostasis and regulates thrombosis. J Clin Invest 124: 4281–93, 2014. doi: 10.1172/JCI74630.

[30] Murphy AJ, Bijl N, Yvan-Charvet L, Welch CB, Bhagwat N, Reheman A, Wang Y, Levine R, Ni H, Tall AR, Wang N. Cholesterol efflux in megakaryocyte progenitors suppresses platelet production and thrombosis. Nat Med 19: 586–94, 2013. doi: 10.1038/nm.3150.

[31] Wang Y, Andrews M, Lang S, Jin JW, Cameron-Vendrig A, Zhu G, Reheman A, Ni H. Platelets in thrombosis and hemostasis. Old topic with new mechanisms. Cardiovascular & haematological disorders. Drug Targets 12: 126–132, 2012.

[32] Astrup J, Siesjo BK, Symon L. Thresholds in cerebral ischemia—the ischemic penumbra. Stroke 12(6): 723–5, 1981.

[33] Heiss WD. The ischemic penumbra: correlates in imaging and implications for treatment of ischemic stroke. The Johann Jacob Wepfer award 2011. Cerebrovasc Dis 32(4): 307–20, 2011. doi: 10.1159/000330462.

[34] Davalos A, Blanco M, Pedraza S, Leira R, Castellanos M, Pumar J M, et al. The clinical-DWI mismatch: a new diagnostic approach to the brain tissue at risk of infarction. Neurology 62(12): 2187–92, 2004.

[35] Group TNIoNDaSr-PSS. Tissue plasminogen activator for acute ischemic stroke. The National Institute of Neurological Disorders and Stroke rt-PA Stroke Study Group. N Engl J Med 333(24): 1581–7, 1995.

[36] Hacke W, Kaste M, Bluhmki E, Brozman M, Dávalos A, Guidetti D, Larrue V, Lees KR, Medeghri Z, Machnig T, Schneider D, von Kummer R, Wahlgren N, Toni D, ECASS Investigators. Thrombolysis with alteplase 3 to 4.5 hours after acute ischemic stroke. N Engl J Med 359(13): 1317–29, 2008.

[37] Del Zoppo GJ, Saver JL, Jauch EC, Adams, HP, Jr. American Heart Association Stroke Council Expansion of the time window for treatment of acute ischemic stroke with intravenous tissue plasminogen activator: a science advisory from the American Heart Association/American Stroke Association. Stroke 40(8): 2945–8, 2009.

[38] Fugate JE, Rabinstein AA. Absolute and relative contraindications to IV rt-PA for acute ishcemic stroke. Neurohospitalist 5(3): 110–121, 2015. doi: 10.1177/1941874415578532.

[39] Mishra NK, Ahmed N, Andersen G, et al. Thrombolysis in very elderly people: controlled comparison of SITS International Stroke Thrombolysis Registry and Virtual International Stroke Trials Archive. BMJ 341: c6046, 2010.

[40] Berruschot J, Rother J, Glahn J, Kucinski T, Fiehler J, Thomalla G. Outcome and severe hemorrhagic complications of intravenous thrombolysis with tissue plasminogen activator in very old (> or =80 years) stroke patients. Stroke 36(11): 2421–5, 2005.

[41] Fiehler J, Albers GW, Boulanger JM, et al. Bleeding risk analysis in stroke imaging before thrombolysis (BRASIL): pooled analysis of T2-weighted magnetic resonance imaging data from 570 patients. Stroke 38(10): 2738–44, 2007.

[42] Katzan IL, Furlan AJ, Lloyd LE, et al. Use of tissue-type plasminogen activator for acute ischemic stroke: the Cleveland area experience. JAMA 283(9): 1151–8, 2000.

[43] Jauch EC, Saver JL, Adams HP, Jr, et al. Guidelines for the early management of patients with acute ischemic stroke: a guideline for healthcare professionals from the American Heart Association/American Stroke Association. Stroke 44(3): 870–947, 2013.

[44] Tissue plasminogen activator for acute ischemic stroke. The National Institute of Neurological Disorders and Stroke rt-PA Stroke Study Group. N Engl J Med 333(24): 1581–7, 1995.

[45] Shinton RA, Gill JS, Melnick SC, Gupta AK, Beevers DG. The frequency, characteristics and prognosis of epileptic seizures at the onset of stroke. J Neurol Neurosurg Psychiatry 51(2): 273–6, 1988.

[46] Bluhmki E, Chamorro A, Davalos A, Machnig T, Sauce C, Wahlgren N, et al. Stroke treatment with alteplase given 3.0–4.5 h after onset of acute ischaemic stroke (ECASS III): additional outcomes and subgroup analysis of a randomised controlled trial. Lancet Neurol 8(12): 1095–102, 2009.

[47] Iguchi Y, Kimura K, Sakai K, Matsumoto N, Aoki J, Yamashita S, et al. Hyper-acute stroke patients associated with aortic dissection. Intern Med 49(6): 543–7, 2010.

[48] Anan C, Oomura M, Saeki T, Ikeda T, Sato C, Yamada K. Fatal intraperitoneal bleeding after intravenous administration of tissue plasminogen activator. J Stroke Cerebrovasc Dis 24(7): e177–8, 2015. doi: 10.1016/j.jstrokecerebrovasdis.2015.03.025.

[49] Saqqur M, Uchino K, Demchuk AM, Molina CA, Garami Z, Calleja S, et al. Site of arterial occlusion identified by transcranial Doppler predicts the response to intravenous thrombolysis for stroke. Stroke. 38(3): 948–54, 2007.

[50] Investigators TIS. Combined intravenous and intra-arterial recanalization for acute ischemic stroke: the Interventional Management of Stroke Study. Stroke 35(4): 904–11, 2004.

[51] Broderick JP, Palesch YY, Demchuk AM, Yeatts SD, Khatri P, Hill MD, et al. Endovascular therapy after intravenous t-PA versus t-PA alone for stroke. N Engl J Med 368(10): 893–903, 2013. doi: 10.1056/NEJMoa1214300.

[52] Berkhemer OA, Fransen PS, Beumer D, van den Berg LA, Lingsma HF, Yoo AJ, et al. A randomized trial of intraarterial treatment for acute ischemic stroke. N Engl J Med 372(1): 11–20, 2015. doi: 10.1056/NEJMoa1411587.

[53] Campbell BC, Mitchell PJ. Endovascular therapy for ischemic stroke. N Engl J Med 372(24): 2365–6, 2015. doi: 10.1056/NEJMc1504715.

[54] Goyal M, Demchuk AM, Menon BK, Eesa M, Rempel JL, Thornton J, et al. Randomized assessment of rapid endovascular treatment of ischemic stroke. N Engl J Med 372(11): 1019–30, 2015. doi: 10.1056/NEJMoa1414905.

[55] Jovin TG, Chamorro A, Cobo E, de Miquel MA, Molina CA, Rovira A, et al. Thrombectomy within 8 hours after symptom onset in ischemic stroke. N Engl J Med 372(24): 2296–306, 2015. doi: 10.1056/NEJMoa1503780.

[56] Saver JL, Goyal M, Bonafe A, Diener HC, Levy EI, Pereira VM, et al. Stent-retriever thrombectomy after intravenous t-PA vs. t-PA alone in stroke. N Engl J Med 372(24): 2285–95, 2015. doi: 10.1056/NEJMoa1415061.

[57] Anderson CS, Robinson T, Lindley RI, Arima H, Lavados PM, Lee TH, Broderick JP, Chen X, Chen G, Sharma VK, Kim JS, Thang NH, Cao Y,Parsons MW, Levi C, Huang Y, Olavarría VV, Demchuk AM, Bath PM, Donnan GA, Martins S, Pontes-Neto OM,

Silva F, Ricci S, Roffe C, Pandian J, Billot L, Woodward M, Li Q, Wang X, Wang J, Chalmers J. Low-dose versus standard-dose intravenous alteplase in acute ischemic stroke. N Engl J Med 2016, May 10 [Epub ahead of print].

[58] Granger CB, Alexander JH, McMurray JJ, et al. Apixaban versus warfarin in patients with atrial fibrillation. N Engl J Med 365(11): 981–92, 2011.

[59] Wahlgren N, Moreira T, Michel P, Steiner T, Jansen O, Cognard C, Mattle HP, van Zwam W, Holmin S, Tatlisumak T, Petersson J, Caso V, Hacke W, Mazighi M, Arnold M, Fischer U, Szikora I, Pierot L, Fiehler J, Gralla J, Fazekas F, Lees KR; ESO-KSU, ESO, ESMINT, ESNR and EAN. Mechanical thrombectomy in acute ischemic stroke: consensus statement by ESO-Karolinska Stroke Update 2014/2015, supported by ESO, ESMINT, ESNR and EAN. Int J Stroke 11(1): 134–47, 2016. doi: 10.1177/1747493015609778.

[60] Zhu G, Michel P, Aghaebrahim A, Patrie JT, Xin W, Eskandari A, et al. Prediction of recanalization trumps prediction of tissue fate: the penumbra: a dual-edged sword. Stroke J Cerebral Circ 44: 1014–9, 2013. doi: 10.1161/STROKEAHA.111.000229.

[61] EC/IC Study Group. Failure of EC-IC bypass to reduce the risk of ischemic stroke. N Engl J Med 313: 1191–200, 1985.

[62] Lavallée PC, Mazighi M, Saint-Maurice JP, Meseguer E, Abboud H, Klein IF. Stent-assisted endovascular thrombolysis versus intravenous thrombolysis in internal carotid artery dissection with tandem internal carotid and middle cerebral artery occlusion. Stroke 38: 2270–4, 2007.

[63] Inoue T, Tamura A, Tsutsumi K, Saito I, Saito N. Surgical embolectomy for large vessel occlusion of anterior circulation. Br J Neurosurg 27: 783–90, 2013. doi: 10.3109/02688697.2013.793286.

[64] Powers WJ, Clarke WR, Grubb RL, Videen TO, Adams HP, Derdeyn CP. Extracranial-intracranial bypass surgery for stroke prevention in hemodynamic cerebral ischemia: the carotid occlusion surgery study randomized trial. JAMA 306: 1983–92, 2011. doi: 10.1001/jama.2011.1610.

[65] Fusco MR, Harrigan MR. Cerebrovascular dissections—a review part I: spontaneous dissections. Neurosurgery 68: 242, 2011. doi: 10.1227/NEU.0b013e3182012323.

[66] Kim YS, Garami Z, Mikulik R, Molina CA, Alexandrov AV. Early recanalization rates and clinical outcomes in patients with tandem internal carotid artery/middle cerebral artery occlusion and isolated middle cerebral artery occlusion. Stroke 36: 869–71, 2005.

[67] Rubiera M, Ribo M, Delgado-Mederos R, Santamarina E, Delgado P, Montaner J. Tandem internal carotid artery/middle cerebral artery occlusion: an independent predictor of poor outcome after systemic thrombolysis. Stroke 37: 2301–5, 2006.

[68] Nussbaum ES, Janjua TM, Defillo A, Lowary JL, Nussbaum LA. Emergency extracranial-intracranial bypass surgery for acute ischemic stroke. J Neurosurg 112: 666–73, 2010.

[69] Amin-Hanjani S, Barker FG, Charbel FT, Connolly ES, Morcos JJ, Thompson BG. Cerebrovascular section of the American Association of Neurological Surgeons; Congress of Neurological Surgeons. Extracranial-intracranial bypass for stroke-is this the end of the line or a bump in the road? Neurosurgery 71: 557–61, 2012.

[70] Kanamaru K, Araki T, Kawakita F, Hamada K, Kanamaru H, Matsuura K, Sato A, Suzuki H. STA-MCA bypass for the treatment of ischemic stroke. Acta Neurochir Suppl 112: 55–7, 2011. doi: 10.1007/978-3-7091-0661-7_10.

[71] Carter BS, Ogilyv CS, Candia GJ, et al. One-year outcome after decompressive surgery for massive nondominant hemispheric infarction. Neurosurgery 40: 1168–76, 1997.

[72] Schwab S, Steiner T, Aschoff A, et al. Early hemicraniectomy in patients with complete middle cerebral artery infarction. Stroke 29: 1888–93, 1998.

[73] Bruni EJ, Montemurro DG, editors. Human Neuroanatomy: A Text, Brain Atlas, and Laboratory Dissection Guide. Oxford University Press; 2009. p. 33–51. ISBN: 978-0-19-537142-0.

[74] Tanrikulu L, Oez-Tanrikulu A, Weiss C, Scholz T, Schiefer J, Clusmann H, Schubert GA. The bigger, the better? About the size of decompressive hemicraniectomies. Clin Neurol Neurosurg 135: 15–21, 2015. doi: 10.1016/j.clineuro.2015.04.019. Epub 2015, May 5.

[75] Zweckberger K, Juettler E, Bösel J, Unterberg WA. Surgical aspects of decompression craniectomy in malignant stroke: review. Cerebrovasc Dis 38(5): 313–23, 2014. doi: 10.1159/000365864.

[76] Inamasu J, Kaito T, Watabe T, Ganaha T, Yamada Y, Tanaka T, Imizu S, Hayashi T, Hayakawa M, Kato Y, Hirose Y. Decompressive hemicraniectomy for malignant hemispheric stroke in the elderly: comparison of outcomes between individuals 61–70 and >70 years of age. J Stroke Cerebrovasc Dis 22(8): 1350–4, 2013.

[77] Schaller B, Graf R, Sanada Y, Rosner G, Wienhard K, Heiss WD. Hemodynamic and metabolic effects of decompressive hemicraniectomy in normal brain. An experimental PET-study in cants. Brain Res 982(1): 31–7, 2003.

[78] Vahedi K, Vicaut E, Mateo J, Kurtz A, Orabi M, Guichard JP, Boutron C, Couvreur G, Rouanet F, Touzé E, Guillon B, Carpentier A, Yelnik A, George B, Payen D, Bousser MG; DECIMAL Investigators. Sequential-design, multicenter, randomized, controlled trial of early decompressive craniectomy in malignant middle cerebral artery infarction (DECIMAL Trial). Stroke 38(9): 2506–17, 2007. doi: 10.1161/STROKEAHA.107.485235.

[79] Cappabianca P, Califano L, Iaconetta G, editors. Cranial, Craniofacial and Skull Base Surgery. Springer-Verlag Italia; 2010. p. 159–165. doi: 10.1007/978-88-470-1167-0.

[80] Lipsman N, Mainprize TG, Schwartz ML, Hynynen K, Lozano AM. Intracranial applications of magnetic resonance-guided focused ultrasound. Neurotherapeutics 11(3): 593–605, 2014. doi: 10.1007/s13311-014-0281-2.

Chapter 8

Cryptogenic Stroke

Rubens J. Gagliardi and Vivian D.B. Gagliardi

Additional information is available at the end of the chapter

http://dx.doi.org/10.5772/65045

Abstract

Introduction: To emphasize the importance of this kind of stroke, to focus on secondary stroke prevention and to recognize that the etiology of stroke is fundamental for proper prevention. In this chapter, the history of this stroke subtype is described and its actual specific denomination: embolic stroke undetermined source (ESUS).

Objectives: To define "cryptogenic stroke," the main characteristics and therapeutics proposals.

Discussion: The following main characteristics of this kind of stoke are presented here: the incidence in several countries and international statistics, the specific physiopathology of this kind of stroke, the different methods for its correct diagnosis and the importance of exhaustive cardiac investigation, the main cause of ESUS with special focus in the importance of paroxysmal atrial fibrillation. The new therapeutic options (anticoagulants versus antiplatelets) are presented and discussed based on the recent trials.

Conclusion: Importance of correct definition of the stroke etiology for its appropriate secondary prevention; would anticoagulation be better than antiaggregation for adequate prevention? We look forward to the results of recent trials in this field.

Keywords: stroke, cryptogenic stroke, cerebral embolism, embolic stroke of undetermined source (ESUS), anticoagulants, atrial fibrillation

1. Introduction

Cryptogenic stroke is a kind of stroke without a known cause, with a negative screening for a definite cause, such as cardioembolism, atherothrombosis, arterial dissection, and lacunar stroke [1]. This term was introduced in 1988 [1] and has gained importance because of the need to clarify the stroke cause for its effective treatment and secondary prevention. The definition of the stroke etiology is of great importance since it is directly related to its prognosis and treatment and guides the secondary prevention strategy.

Known atherothrombotic stroke responds reasonably well to antiplatelet (AG), and cardioembolic stroke responds better to anticoagulant than to AG, and therefore, there should be a careful etiological definition. The risk of recurrence of a cryptogenic stroke is high [2, 3], because it surely is not being adequately prevented. Recently, the term ESUS ("embolic stroke undetermined source") has been used to describe these cases [4], since most of these cases of cryptogenic strokes are embolic with an undetermined the source of embolism.

1.1. Etiologic stroke classification

There are several classifications and scales to help determine the etiologic diagnosis of stroke. The TOAST (Trial of Org 10172 in Acute Stroke Treatment) Subtype Classification System [1] has been widely used and divides the acute ischemic stroke in five subtypes according to their causes: atherosclerosis of large arteries (carotid and cerebral), cardioembolic, occlusion of small vessels (lacunar), certain other causes (e.g., thrombophilias), and undetermined cause (cryptogenic stroke). The prevalence of cryptogenic strokes varies from 20 to 40% of all subtypes of stroke in most studies [2, 3].

Recently, researchers have discussed deeply on why the incidence of this event has remained high over the years. Often the investigation is incomplete, but in many cases, this investigation is adequate, and yet it is not possible to identify the cause of the stroke. In these cases, the first suspicion should be for a transient or reversible mechanism [4, 5].

2. Physiopathology

Many different pathophysiological mechanisms have been proposed as possible causes for a cryptogenic stroke [4]:

- Cardioembolic sources, such as mitral annular calcification, aortic valve stenosis, aortic valve calcification, atrial asystole and sick sinus syndrome, atrial high rate episodes, atrial appendage stasis with reduced flow velocities or spontaneous echodensities atrial structural abnormalities, atrial septal aneurysm, Chiari network, moderate systolic or diastolic dysfunction (global or regional), ventricular non-compaction, endomyocardial fibrosis, covert paroxysmal atrial fibrillation.

- Cancer-associated emboli: covert nonbacterial thrombotic endocarditis, tumor emboli from occult cancer.

- Arteriogenic emboli: aortic arch atherosclerotic plaques, cerebral artery non-stenotic plaques with ulceration.

http://dx.doi.org/10.5772/65045

– Paradoxical embolism: patent foramen ovale, atrial septal defect, pulmonary arteriovenous fistula.

The cardioembolic mechanisms as possible genesis of cryptogenic stroke have been deeply discussed [4, 6], believing that they are often are not recorded, either for lack of relevant research or the characteristic paroxysms (as in paroxysmal atrial fibrillation), which may make this arrhythmia not evident at the time of investigation. The cardioembolic causes has been the subject of deep and extensive discussions in recent years, with special attention to atrial fibrillation (AF) and patent foramen ovale (PFO), due to its high prevalence in the general population.

2.1. Atrial fibrillation

Atrial fibrillation is an example of a transient cause that corresponds to 10% of all stroke and is estimated to be responsible for 50% of the cryptogenic stroke. The AF is paroxysmal in 30% of patients with stroke and therefore is often not identified within the first days or weeks after a stroke, as seen in several trials. It is known that the investigation of AF can present false negatives because of the possible paroxysmal rhythm, which suggests the need for long-term monitoring. Several studies have proven that long-term monitoring [7–9] for atrial fibrillation increases the chances of detecting paroxysmal AF. Several devices have been proven for this, including outpatient mobile telemetry and the outpatient transtelephonic monitoring, implantable loop recorder. Culebras et al. [8] describe in the 2014 consensus of the American Academy of Neurology evidence of the work of the last decade analyzing the effectiveness of these mechanisms to detect AF (ECG, Holter, event loop, outpatient telemetry / hospital, outpatient transtelephonic monitoring ECGs series) and showed a tendency that the higher monitoring time is related to the higher detection rate of the AF.

For example, the study CRYSTAL AF [9] in 2014 studied the presence of AF in patients with transient ischemic attack (TIA) or stroke cryptogenic for 6 and 12 months, using a insertable cardiac monitor, a previously validated device for AF detection which is implanted in the patient and records an electrocardiographic lead. This study showed that when compared to control groups, AF was observed in 8.9% of patients within 6 months of evaluation, compared to 1.4% in control patients ($p < 0.001$) and 12.4% of patients 12-month assessment, against 2.0% in the control group ($p < 0.001$). Thus, it is clear that patients with cryptogenic stroke should have a more comprehensive research, in addition to ECG and Holter, since there is evidence that device is most effective in detecting paroxysmal AF.

A potential biomarker for determining the risk of AF occurring after cryptogenic stroke could be the dosage of brain natriuretic peptide (sBNP) serum levels [10], which are high in AF, and therefore could be useful for the monitoring of these patients; however, this is not consensual yet and needs further confirmation.

2.2. Patent foramen ovale

Another situation often associated with cryptogenic stroke is the presence of patent foramen ovale (PFO). This is a common anatomic abnormality in the general population—an estimated prevalence of 26% [11]. The PFO appears to be a risk factor for stroke in young adults; one meta-analysis showed that patients younger than 55 years have higher rates in the presence of PFO than the control population, and the same does not occur in patients older than 55 years [11].

The presence of PFO may lead to cerebral ischemia by several mechanisms [6]:

- Paroxysmal embolism of peripheral venous system;
- Embolization of thrombi in the atrial septum;
- Embolization of thrombi formed by paroxysmal arrhythmias.

The presence of PFO may be associated with the occurrence of atrial septal aneurysm (ASA), Chiari network, or other atrial septal defects. The presence of PFO and its relationship to stroke can be difficult to determine. The SPARC study [12] suggests that the presence of an isolated PFO, adjusted to age and comorbidities, is not considered a risk factor for cerebrovascular events; however, the risk of stroke in patients with PFO and ASA is four times higher than in patients without ASA. Other features such as the right-left shunt at rest and septal hypermobility are related to higher risk of stroke than isolated PFO [13].

The diagnosis of PFO is performed by echocardiography; evaluation by transcranial Doppler can aid the diagnosis in a first approach as it can demonstrate right-left communication (shunts) when detecting microembolic signals; however, this rating is less sensitive to small PFOs and does not evaluate cardiac structure anatomically, so that echocardiography is still the method of choice [6]. The gold standard investigation for PFO is the Transesophageal echocardiography (TEE) [6].

There is no consensus regarding the treatment of PFO, and its approach includes the use of antiplatelet agents, anticoagulants, closing by percutaneous, or surgical closure device. Clinical treatment with warfarin or acetylsalicylic acid (ASA) is indicated as secondary prophylaxis in cryptogenic stroke in patients with PFO—there is no evidence of superiority of one treatment compared to another. There is still no clear benefit of PFO closure therapy because it is not yet clear which the patient that best benefits from this approach, nor what kind of approach would be superior [14, 15].

3. Etiological investigation

There is no consensus about the etiological investigation stroke, but recent studies cite that the investigation should include performing computed tomography (CT) or magnetic resonance imaging (MRI) of the brain, 12-lead ECG, cardiac monitoring for 24 h (Holter), transthoracic echocardiogram, screening for thrombophilia in patients younger than 55 years, angio-CT/ angio MRI/or cervical and intracranial digital angiography, ultrasonography Doppler of cervical, and vertebral arteries.

In cases where the cause for the stroke is unknown despite adequate research, it is suggested to expand the investigation of possible cardioembolic events, given their greater frequency in the general population. To this end, it is suggested performing transcranial Doppler, transesophageal echocardiography-TEE (which is the gold standard for cardiac anatomic evaluation), and an increased time heart rhythm study (greater than 24 h), as discussed previously. The TEE should also evaluate the presence of aortic arch atheroma, as cryptogenic stroke patients have an increased prevalence of atherosclerotic disease of the aorta, which could lead to an embolic stroke [16]. The transcranial Doppler may detect microembolic signs [17], which could be related to PFO or pulmonary arteriovenous fistula for example.

Some authors also suggest including pelvic magnetic resonance venography in patients with cryptogenic stroke and PFO, as deep vein thrombosis could be a source of paradoxical embolism in these patients [18].

There seem to be a statistically significant clinical and radiological difference between patients with cryptogenic stroke and PFO, AF, and aortic arch atheroma. Ryoo et al. [16] described in one study that patients with PFO had healthy vascular risk and more posterior circulation involvement; AF-related events present with higher NIHSS scores and larger lesions than other groups; and aortic arch atheroma was related to small lesions in multiple territories. Although this needs further studies, these patterns could help guiding the investigation.

In young patients with cryptogenic stroke and already investigated for thrombophilias, supplementation with genetic study to thrombophilic disease appears to have no benefit [15]. Studying this situation showed no statistically significant increase in the prevalence of Stroke related to genetic polymorphisms in young patients investigated for thrombophilic causes, including evaluation of factor V gene Leiden, prothrombin gene, angiotensin-converting enzyme gene, gene of 5,10-metilenotetrahidrofolate-reductase (MTHFR), endothelial nitric oxide synthetase gene (ecNOS) activating factor gene of plasminogen activator (tPA) inhibitor factor-1 gene of plasminogen activator (PAI-1), and HaeIII polymorphism of β-fibrinogen gene [19].

4. Treatment

Considering that the correct secondary stroke prevention depends on the precise knowledge of the etiology of the stroke, it is very important to define it. Unfortunately, until now, there is no definition about the best management of secondary prevention in cryptogenic stroke.

The consensus of the American Stroke Association/American Heart Association 2008 specifically recommends antiplatelet indication for the treatment of cryptogenic stroke. However, more recent consensus does not specifically comment on managing this stroke subtype [4].

There are few studies analyzing this issue. The WARSS study [20] showed that in a sample of patients with cryptogenic stroke, the rate of recurrence of the event or death was statistically lower in patients who used warfarin (target INR between 1.4 and 2.8) than in patients receiving acid acetylsalicylic (ASA) at a dose of 325 mg/day. Recently, some authors as Hart et al. [4] suggest the introduction of anticoagulant treatment for secondary prophylaxis in patients with undetermined etiology stroke. Ongoing trials such as the RES-PECT ESUS [21] studies and NAVIGATE ESUS [22] are comparing the use of acetylsalicylic acid to the use of novel oral anticoagulants and should help to determine the choice of treatment in the future (**Table 1**).

Trial	Drug	Started
RES-PECT ESUS [21]	Dabigatran vs. ASA	2015
NAVIGATE ESUS [22]	Rivaroxaban vs. ASA	2015

ASA, acetylsalicylic acid.

Table 1. Ongoing trials comparing ASA vs. the new oral anticoagulants in ESUS patients.

Author details

Rubens J. Gagliardi[1,2] and Vivian D.B. Gagliardi[3*]

*Address all correspondence to: rubensjg@apm.org.br and viviandbg@gmail.com

1 Neurology, School of Medical Sciences, Santa Casa de Sao Paulo, Sao Paulo, SP, Brazil

2 Brazilian Academy of Neurology, Brazil

3 Federal University of São Paulo, Sao Paulo, SP, Brazil

References

[1] Adams HP Jr, Bendixen BH, Kappelle LJ, Biller J, Love BB, Gordon DL, Marsh EE 3rd. Classification of subtype of acute ischemic stroke. Stroke. 1993;24:35–41. doi: 10.1161/01.STR.24.1.35

[2] Sacco RL, Ellenberg JH, Mohr JP, Tatemichi TK, Hier DB, Price TR, Wolf PA. Infarcts of undetermined cause: the NNCDS Stroke Data Bank. Ann Neurol. 1989;25:382–390. doi: 10.1002/ana.410250410

[3] Rosamond WD, Folsom AR, Chambless LE, et al. Stroke incidence and survival among middle-aged adults: 9-year follow-up of the Atherosclerosis Risk in Communities (ARIC) cohort. Stroke. 1999;30:736–743. doi:10.1161/01.STR.30.4.736

[4] Hart RG, Diener HC, Coutts SB, Easton JD, Granger CB, O'Donnell MJ, Sacco RL, Connolly SJ; Cryptogenic Stroke/ESUS International Working Group. Cryptogenic Stroke/ESUS International Working Group. Embolic strokes of undetermined source:

a case for a new clinical construct. Lancet Neurol. 2014;13:429–438. doi:http://dx.doi.org/10.1016/S1474-4422(13)70310-7

[5] Bang OY, Lee PH, Joo SY, Lee JS, Joo IS, Huh K. Frequency and mechanisms of stroke recurrence after cryptogenic stroke. Ann Neurol. 2003;54:227–234. doi:10.1002/ana.10644

[6] Guernici F, Acciarresi M, Agnelli G, Paciaroni M. Cryptogenic stroke: time to determine aetiology. J Thromb Haemost. 2008;6:549–554. doi:10.1111/j.1538-7836.2008.02903.x.

[7] Jabaudon D, Sztajzel J, Sievert K, Landis T, Sztajzel R. Usefulness of ambulatory 7-day ECG monitoring for the detection of atrial fibrillation and flutter after acute stroke and transient ischemic attack. Stroke. 2004;35:1647–1651. doi:10.1161/01.STR.0000131269.69502.d9

[8] Culebras A, Messe SR, Chatuverdi S, Kase CS, Gronseth G. Summary of evidence-based guideline update: prevention of stroke in nonvalvular atrial fibrillation: report of the Guideline Development Subcommittee of the American Academy of Neurology. Neurology. 2014;82:716–724. doi:10.1212/WNL.0000000000000145

[9] Sanna T, Diener HC, Passman RS, et al. Cryptogenic stroke and underlying atrial fibrillation. N Eng J Med. 2014;370:2478–2486. doi:10.1056/NEJMoa1313600

[10] Rodrigues-Yañez M, Arias-Rivas S, Santamaria-Cadavid M, Sobrino T, Castillo J, Blanco M. High pro-BNP levels predict the occurrence of atrial fibrillation after cryptogenic stroke. Neurology. 2013;81:444–447. doi:10.1212/WNL.0b013e31829d8773

[11] Overell JR, Bone I, Lees KR. Interatrial septal abnormalities and stroke: a meta-analysis of case-control studies. Neurology. 2000;55:1172–1179. doi:http://dx.doi.org/10.1212/WNL.55.8.1172

[12] Meissner I, Whisnant JP, Khandheria BK, Spittell PC, O'Fallon WM, Pascoe RD, Enriquez-Sarano M, Seward JB, Covalt JL, Sicks JD, Wiebers DO. Prevalence of potential risk factors for stroke assessed by transesophageal echocardiography and carotid ultrasonography: the SPARC study. Mayo Clin Proc. 1999;74:862–869. doi:http://dx.doi.org/10.4065/74.9.862

[13] Roth C, Alli O. Patent foramen ovale and cryptogenic stroke: many unanswered questions. Cleve Clin J Med. 2014;81(7):417–424. doi:10.3949/ccjm.81a.13144

[14] Thaler DE, Ruthazer R, Weimar C, Mas JL, Serena J, Di Angelantonio E, Papetti F, Homma S, Mattle HP, Nedeltchev K, Mono ML, Jaigobin C, Michel P, Elkind MS, Di Tullio MR, Lutz JS, Griffith J, Kent DM. Recurrent stroke predictors differ in medically treated patients with pathogenic vs other PFOs. Neurology. 2014;83:221–226. doi: 10.1212/WNL.0000000000000589

[15] Thaler DE, Ruthazer R, Weimar C, Serena J, Mattle HP, Nedeltchev K, Mono ML, Di Angelantonio E, Elkind MS, Di Tullio MR, Homma S, Michel P, Meier B, Furlan AJ, Lutz JS, Kent DM. Determinants of antithrombotic choice for patent foramen ovale in

cryptogenic stroke. Neurology. 2014;83:1954–1957. doi:10.1212/WNL.0000000000001007

[16] Ryoo S, Chung JW, Lee MJ, Kim SJ, Lee JS, Gyeong Moon Kim, Chin?Sang Chung, Lee KH, Hong JM, Bang OY. An approach to working up cases of embolic stroke of undetermined source. J Am Heart Assoc. 2016;5(3):1–10. doi:10.1161/JAHA.115.002975

[17] Shariat A, Yaghoubi E, Nemati R, Moaref AR, Aghasadeghi K, Borhani Haghighi A. Microembolic signals in patients with cryptogenic stroke with or without patent foramen ovale. J Stroke Cerebrovasc Dis. 2012;21:662–666. doi:10.1016/j.jstrokecerebrovasdis.2011.02.015.

[18] Liberman AL, Daruwalla VJ, Collins JD, Maas MB, Botelho MP, Ayache JB, Carr J, Ruff I, Bernstein RA, Alberts MJ, Prabhakaran S. Diagnostic yield of pelvic magnetic resonance venography in patients with cryptogenic stroke and patent foramen ovale. Stroke. 2014;45:2324–2329. doi:10.1161/STROKEAHA.114.005539

[19] Austin H, Chimowitz MI, Hill HA, Chaturvedi S, Wechsler LR, Wityk RJ, Walz E, Wilterdink JL, Coull B, Sila CA, Mitsias P, Evatt B, Hooper WC; Genetics and Stroke in the Young Study Group. Cryptogenic stroke in relation to genetic variation in clotting factors and other genetic polymorphisms among young men and women. Stroke. 2002;33:2762–2768. doi:10.1161/01.STR.0000038094.79901.3B

[20] Hankey GJ. Warfarin-Aspirin Recurrent Stroke Study (WARSS) trial—is warfarin really a reasonable therapeutic alternative to aspirin for preventing recurrent noncardioembolic ischemic stroke? Stroke. 2002;33:1723–1726. doi:10.1161/01.STR.0000016922.22707.27

[21] Diener HC, Easton JD, Granger CB, Cronin L, Duffy C, Cotton D, Brueckmann M, Sacco RL. Design of randomized, double-blind, evaluation in secondary stroke prevention comparing the efficacy and safety of the oral thrombin inhibitor dabigatran etexilate vs. acetylsalicyclic acid in patient with embolic stroke of undetermined source (RE-SPEcT ESUS). Int J Stroke. 2015;10:1309–1312. doi:10.1111/ijs.12630

[22] Ameriso S, Lavados P, Arauz A, Gagliardi RJ, Shoamanesh A, Pater C, Mundl H, Berkowitz SD, Connolly SJ, Hart RG. NAVIGATE ESUS: Phase-III RCT assessing prevention of stroke and systemic embolism in patients with embolic stroke of undetermined source. J Neurol Sci. 2015;357(1):e364–e365. doi:http://dx.doi.org/10.1016/j.jns.2015.08.1308

Chapter 9

Updates in Mechanical Thrombectomy

Robert C. Rennert, Arvin R. Wali, Christine Carico,
Jeffrey Scott Pannell and Alexander A. Khalessi

Additional information is available at the end of the chapter

http://dx.doi.org/10.5772/64398

Abstract

Strokes are a major source of morbidity and mortality worldwide. The long-standing gold standard in stroke therapy, intravenous administration of tissue plasminogen activator (tPA), is limited by strict timing parameters and modest efficacy in large strokes caused by thrombi in the proximal cerebral vasculature. Multiple recent randomized controlled trials have demonstrated the efficacy of mechanical thrombectomy for patients with large vessel occlusions (LVOs). Recent clinical guidelines have been updated to include mechanical thrombectomy as a standard of care in properly selected stroke patients, with ongoing and future studies working to refine the optimal clinical and technical variables of this approach.

Keywords: mechanical thrombectomy, large vessel occlusion, stroke, stent-retriever, endovascular

1. Large vessel ischemic stroke: an opportunity for improvement

Strokes are the third leading cause of death globally and the leading cause of acquired adult disability [1, 2]. There are approximately 700,000 strokes annually in the United States and 4.5 million stroke survivors suffering from disability and loss of independence [3]. Proximal large vessel occlusions (LVOs) are particularly devastating, with an approximate 60–80% risk of 90-day mortality or severe morbidity [4, 5]. Costs associated with the treatment of stroke patients are more than 22 billion dollars annually [3, 6]. With an aging global population, the incidence of stroke is expected to increase over time, making improvements in detection, treatment, and management essential.

The pathophysiology of ischemic strokes, which accounts for 85–90% of all strokes, is an ischemic cascade in the cerebral vasculature that leads to cellular bioenergetic failure. This injury is caused by cerebral hypoperfusion and subsequent excitotoxicity, oxidative stress, blood-brain barrier dysfunction, and post-ischemic inflammation that culminate in the death of neurons, glia, and endothelial cells [2]. Therapies targeting these deleterious pathways have been shown to improve cerebral perfusion and decrease secondary injury [7, 8], although rapid restoration of blood flow to affected areas remains the ultimate goal in stroke treatment.

Evidence-based indications (all criteria met)
Pre-stroke mRS 0–1
Acute ischemic stroke of ICA or proximal MCA receiving tPA within 4.5 hours
Age ≥ 18 years
NIHSS/ASPECTS ≥ 6
Thrombectomy initiated within 6 hours of symptom onset
Thrombectomy may be considered (no definitive data and imaging to determine infarct core/penumbra may be helpful)
>6 hours from symptom onset
Patients with contraindications to tPA
Distal MCA, ACA, and posterior circulation occlusions
<18 years of age
Pre-stroke mRS > 1, NIHSS/ASPECTS < 6

Abbreviations: ACA, anterior cerebral artery; ASPECTS, Alberta Stroke Program Early CT score; ICA, internal cerebral artery; MCA, middle cerebral artery; mRS, modified Rankin Scale; NIHSS, National Institutes of Health Stroke Scale; tPA, tissue plasminogen activator.

Table 1. Summary of current indications for mechanical thrombectomy for stroke.

The long-standing gold standard for restoration of blood flow to ischemic brain is intravenous administration of the thrombolytic agent tissue plasminogen activator (tPA) within 3–4.5 hours of symptom onset [9, 10]. Tissue plasminogen activator leads to a 30% decreased risk of having no or minimal disability at 30 days [11]. However, strict parameters for tPA administration, such as its narrow treatment window and requirement that the patient has no recent surgeries, recent stroke, or prior hemorrhagic stroke, leave tPA underutilized. Only 3–5% of all stroke patients receive tPA, and less than half of patients that would be eligible for tPA actually receive treatment [12]. tPA is also associated with a 6% rate of hemorrhagic strokes and a 2% risk of systemic hemorrhage [13]. Most importantly, in high-risk patients with LVO, tPA has only modest rates of early reperfusion and thus limited efficacy [4, 5, 14, 15]. The limitations and risks of medical stroke therapies, particularly in patients with LVO, have led to the exploration of other reperfusion techniques by mechanical clot removal (thrombectomy). Recently, multiple large randomized trials demonstrated improved outcomes in patients with LVO [5, 16–19]. Based on this data, mechanical thrombectomy is now a standard of care in appropriately selected stroke patients with LVO (**Table 1**) [20]. This chapter focuses on the theory, technical aspects, current data, and future directions of mechanical thrombectomy for stroke.

2. Introduction to mechanical thrombectomy

Mechanical thrombectomy employs direct arterial access to physically remove a thrombus from the cerebral circulation, providing in theory immediate and definitive reversal of hypoperfusion. While intuitively appealing, optimizing the technical aspects of this approach has delayed its widespread implementation. Early-generation devices included the MERCI Retriever (Concentric Medical Inc/Stryker Corp., Kalamazoo, MI), a flexible helical nitinol wire that is deployed through a microcatheter into the clot under balloon vessel occlusion and large-bore direct aspiration catheters with or without mechanical clot separators (Penumbra, Inc., Alameda, CA). Intra-arterial application of tPA directly to the site of the lesion was also explored in parallel to the above early techniques.

Initial randomized clinical trials with these devices/techniques demonstrated their safety but failed to show their superiority to intravenous tPA [4, 21, 22]. Potential reasons for the non-superiority of endovascular interventions in these trials include prolonged durations between symptom onset and intervention, poor patient selection as LVO was not in the selection criteria, and suboptimal recanalization rates likely resulting from use of early generation thrombectomy devices.

Newer generation stent retrievers, such as Solitaire FR (Covidien, Ltd., Mansfield, OH) and TREVO (Stryker Corp.), act as stents that are deployed within the clot and then retrieved to complete the thrombectomy. These devices have demonstrated superiority to older products like MERCI [23, 24] and are associated with significantly reduced endothelial damage [25]. Multiple large randomized trials have recently been published demonstrating improved outcomes in patients with LVO treated with stent retrievers as compared to intravenous tPA [5, 16–19], with clinical guideline updates including these therapies as standard of care.

3. Updated clinical data on mechanical thrombectomy

The American Heart Association (AHA)/American Stroke Association (ASA) released a set of updated guidelines for the management of patients with acute ischemic disease regarding endovascular treatment in 2015 after recent randomized controlled trial data clearly demonstrated the safety and efficacy of mechanical thrombectomy as compared to tPA for large vessel occlusion [20]. A summary of this clinical data follows and is highlighted in **Table 2**.

The Multicenter Randomized Clinical Trial of Endovascular Treatment for Acute Ischemic Stroke in the Netherlands (MR CLEAN) enrolled 500 patients with anterior cerebral circulation arterial occlusion and an National Institutes of Health Stroke Scale (NIHSS) score ≥2, who could be treated endovascularly within 6 hours of symptom onset [5]. The effects of intra-arterial treatment plus standard medical therapy (intervention) versus standard medical therapy alone (control; including intravenous tPA, if eligible) were assessed. Mechanical thrombectomy was performed in 195 of 233 patients randomized to the intervention group, with retrievable stents used in 190 of these 195 patients. A modified thrombolysis in cerebral infarction (TICI) score of 2b or 3 (indicating >50% or complete distal reperfusion, respectively) was achieved in 58.7% of patients in the intervention group. This study reported a 13.5% increase in functional independence in the intervention group (32.6 versus 19.1, $p < 0.05$ as determined by the primary study outcome 90-day modified Rankin Scale [mRS] ≤ 2), with no significant difference in mortality or intracerebral hemorrhage rates. Secondary outcomes of the 5- and 7-day NIHSS score, the absence of residual occlusion at 24 hours, and the infarct volume were also improved in the intervention group.

The Endovascular Treatment for Small Core and Anterior Circulation Proximal Occlusion with Emphasis on Minimizing CT to Recanalization Times (ESCAPE) trial enrolled 316 patients with proximal anterior circulation occlusions, moderate-to-good collateral circulation, and a small infarct core, up to 12 hours after symptom onset [16]. The effects of intra-arterial treatment plus standard medical therapy (intervention) versus standard medical therapy alone (control; including intravenous tPA, if eligible) were assessed. This study was terminated early after an interim analysis demonstrated clear treatment efficacy. One hundred and fifty-one of the 165 patients assigned to the intervention group received intra-arterial therapy, with retrievable stents used in 130 of these patients. A modified TICI 2b or 3 score was achieved in 72.4% of patients in the intervention group. This study reported a 23.7% increase in functional independence (90-day mRS ≤ 2) with intervention (53.0 versus 29.3%, $p < 0.05$; a primary study outcome) and a decrease in 90-day mortality (10.4 versus 19.0%; $p = 0.04$). Secondary quality of life outcomes including 90-day Barthel Index (BI), NIHSS, and EuroQoL Group 5-Dimension Self-Report Questionnaire (EQ-5D) all favored the intervention group as well.

The Solitaire FR with the Intention for Thrombectomy as Primary Endovascular Treatment of Acute Ischemic Stroke (SWIFT PRIME) trial enrolled 196 patients with confirmed proximal anterior circulation occlusions and the absence of a large ischemic core that could be treated within 6 hours of symptom onset [17]. The effects of intravenous tPA (control) versus intravenous tPA plus stent-retriever thrombectomy (intervention) were assessed. This study was terminated early after an interim analysis demonstrated clear treatment efficacy. The intervention group of 98 patients had a median time from qualifying imaging to groin puncture of 57 minutes. At the end of the procedure, the rate of substantial reperfusion was 88%. This study reported a 25% increase in functional independence (90-day mRS ≤ 2) with intervention (60 versus 35%, $p < 0.001$; a primary study outcome). Secondary outcomes including 27-hour successful reperfusion and NIHSS were also significantly improved in the intervention group. There were no significant differences between the intervention and control group in 90-day mortality or symptomatic intracranial hemorrhage.

Trial name	Year	Study design	Groups	Number of patients	Study criteria	Interventional outcome	Clinical outcome	Reference
Multicenter Randomized Clinical Trial of Endovascular Treatment for Acute Ischemic Stroke in the Netherlands (MR CLEAN)	2015	Rando-mized, contr-olled	Intra-arterial treatment + usual care versus usual care alone	500 (233 intra-arterial treatment [81% stent retriever]; 267 control)	Proximal anterior circulation occlusions, NIHSS ≥ 2, treated within 6 hours	58.7% TICI 2b or 3 score with intervention	13.5% increase in rate of functional independence (90-day mRS ≤ 2) with intra-arterial intervention (32.6 versus 19.1%; $p < 0.05$). No significant difference in mortality or symptomatic intracerebral hemorrhage	[5]
Endovascular Treatment for Small Core and Anterior Circulation Proximal Occlusion With Emphasis on Minimizing CT to Recanalization Times (ESCAPE)	2015	Rando-mized, contr-olled	Intra-arterial treatment + usual care versus usual care alone	316 (165 intra-arterial treatment [78% stent retriever]; 150 control)	Proximal anterior circulation occlusions, moderate-to-good collateral circulation, small infarct core, treated within 12 hours	72.4% TICI 2b or 3 score with intervention	23.7% increase in functional independence (90-day mRS ≤ 2) with intra-arterial intervention (53.0 versus 29.3%, $p < 0.05$) and a decrease in 90-day mortality (10.4 versus 19.0%; $p = 0.04$)	[16]
Solitaire FR With the Intention for Thrombectomy as Primary	2015	Rando-mized, contr-olled	Stent-retriever thrombectomy + usual care	196 (98 stent retriever; 98 control)	Proximal anterior circulation occlusions,	88% rate of substantial reperfusion	25% increase in functional independence (90-day mRS ≤ 2)	[17]

Trial name	Year	Study design	Groups	Number of patients	Study criteria	Interventional outcome	Clinical outcome	Reference
Endovascular Treatment of Acute Ischemic Stroke (SWIFT PRIME)			versus usual care alone		no large ischemic core, treated within 6 hours		with intervention (60 versus 35%, $p < 0.001$). No significant difference in 90-day mortality or symptomatic intracranial hemorrhage	
Extending the Time for Thrombolysis in Emergency Neurological Deficits – Intra-Arterial (EXTEND-IA)	2015	Rando-mized, contr-olled	Stent-retriever thrombectomy + usual care versus usual care alone	70 (35 stent retriever; 35 control)	Proximal anterior circulation occlusions, no large ischemic core, treated within 6 hours	86% TICI 2b or 3 score with intervention	31% increase in functional independence (90-day mRS ≤ 2) with intervention (71 versus 40%; $p = 0.01$). No significant difference in 90-day mortality or symptomatic intracranial hemorrhage	[18]
Endovascular Revascularization With Solitaire Device Versus Best Medical Therapy in Anterior Circulation Stroke Within 8 Hours (REVASCAT)	2015	Rando-mized, contr-olled	Stent-retriever thrombectomy + usual care versus usual care alone	206 (103 intervention [98 stent retriever]; 103 control)	Proximal anterior circulation occlusions, no large ischemic core, treated within 8 hours	65.7% TICI 2b or 3 score with intervention	15.5% increase in functional independence (90-day mRS ≤ 2) with intervention (43.7 versus 28.2%, $p < 0.05$). No significant difference in 90-	[19]

Trial name	Year	Study design	Groups	Number of patients	Study criteria	Interventional outcome	Clinical outcome	Reference
							day mortality or symptomatic intracranial hemorrhage	

Abbreviations: mRS, modified Rankin Scale; TICI, thrombolysis in cerebral infarction score.

Table 2. Summary of randomized controlled trials for mechanical thrombectomy in stroke.

The Extending the Time for Thrombolysis in Emergency Neurological Deficits – Intra-Arterial (EXTEND-IA) trial was designed similarly to SWIFT PRIME and enrolled 70 patients with confirmed proximal anterior circulation occlusions and the absence of a large ischemic core that could be treated within 6 hours of symptom onset [18]. Again, the effects of intravenous tPA (control) versus intravenous tPA plus stent-retriever thrombectomy (intervention) were assessed, and this study was also terminated early after an interim analysis demonstrated clear treatment efficacy. The 35 patients in the intervention group had a median time from qualifying imaging to groin puncture of 93 minutes. A modified TICI 2b or 3 score was achieved in 86% of patients in the intervention group. This study reported a significant increase in ischemic territory reperfusion at 24 hours with intervention (median 100 versus 37%; $p < 0.001$) and increased neurologic improvement at 3 days (80 versus 37%; $p < 0.01$). They also report a 31% increase in functional independence (90-day mRS ≤ 2) with intervention (71 versus 40%; $p = 0.01$), with no significant difference in rate of symptomatic intracerebral hemorrhage or death.

The Endovascular Revascularization with Solitaire Device Versus Best Medical Therapy in Anterior Circulation Stroke within 8 Hours (REVASCAT) trial enrolled 206 patients with occlusion of the proximal anterior circulation and the absence of a large ischemic core who could be treated within 8 hours of symptom onset [19]. The effects of stent-retriever thrombectomy plus standard medical therapy (intervention) versus standard medical therapy alone (control; including intravenous tPA, if eligible) were assessed. This study was terminated early after an interim analysis demonstrated clear treatment efficacy. Ninty-eight of the 103 patients in the intervention group underwent thrombectomy, with a median time from stroke onset to groin puncture of 269 minutes. A modified TICI 2b or 3 score was achieved in 65.7% of patients in the intervention group. This study reported a 15.5% increase in functional independence (90-day mRS ≤ 2) with intervention (43.7 versus 28.2%, $p < 0.05$; a primary study outcome). Secondary functional outcomes including 90-day BI, NIHSS, and EQ-5D all favored the intervention group, as did the median 24-hour infarct volume. There were no significant differences between the intervention and control groups in 90-day mortality or symptomatic intracranial hemorrhage.

These five trials clearly demonstrate the therapeutic efficacy of mechanical thrombectomy with stent retrievers in stroke patients with LVO. The dramatic results from these studies (with multiple trials being stopped early for treatment efficacy) demanded a rapid update of clinical guidelines.

4. Updates of stoke treatment guidelines: role of mechanical thrombectomy

In response to the above trials and other recent smaller studies, in 2015 the American Heart Association (AHA) and American Stroke Association (ASA) released a focused update of the 2013 guidelines for the endovascular treatment of patients presenting with acute ischemic stroke [20].

These updated guidelines fall under several classifications of recommendation and levels of evidence. Class I recommendations imply that the benefits of the suggested procedure well outweighs the potential risks, and therefore indicate that the treatment should be administered. Class IIa recommendations indicate a moderate outweighing of benefit over risk and suggest that a treatment is reasonable to consider performing, but further studies are needed to ensure appropriate clinical application. Class IIb recommendations indicate that the benefits of the procedure may or may not outweigh its associated risks, and these procedures may be considered, although higher classifications of treatment recommendations take priority. Evidence pertaining to individual recommendations is stratified by level, indicating the strength of supporting data. Level A indicates that multiple populations have been evaluated and that data supporting the recommendation has been derived from multiple trials. Level B indicates that fewer populations have been evaluated or that the data supporting the recommendation has been derived from a single trial. Level C data indicates that the only data supporting the recommendation are the opinions of experts, case studies, or current standard of care [26].

A summary of the AHA/ASA 2015 guidelines detailing recommendations for treatment of patients using mechanical thrombectomy is as follows [20]. If patients meet all of the following criteria, mechanical thrombectomy using stent retriever is indicated and should be performed (Class I, Level of Evidence A): (a) prestroke mRS (modified Rankin Scale) score of 0 or 1, (b) presentation of acute ischemic stroke and receiving intravenous tPA within 4.5 hours of symptom onset, (c) causative occlusion of internal carotid artery or proximal MCA (M1), (d) age of at least 18 years, (e) NIHSS score of at least 6, (f) Alberta Stroke Program Early CT score (ASPECTS) of at least 6, and (g) treatment that can be initiated within 6 hours of symptom onset.

Importantly, eligible patients should receive tPA even if endovascular treatments are being considered, and contrary to previous guidelines, observation of patients after administration of tPA for clinical response is no longer required nor recommended prior to initiation of endovascular treatment (Class III, Level of Evidence B [randomized data]). Additionally, the ASA states that the use of stent retrievers is preferable to the MERCI device (Class I, Level of Evidence A) and that the use of alternate mechanical thrombectomy devices aside from stent retrievers may be acceptable in some cases (Class IIb, Level of Evidence B [non-randomized data]) [20].

The new guidelines have also stipulated that the ultimate goal of mechanical thrombectomy should be a modified TICI score of 2b/3 in angiographic imaging (Class I, Level of Evidence A), as early as possible and within 6 hours of stroke onset (Class I, Level of Evidence B [randomized]) [20]. If mechanical thrombectomy following intravenous tPA administration is not adequate to achieve this angiographic result, the use of additional adjuncts including intra-arterial fibrinolysis is indicated to maximize the angiographic result (Class IIb, Level of Evidence B [randomized]). The treatment efficacy of mechanical thrombectomy initiated longer than 6 hours from symptom onset is unknown; however, additional trials are needed to determine the clinical benefit in this setting [20].

While adhering to the above recommendations is ideal for maximal clinical benefit, acute ischemic stroke patients are heterogeneous. The ASA thus included alternate recommendations for patient subpopulations/clinical situations not covered above. These expanded recommendations are as follows [20]. The use of stent retrievers alone is reasonable in patients presenting with anterior circulation occlusion even when intravenous tPA is contraindicated (i.e., outside of time window, prior stroke, head trauma, hemorrhagic coagulopathy, etc.) (Class IIa, Level of Evidence C). However, there is currently inadequate data definitively determining the clinical efficacy of monotherapy alone for this patient cohort. Intra-arterial fibrinolysis may be considered in these patients, but the clinical benefit of this approach has also yet to be established (Class IIb, Level of Evidence C).

Although no study-based evidence exists, the ASA recommendations include the use of stent retrievers in patients experiencing causative occlusions of the M2 or M3 portions of the MCA, anterior cerebral artery, vertebral arteries, basilar arteries, and posterior cerebral arteries, if treatment can be initiated within 6 hours of symptom onset (Class IIa, Level of Evidence C). Stent retrievers may also be appropriate in treatment of patients under 18 years of age with occlusion of large vessels and patients with an mRS score of >1, an ASPECTS score <6, or an NIHSS score <6 who present with causative occlusions of the internal carotid artery or proximal MCA (M1) (Class IIb, Level of Evidence C). However, randomized trials are required to provide data on the clinical efficacy of stent-retriever usage in such patients.

Additionally, the updated guidelines discuss multiple technical aspects of endovascular intervention in strokes [20]. Specifically, they state the use of a proximal balloon guide catheter or a large-bore distal access catheter to provide flow stasis, and/or simultaneous aspiration as opposed to a cervical guide catheter alone during stent-retriever thrombectomy may be beneficial (Class IIa, Level of Evidence C). Future studies are nonetheless needed to determine the optimal technical approach with regard to recanalization and distal embolization rates. They also state that angioplasty and stenting of proximal cervical atherosclerotic stenoses or occlusions at the time of thrombectomy are reasonable (Class IIb, Level of Evidence C), although the utility of this intervention is currently unknown.

Lastly, the guidelines addressed the issue of conscious sedations versus general anesthesia during mechanical thrombectomy. However, given a lack of randomized trial data, they state that anesthetic selection should be patient-based after considering individual risk factors, tolerance of procedure, other clinical characteristics, and evaluation of a patient's medical history [20].

5. Future considerations in mechanical thrombectomy

Despite being the new gold standard for large vessel acute stroke, there remain multiple unknown technical and clinical variables regarding the optimization of mechanical thrombectomy for strokes. As alluded to in the above guideline summary, outstanding clinical questions requiring further study include the use of adjunct imaging modalities to further define an acceptable pre-intervention ischemic core/penumbra (e.g., CT-perfusion/diffusion and perfusion-weighted imaging), the utility of simultaneous lesional catheter aspiration versus standard carotid balloon occlusion, the efficacy of thrombectomy in the posterior circulation, and the maximal acceptable timing of intervention from symptom onset.

Moreover, many technical aspects of the devices employed are still being optimized. Future device designs will center on reduction of the endothelial footprint both by changing device design and optimizing device size relative to the vasculature. Additionally, reduction of embolic complications beyond those afforded by direct lesional aspiration, and increasing first pass success, will be major driving forces behind future iterations of stent-retriever devices.

Guiding these changes is a fundamental inquiry into stroke physiology, and how device characteristics beyond efficacy of clot removal can affect outcomes. For example, an area of ongoing and future study is the potential role of iatrogenic endothelial damage on post-thrombectomy secondary neurologic injury (**Figure 1**). The potential importance of endothelial injury becomes apparent upon close analysis of existing clinical data. Specifically, while the initial equivocal thrombectomy clinical trial data is likely due in part to lower recanalization rates than with more recent studies [4, 5, 16–19, 21, 22], another potential explanation may relate to the increased iatrogenic endothelial injury generated by older thrombectomy devices when studied in both in vitro and in vivo models [25]. When combined with the known deleterious effects of physiologic blood flow disruptions on endothelial cell homeostasis and cytokine signaling [27–37], these findings necessitate future studies to determine how iatrogenic endothelial damage affects secondary neuronal injury in post-thrombectomy stroke patients. This line of study is critical to next generation device design.

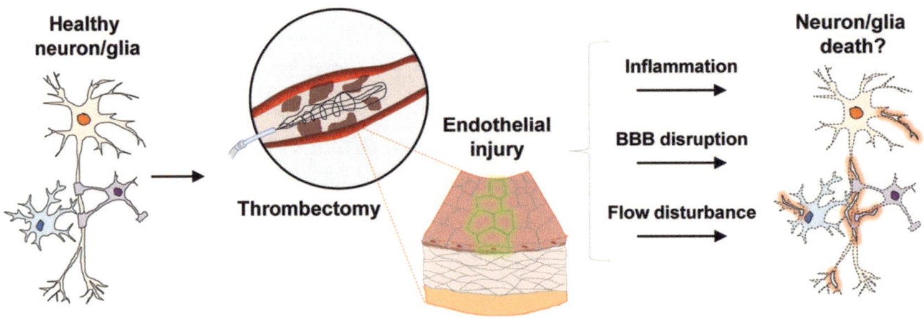

Figure 1. Schematic illustration of the potential negative effects of iatrogenic endothelial damage during thrombectomy on downstream neurons/glia. Proposed deleterious mechanisms include upregulation of inflammatory pathways, blood-brain barrier (BBB) disruption, and flow disturbances. Ongoing work to understand these effects will inform future thrombectomy device design.

http://dx.doi.org/10.5772/64398

In summary, mechanical thrombectomy for selected patients with large vessel acute stroke is the new standard of care based on overwhelming clinical efficacy data. Future studies and technical and procedural refinements will undoubtedly increase the indications for this intervention.

Acknowledgements

The authors acknowledge Victor W. Wong for contributing his original artwork to this chapter.

Author details

Robert C. Rennert, Arvin R. Wali, Christine Carico, Jeffrey Scott Pannell and Alexander A. Khalessi*

*Address all correspondence to: akhalessi@ucsd.edu

Department of Neurosurgery, University of California – San Diego, La Jolla, California, USA

References

[1] Redon J, Olsen MH, Cooper RS, Zurriaga O, Martinez-Beneito MA, Laurent S, et al. Stroke mortality and trends from 1990 to 2006 in 39 countries from Europe and Central Asia: implications for control of high blood pressure. Eur Heart J 2011;32:1424–1431.

[2] Brouns R, De Deyn PP. The complexity of neurobiological processes in acute ischemic stroke. Clin Neurol Neurosurg 2009;111:483–495.

[3] Joo H, George MG, Fang J, Wang G. A literature review of indirect costs associated with stroke. J Stroke Cerebrovasc Dis 2014;23:1753–1763.

[4] Broderick JP, Palesch YY, Demchuk AM, Yeatts SD, Khatri P, Hill MD, et al. Endovascular therapy after intravenous t-PA versus t-PA alone for stroke. N Engl J Med 2013;368:893–903.

[5] Berkhemer OA, Fransen PS, Beumer D, van den Berg LA, Lingsma HF, Yoo AJ, et al. A randomized trial of intraarterial treatment for acute ischemic stroke. N Engl J Med 2015;372:11–20.

[6] Camak DJ. Addressing the burden of stroke caregivers: a literature review. J Clin Nurs 2015;24:2376–2382.

[7] Doyle KP, Simon RP, Stenzel-Poore MP. Mechanisms of ischemic brain damage. Neuropharmacology 2008;55:310–318.

[8] Lee Y, Lee SR, Choi SS, Yeo HG, Chang KT, Lee HJ. Therapeutically targeting neuroinflammation and microglia after acute ischemic stroke. Biomed Res Int 2014;2014:297241.

[9] Hacke W, Donnan G, Fieschi C, Kaste M, von Kummer R, Broderick JP, et al. Association of outcome with early stroke treatment: pooled analysis of ATLANTIS, ECASS, and NINDS rt-PA stroke trials. Lancet 2004;363:768–774.

[10] Del Zoppo GJ, Saver JL, Jauch EC, Adams HP, Council AHAS. Expansion of the time window for treatment of acute ischemic stroke with intravenous tissue plasminogen activator: a science advisory from the American Heart Association/American Stroke Association. Stroke 2009;40:2945–2948.

[11] Chapman SN, Mehndiratta P, Johansen MC, McMurry TL, Johnston KC, Southerland AM. Current perspectives on the use of intravenous recombinant tissue plasminogen activator (tPA) for treatment of acute ischemic stroke. Vasc Health Risk Manag 2014;10:75–87.

[12] Hargis M, Shah JN, Mazabob J, Rao CV, Suarez JI, Bershad EM. Barriers to administering intravenous tissue plasminogen activator (tPA) for acute ischemic stroke in the emergency department: a cross-sectional survey of stroke centers. Clin Neurol Neurosurg 2015;135:79–84.

[13] Miller DJ, Simpson JR, Silver B. Safety of thrombolysis in acute ischemic stroke: a review of complications, risk factors, and newer technologies. Neurohospitalist 2011;1:138–147.

[14] del Zoppo GJ, Poeck K, Pessin MS, Wolpert SM, Furlan AJ, Ferbert A, et al. Recombinant tissue plasminogen activator in acute thrombotic and embolic stroke. Ann Neurol 1992;32:78–86.

[15] Bhatia R, Hill MD, Shobha N, Menon B, Bal S, Kochar P, et al. Low rates of acute recanalization with intravenous recombinant tissue plasminogen activator in ischemic stroke: real-world experience and a call for action. Stroke 2010;41:2254–2258.

[16] Goyal M, Demchuk AM, Menon BK, Eesa M, Rempel JL, Thornton J, et al. Randomized assessment of rapid endovascular treatment of ischemic stroke. N Engl J Med 2015;372:1019–1030.

[17] Saver JL, Goyal M, Bonafe A, Diener HC, Levy EI, Pereira VM, et al. Stent-retriever thrombectomy after intravenous t-PA vs. t-PA alone in stroke. N Engl J Med 2015;372:2285–2295.

[18] Campbell BC, Mitchell PJ, Kleinig TJ, Dewey HM, Churilov L, Yassi N, et al. Endovascular therapy for ischemic stroke with perfusion-imaging selection. N Engl J Med 2015;372:1009–1018.

[19] Jovin TG, Chamorro A, Cobo E, de Miquel MA, Molina CA, Rovira A, et al. Thrombectomy within 8 hours after symptom onset in ischemic stroke. N Engl J Med 2015;372:2296–2306.

[20] Powers WJ, Derdeyn CP, Biller J, Coffey CS, Hoh BL, Jauch EC, et al. 2015 American Heart Association/American Stroke Association Focused update of the 2013 guidelines for the early management of patients with acute ischemic stroke regarding endovascular treatment: a guideline for healthcare professionals from the American Heart Association/American Stroke Association. Stroke 2015;46:3020–3035.

[21] Kidwell CS, Jahan R, Gornbein J, Alger JR, Nenov V, Ajani Z, et al. A trial of imaging selection and endovascular treatment for ischemic stroke. N Engl J Med 2013;368:914–923.

[22] Ciccone A, Valvassori L, Nichelatti M, Sgoifo A, Ponzio M, Sterzi R, et al. Endovascular treatment for acute ischemic stroke. N Engl J Med 2013;368:904–913.

[23] Saver JL, Jahan R, Levy EI, Jovin TG, Baxter B, Nogueira RG, et al. Solitaire flow restoration device versus the Merci Retriever in patients with acute ischaemic stroke (SWIFT): a randomised, parallel-group, non-inferiority trial. Lancet 2012;380:1241–1249.

[24] Nogueira RG, Lutsep HL, Gupta R, Jovin TG, Albers GW, Walker GA, et al. Trevo versus Merci retrievers for thrombectomy revascularisation of large vessel occlusions in acute ischaemic stroke (TREVO 2): a randomised trial. Lancet 2012;380:1231–1240.

[25] Teng D, Pannell JS, Rennert RC, Li J, Li YS, Wong VW, et al. Endothelial trauma from mechanical thrombectomy in acute stroke: in vitro live-cell platform with animal validation. Stroke 2015;46:1099–1106.

[26] Agency for Healthcare Research and Quality (AHRQ). Assessing Cardiovascular Risk: Guideline Synthesis. AHRQ. http://www.medscape.com/viewarticle/759314_9. Published: March 1, 2012. Accessed: March 17, 2016.

[27] Galbraith CG, Skalak R, Chien S. Shear stress induces spatial reorganization of the endothelial cell cytoskeleton. Cell Motil Cytoskeleton 1998;40:317–330.

[28] Wu CC, Li YS, Haga JH, Kaunas R, Chiu JJ, Su FC, et al. Directional shear flow and Rho activation prevent the endothelial cell apoptosis induced by micropatterned anisotropic geometry. Proc Natl Acad Sci U S A 2007;104:1254–1259.

[29] Chen BP, Li YS, Zhao Y, Chen KD, Li S, Lao J, et al. DNA microarray analysis of gene expression in endothelial cells in response to 24-h shear stress. Physiol Genomics 2001;7:55–63.

[30] Butler PJ, Norwich G, Weinbaum S, Chien S. Shear stress induces a time- and position-dependent increase in endothelial cell membrane fluidity. Am J Physiol Cell Physiol 2001;280:C962–969.

[31] Hu YL, Lu S, Szeto KW, Sun J, Wang Y, Lasheras JC, et al. FAK and paxillin dynamics at focal adhesions in the protrusions of migrating cells. Sci Rep 2014;4:6024.

[32] Zhou J, Li YS, Wang KC, Chien S. Epigenetic mechanism in regulation of endothelial function by disturbed flow: Induction of DNA hypermethylation by DNMT1. Cell Mol Bioeng 2014;7:218–224.

[33] Wang KC, Nguyen P, Weiss A, Yeh YT, Chien HS, Lee A, et al. MicroRNA-23b regulates cyclin-dependent kinase-activating kinase complex through cyclin H repression to modulate endothelial transcription and growth under flow. Arterioscler Thromb Vasc Biol 2014;34:1437–1445.

[34] Hur SS, del Alamo JC, Park JS, Li YS, Nguyen HA, Teng D, et al. Roles of cell confluency and fluid shear in 3-dimensional intracellular forces in endothelial cells. Proc Natl Acad Sci U S A 2012;109:11110–11115.

[35] del Alamo JC, Norwich GN, Li YS, Lasheras JC, Chien S. Anisotropic rheology and directional mechanotransduction in vascular endothelial cells. Proc Natl Acad Sci U S A 2008;105:15411–15416.

[36] Wang Y, Chang J, Chen KD, Li S, Li JY, Wu C, et al. Selective adapter recruitment and differential signaling networks by VEGF vs. shear stress. Proc Natl Acad Sci U S A 2007;104:8875–8879.

[37] Zhou J, Wang KC, Wu W, Subramaniam S, Shyy JY, Chiu JJ, et al. MicroRNA-21 targets peroxisome proliferators-activated receptor-alpha in an autoregulatory loop to modulate flow-induced endothelial inflammation. Proc Natl Acad Sci U S A 2011;108:10355–10360.

Chapter 10

Large Artery Occlusive Disease

John W. Cole and Christopher A. Stack

Additional information is available at the end of the chapter

http://dx.doi.org/10.5772/65047

Abstract

Extracranial and intracranial large artery atherosclerosis is often identified as a potential etiologic cause for ischemic stroke and transient ischemic attack (TIA). Given the high prevalence of large artery atherosclerosis in the general population, optimally treating each patient to minimize future stroke risk is paramount. To optimally define treatment, as based upon the individual patient's history, examination, and anatomical imaging findings, clinicians can compartmentalize this disease entity into four distinct clinical scenarios: 1(a) asymptomatic and 1(b) symptomatic extracranial carotid stenosis, (2) intracranial atherosclerosis, and (3) atherosclerotic vertebrobasilar disease. In this chapter, we work to provide a framework for clinicians evaluating and treating such patients.

Keywords: ischemic stroke, large artery atherosclerosis, risk factors, prevention, treatment, extracranial, intracranial, atherosclerosis, carotid stenosis, carotid endarterectomy, carotid angioplasty, stenting

1. Introduction

Large artery atherosclerosis (LAA) of the head and neck is responsible for approximately 15% of all ischemic strokes. The identification and appropriate treatment of such atherosclerotic lesions is an essential skill for all physicians diagnosing and treating stroke patients. Broadly, LAA lesions can be classified into four distinct clinical scenarios as based upon the individual patient's anatomical and clinical findings, and these include the following: 1(a) asymptomatic and 1(b) symptomatic extracranial carotid stenosis, (2) intracranial atherosclerotic disease, and (3) atherosclerotic disease of the vertebrobasilar system. While each of these scenarios' anatomical lesion locations differs, it is important to note that they all share the same risk-factor profiles and somewhat overlapping treatment options. In short, continuous vascular risk-factor optimization via sustained behavioral modifications and intensive medical therapy is critical to prevent stroke in the setting of LAA. In fact, specific to the settings of intracranial and vertebrobasilar atherosclerosis, as well as asymptomatic carotid atherosclerosis, risk-factor modification is the *primary* treatment option. In symptomatic patients with extracranial atherosclerosis treatment, options also include revascularization procedures including carotid endarterectomy (CEA) and carotid artery stenting (CAS). Appropriate patient selection and timing of such revascularization procedures must be considered. Options in symptomatic intracranial occlusive disease also include stenting vs. medical therapy, but again medical therapy is the primary treatment modality. Across each of these four clinical situations, the results of numerous randomized and nonrandomized clinical trials have led to periodically updated meta-analyses and consensus guidelines that provide evidence-based recommendations for practicing clinicians. While each of these four clinical situations could easily be (and are often) the subject of independent reviews, in this chapter we aim to provide a framework for clinicians evaluating and treating patients across these four clinical scenarios, emphasizing key considerations, clinical trial evidence, and the most recent professional and societal guidelines.

2. Common considerations across all cases of large artery atherosclerosis

Clinical presentation: Defining an ischemic stroke or transient ischemic attack (TIA) as causally related to LAA lesion can be difficult, as each individual patient's symptomatology and workup results can be quite varied. First, it is important to determine if the identified LAA lesion is proximal to a vascular territory that corresponds to the patients' stroke on imaging or symptoms in the setting of a TIA. For example, vague TIA symptoms such as 'transient dizziness or lightheadedness' could potentially infer a posterior circulation etiology but do not necessitate this fact. Such symptoms could also occur in the setting of cardiac arrhythmias or dehydration. More definitive symptoms such as transient diplopia or dysmetria increase the likelihood of a posterior circulation TIA. Again, vague symptoms such as 'transient dizziness or lightheadedness' should also not be utilized to classify a patient as 'symptomatic' for the purposes of managing anterior circulation carotid artery stenosis. To optimize anatomical localization (anterior vs. posterior circulation) in the setting of both stroke and TIA, clinicians must take a detailed history asking about symptoms (e.g., weakness, sensory changes, vision changes, balance problems, etc.) and whether these occurred in isolation or previously, both over the near and long term. Positive imaging demonstrating a clearly defined stroke can make the LAA etiologic diagnosis easier, assuming that the stroke is located in a vascular territory distal to a highly stenosed vessel and/or an irregularly calcified plaque. Stroke in a 'watershed' pattern distal to an LAA lesion might infer a hypoperfusional etiology, which may be related to acute changes in blood pressure (BP). However, similar imaging findings can also be seen in the setting of acute changes to an LAA plaque morphologically via plaque rupture or an embolus from a more proximal source reducing lumen diameter; such situations can impede flow distally resulting in reduced perfusion. Tandem lesions in the same vascular territory can also yield brain regions more at risk for hypoperfusion, as often there are sequential pressure drops across each LAA lesion. Such findings complicate management, as predicting whether an acute intervention would help reduce risk becomes more difficult. Further, guideline recommendations in such settings are limited. In summary, LAA can lead to two primary mechanisms of ischemic symptomatology: embolic phenomena and regional brain hypoperfusion. Clearly embolic phenomena should be considered as symptomatic, necessitating clinicians to consider the potential revascularization procedures as to be discussed later in this chapter. Stroke in the setting of LAA hypoperfusional states, while symptomatic, offers additional choices such as intensive medical therapy or permissive hypertension (HTN), thereby allowing the individual patient time to develop improved collateral circulatory pathways, potentially reducing the need for a revascularization procedure.

Workup: All stroke and suspected TIA patients warrant an expedited evaluation that can be simply defined as from '*heart to head*.' In other words, evaluations of the heart, the proximal aorta, the vasculature of the head and neck, as well as clinical and laboratory testing related to vascular risk factors, should be performed on an *inpatient* basis. While it is beyond the scope of this chapter to provide detailed testing recommendations, ideally a transthoracic echocardiogram (TTE) and vessel imaging of the head and neck by computed tomographic angiography (CTA) or magnetic resonance angiography (MRA) should be performed in all stroke and TIA patients. If LAA disease is identified, further testing to better define the severity of the stenosis should be considered; such testing might include carotid Doppler studies to determine flow velocities or a gadolinium (GAD)-enhanced magnetic resonance angiography (MRA) of the vasculature in question, among others. While a catheter-based cerebral angiogram can be considered, this invasive test has its own procedural risk and should be reserved for select patients, potentially including those with an 'intention to treat' via CAS. Of note, there is considerable clinical interest and ongoing research regarding the stability and embolic potential of LAA lesions, this in an effort to identify those patients at the greatest risk for stroke. Currently employed techniques include transcranial Doppler (TCD) microembolus detection, ulceration assessment using three-dimensional ultrasound, plaque echolucency measures, intraplaque hemorrhage on MRI, and plaque inflammation evaluations via hybrid-imaging techniques combining positron emission tomography (PET) and MRI [1]. Of these, TCD embolus detection is a relatively straightforward test that can be utilized to assist in individual patient risk stratification.

Vascular risk factors: Across all locations of LAA discussed in this chapter, continuous lifelong vascular risk-factor optimization via sustained behavioral (lifestyle) modifications and intensive medical therapy is critical for stroke prevention. This point cannot be emphasized enough. Over approximately the last 10 or so years, our understanding of the importance of medical management in the setting of atherosclerosis has markedly improved. Population-wide improved control of hypertension, dyslipidemia, and diabetes coupled with a reduction in tobacco use has resulted in a decline in stroke mortality from the third leading cause of death to the fifth cause of death in the USA [2]. Clinicians should take pride in these facts, as these improvements are based upon their efforts implementing professional societal position statements and guidelines. As such, maintaining a working knowledge of these evolving guidelines and position statements is a critical tool for physicians and other health professionals working to reduce stroke risk. The reduction of cardiovascular disease (CVD) and stroke related to lifestyle management, treatment of blood cholesterol, and management of obesity was the focus of statements in 2013 by the American College of Cardiology (ACC) and the American Heart Association (AHA) [3–6]. They also released a statement regarding hypertension management in collaboration with the Centers for Disease Control (CDC) [7]. Other professional societies, including the Eighth Joint National Committee (JNC 8) and the American Society of Hypertension/International Society of Hypertension, released separate statements about minimizing cardiovascular risk and complications with optimization of blood pressure [8, 9]. The American Heart Association and the American Stroke Association (ASA) also released new Guidelines for the Primary Prevention of Stroke in 2014 [10] and Guidelines for the Prevention of Stroke in Patients with Stroke and Transient Ischemic Attack [11]. These recent stroke-prevention guidelines offer individualized approach to lifestyle modification including physical activity, diet and nutrition, smoking cessation, obesity, and dyslipidemia. Taken in aggregate, these new guidelines offer up-to-date comprehensive evidence-based recommendations for the primary and secondary prevention of stroke, including those related to LAA. While it is beyond the scope of this chapter to cover all the current recommendations regarding vascular risk-factor control in detail, a few specifics as related to LAA are warranted.

3. Vascular risk-factor control via intensive medical therapy

Based upon the results of numerous recent clinical trials, and as incorporated into the aforementioned recent guidelines, 'intensive (or best) medical therapy' is emphasized for all LAA patients. While the precise definition of intensive medical therapy can be debated, **Table 1** (adapted from [12]) summarizes the key elements. Intensive medical therapy includes smoking cessation, diet, exercise, and control of blood pressure (including diagnosis of the physiological drivers of resistant hypertension by measuring plasma renin and aldosterone [13], dual antiplatelet therapy, and intensive lipid-lowering therapy, not just achieving a target level of fasting low-density lipoprotein (LDL) cholesterol). Overall, the goals of these therapies are to first stop, and then reverse plaque progression. Such regimens clearly are effective. One study demonstrated that by implementing a regimen similar to that as outlined in **Table 1**, they were able to reduce the risk of stroke and myocardial infarction by more than 80% among patients with asymptomatic carotid stenosis [14]. Similarly, the Stenting and Aggressive Medical Management for Prevention of Recurrent Stroke in Intracranial Stenosis (SAMPPRIS) trial [15] demonstrated that "aggressive" medical therapy resulted in better outcomes than with stenting among patients with intracranial stenosis. Several other examples exist.

Antiplatelet agents, including aspirin and clopidogrel, are routinely used for primary and secondary stroke prevention in the setting of LAA. In higher-risk individuals, whose 10-year risk of stroke is greater than 10% and whose risk of stroke outweighs the risks associated with aspirin therapy, the new Guidelines for the Primary Prevention of Stroke recommend the daily use of aspirin [10]. A cardiovascular risk calculator to assist in estimating 10-year risk can be found online at http://my.americanheart.org/cvriskcalculator. Of note, in lower-risk individuals, aspirin is not recommended for primary stroke prevention, or in individuals with diabetes that do not have other high-risk factors. For those using aspirin, the faithful daily use of low-dose aspirin is deemed sufficient. Since coated aspirin is less efficacious than uncoated aspirin in ~40% of individuals, uncoated aspirin is recommended [16]. Clopidogrel alone reduces stroke by only 1.7% greater than aspirin [17] and is thus only marginally better than aspirin, whereas combined aspirin/dipyridamole is no better than clopidogrel [18]. The SAMPPRIS study indicated that the combination of clopidogrel and aspirin is more efficacious for secondary stroke prevention than aspirin alone, with a reduction of stroke by 32% (hazard ratio (HR): 0.68; 95% confidence interval (CI): 0.57–0.81; $p < 0.001$) and no increase in major hemorrhage [19]. More recently, the CHANCE investigators demonstrated that the early benefit of clopidogrel-aspirin treatment in reducing the risk of subsequent stroke persisted after 1 year of follow-up [20]. Again, there was no difference in moderate or severe hemorrhage in the combined treatment group vs. the aspirin-alone group (0.3 vs. 0.4%, respectively; $p = 0.44$) [21]. Dual antiplatelet therapy with aspirin and clopidogrel was also used in the SAMPPRIS trial of intracranial arterial stenosis, which demonstrated that aggressive medical management was superior to percutaneous transluminal angioplasty and stenting [15]. Of note, the CHANCE study was performed in China, but the results are thought to be generalizable in Western populations; this hypothesis is currently being evaluated in the ongoing POINT trial [22].

Several recent studies utilizing transcranial Doppler evaluations to evaluate for microemboli found that dual antiplatelet therapy is more efficacious than aspirin alone in the reduction of microemboli for both intracranial [21] and extracranial arterial stenosis [23]. While dual antiplatelet therapy is commonly used for risk reduction in the setting of coronary disease, particularly in the setting of cardiac stenting, it is not widely used in carotid disease as related to the results of one study in which there was an excess of bleeding in the dual therapy group [24]. To reduce the risk of intracerebral hemorrhage (ICH) in the setting of dual therapy, effective blood pressure control is critical, as evidenced by the North American Symptomatic Carotid Endarterectomy Trial (NASCET) in which effective blood pressure control reduced ICH to 0.4% of strokes [25]. Gastrointestinal hemorrhages could theoretically be reduced by the identification and treatment of *Helicobacter pylori* infections prior to dual therapy, although this has yet to be definitively proven. In summary, dual antiplatelet therapy should at least be considered across most settings of LAA, including both symptomatic and asymptomatic carotid stenosis. The optimal duration of therapy remains a topic of study and debate, but as consistent with the SAMPPRIS study, 3 months of dual antiplatelet therapy is reasonable while working to optimize vascular risk factors.

Treatment of dyslipidemia has drastically shifted away from strict LDL goals in accord with the 2013 "ACC/AHA Guideline on the Treatment of Blood Cholesterol to Reduce Atherosclerotic Cardiovascular Risk in Adults" [5]. The guidelines now promote calculating an estimated 10-year risk for atherosclerotic CVD than determining the intensity of statin therapy. Although the new guidelines shift focus away from specific lipid targets, values for total cholesterol, high-density lipoprotein (HDL), age, sex, race, systolic blood pressure (SBP), hypertension treatment, diabetes mellitus (DM), and cigarette smoking are incorporated into the cardiovascular risk calculator (see previously listed link). Statins are the only lipid-modifying therapy with established benefit on ischemic stroke risk. This has been supported by meta-analysis of 78 trials with 266,973 patients demonstrating an odds ratio (OR) of 0.85 [95% CI: 0.78–0.92] for decreased risk of total stroke; however, diet, fibrates, and other treatments did not demonstrate benefit with OR of 0.92 [95% CI: 0.69–1.23], 0.98 [95% CI: 0.86–1.12], and 0.81 [95% CI: 0.61–1.08], respectively [26].

Measure	Intervention
Lifestyle modification	
•All	Show patients images of their plaque, compare the patient's plaque burden with that of healthy persons of the same age and sex, describe the risks associated with that degree of plaque burden and progression and the possibility of plaque regression
•Smoking cessation	Counseling, liberal nicotine replacement, varenicline or bupropion (depending on history of depression)
•Mediterranean diet	Counseling, provision of a booklet-summarizing advice, and providing recipes and links to Internet sites; repeated at follow-up visits as necessary
•Obesity	Counseling on caloric restriction, referral to dietician, bariatric surgery in refractory patients with severe obesity and diabetes or insulin resistance
•Exercise	Recommendations for moderate exercise at least 30 min a day, with advice tailored to the patient's disabilities if any
•Blood pressure	Advice on how to reduce salt intake, limit alcohol intake, avoid licorice, decongestants
Medical therapy	
•Blood pressure control	Physiologically individualized therapy for resistant hypertension based on renin/aldosterone profile 3; switch NSAIDs to sulindac4
•Lipid lowering	Statins dosed according to plaque progression to the highest dose tolerated (with use of CoQ10 to minimize myopathic symptoms), then addition of ezetimibe, and as needed for low HDL/high triglycerides, addition of fibrates and/or niacin
•Antiplatelet agents	Low-dose aspirin, with addition of clopidogrel in patients with severe stenosis or other indicators of high risk
•Anticoagulation	In patients with atrial fibrillation or other potential cardiac sources of emboli
•Insulin resistance	Pioglitazone, reinforcement of lifestyle issues
•Diabetes	Reinforcement of lifestyle changes, referral to diabetes clinic
Other considerations	
•Obstructive Sleep Apnea	Causes night-time high blood pressure. Referral for sleep study and faithful CPAP use.
•Poor dentition	Induces systemic inflammation that can destabilize atherosclerotic plaques. Dental evaluation.
•Gout	Induces systemic inflammation that can destabilize atherosclerotic plaques. Diagnose and treat.

Table 1. Key elements of intensive medical therapy (adapted from Spence [12]).

http://dx.doi.org/10.5772/65047

While a detailed discussion of all lipid-modifying medications is beyond the scope of this review, recent data regarding niacin use are worth mentioning. Niacin has several favorable properties, including increases in HDL cholesterol (HDL-C), decreased plasma levels of lipoprotein(a) (Lp(a)), inhibition of hepatic production of very-low-density lipoprotein (VLDL), and consequently its metabolite LDL [27]. It raises high-density lipoprotein cholesterol (HDL-C) levels by as much as 30–35%, both by reducing lipid transfer of cholesterol from HDL to VLDL and by delaying HDL clearance [27, 28]. While some early trials of niacin suggested secondary prevention benefits, recent large randomized trials of niacin have raised serious concerns about its safety and efficacy in combination with statin therapy, and by extension concerns about niacin monotherapy. AIM-HIGH found no additional benefit with the addition of extended release niacin to patients treated with a statin with cardiovascular disease, decreased HDL-C levels, and increased triglyceride levels [29]. Notably, the placebo arm received 100–200 mg of niacin daily resulting in HDL-C level increase, which may have reduced the ability to detect a statistically significant benefit. Second, the HPS2-THRIVE trial randomly assigned 25,673 adults aged 50–80 with vascular disease to receive extended-release niacin 2 g daily plus laropiprant (a prostaglandin D2 signal blocker used to reduce flushing from niacin) or placebo; all patients received simvastatin 40 mg daily, and if LDL-C reduction was inadequate with simvastatin, ezetimibe of 10 mg daily was added [30]. Patients in this trial had a long run-in phase demonstrating that they could tolerate simvastatin and then the addition of niacin/laropiprant. After a median follow-up of 3.9 years, there was no reduction with niacin/laropiprant in the primary end point of first major vascular event (13.2 vs. 13.7%; risk ratio [RR]: 0.96, 95% CI: 0.90–1.03) and there was also no benefit for this end point in the subgroup of patients with low HDL-C and elevated triglycerides. Despite the run-in period, there was also an increase in serious adverse events in those receiving niacin/laropiprant including myopathy (RR: 3.54), gastrointestinal side effects, and worsened glucose control with both an increase in new cases of diabetes (RR: 1.32) and serious disturbance in diabetes control (11.5 vs. 7.5%, RR: 1.55; most of these led to hospitalization). Given these results, it advised not to administer niacin to most patients receiving statin therapy. Patients who are unable to take other lipid-lowering therapies may consider long-term niacin therapy if their LDL-C is significantly elevated and is lowered substantially by a trial of niacin treatment.

Hypertension (HTN) is a well-documented and highly prevalent modifiable risk factor for stroke. In general, the most effective stroke prevention measure across all populations is the treatment of hypertension. Despite this, the optimal blood pressure (BP) target has not been elucidated and remains a subject of debate. While decreased BP is associated with reduced stroke risk, but this may not be ubiquitous across all patient populations, specifically those with flow limiting LAA, DM, or advanced age. Interestingly, a lack of definitive benefit from BP clinical trials among older populations was used as the basis to raise the systolic BP treatment goal recommendation from 140 to 150 mmHg in the JNC-8 guidelines [31]. Regardless of this highly controversial change, HTN is often undertreated and an individualized, multifaceted approach including lifestyle changes and medical therapy is emphasized.

Diabetes mellitus (DM) is a well-established risk factor for stroke. Optimal glucose control is achieved by reinforcing lifestyle changes (e.g., dietary, regular exercise, and weight loss) and through consistent use of medications. As related to LAA, the Atherosclerosis Risk in Communities (ARIC) Study demonstrated that the presence of DM was a predictor of carotid intima-media thickness (cIMT) progression ($p < 0.01$) [32]. In NOMAS, the duration of diabetes was independently associated with ischemic stroke risk when adjusting for risk factors [33]. The investigators found that the risk increased 3% each annually, and tripled among those with diabetes ≥10 years. Therefore, optimal glucose control is essential to reduce the risk of stroke.

Other emerging factors for LAA have been identified, including elevated homocysteine, fibrinogen, lipoprotein (a), and C-reactive protein levels [34]. Other risk factors implicated include obstructive sleep apnea [35], gout [36, 37], and poor dentition [38]. Future studies should work to verify the results of these preliminary reports while considering any implications for preventative strategies. From a genetic standpoint, a recently published study by the National Institute of Health/National Institute of Neurological Disorders and Stroke (NIH/NINDS) Genetics Network (SiGN) details the largest and most comprehensive genome-wide association (GWA) study of stroke and its subtypes ever performed [39]. This study verified several previous genetic associations with ischemic stroke and identified a new risk locus on chromosome 1p13. Of the replicated loci, it is notable that this report confirms the association between the *HDAC9* locus and LAA ischemic stroke. Interestingly, this same locus (and the same specific variant) that was also reproducibly associated with coronary artery disease suggests a shared underlying causal gene and mechanism. The novel locus identified by SiGN was detected near *TSPAN2* and was also found to be associated with LAA. TSPAN2 is a scaffolding protein expressed in large arteries. This locus has not been reproducibly associated with coronary artery disease in GWA studies, suggesting that *TSPAN2* is potentially specific to ischemic stroke and might therefore provide insight into the pathophysiology of LAA ischemic stroke, rather than just generic atherosclerosis. Studies regarding the mechanistic links between both *HDAC9* and *TSPAN2* with LAA stroke are ongoing. Given the rapid evolution of genomic medicine, it is anticipated that in the near future we will be able to genetically determine disease susceptibility within individuals, families, and populations, thereby allowing preventive stroke therapies as based on individualized genotype.

In summary, the most recent guidelines emphasize intensive medical therapy with a focus on optimal vascular risk-factor control, but now in a more patient-centered approach than in the past. Given that the results from multiple clinical trials drive these recommendations, the applicability of these results at the level of the individual can be confusing, particularly if an individual does not fulfill the clinical trial inclusion criteria driving the recommendations. As such, physicians should consider each patient on an individual basis, working to optimize their risk-factor profile over the long term as based on ever-changing guidelines and information. With so much ongoing research, the optimization of stroke prevention for individuals requires physician diligence to identify risk factors as they emerge and physician maintenance of knowledge to optimally control risk factors in the safest, expeditious, and cost-effective manner possible. While the described multifaceted approach of intensive medical therapy reduces stroke risk in all patients with LAA, broadly classifying LAA patients into one of four clinical scenarios as based upon the individual patient's history, examination, and anatomical imaging findings is a useful way to clarify individual treatment options. These four scenarios

http://dx.doi.org/10.5772/65047

are discussed now and include the following: 1(a) asymptomatic and 1(b) symptomatic extracranial carotid stenosis, (2) intracranial atherosclerosis, and (3) atherosclerotic vertebrobasilar disease.

4. Cervical extracranial carotid atherosclerosis

Carotid atherosclerosis accounts for ~10% of ischemic stroke cases. Although carotid artery stenosis is a risk factor for stroke, not every carotid stenosis carries the same risk for future stroke. Assuming a relevant stenosis is identified, key factors to consider include the degree of stenosis and the stability of the plaque, this in the setting of the individual patient. Clinicians should be geared toward answering two questions: (1) Which patients should opt for revascularization procedures (vs. intensive medical therapy alone) and (2) Which is the appropriate revascularization procedure (carotid endarterectomy [CEA] vs. carotid artery stenting [CAS])?

Assessment of carotid stenosis: When carotid stenosis produces a pressure drop across the lesion and/or a flow reduction distal to the lesion that is hemodynamically significant, this typically equates to 60% diameter reducing stenosis on catheter angiography via the North American method [10]. The formula is Stenosis = $(1 - N/D) \times 100\%$ (N = diameter at the point of maximum stenosis, D = diameter of the diameter of the arterial segment distal to the stenosis where the arterial walls first become parallel) [10]. This is contrasted with the European method, which estimates the stenosis at the internal carotid bulb. Catheter angiography, considered the 'gold standard' for assessing stenosis, historically carried a ≈1% risk of causing a stroke in patients with atherosclerotic disease; however, the complication rate has been dropping with the stroke complication rate now <0.2% [40]. Duplex ultrasound is the most commonly used method to screen the extracranial carotid artery for atherosclerotic stenosis and carries the lowest risks and costs. Of note, Duplex ultrasound may be insensitive to differentiate between high-grade stenosis from complete occlusion, with additional testing required in such situations. MRA, with or without contrast, is another noninvasive method for evaluating arterial anatomy and has the advantage of providing images of both the cervical and intracranial portions of the carotid artery and its proximal intracranial branches. Time of flight (TOF) MRA without contrast may overestimate the degree of stenosis, as such a GAD-enhanced MRA may be more useful, particularly when working to differentiate high-grade stenosis from total occlusion. Clinicians should be mindful that nephrogenic systemic fibrosis is a rare complication among patients with poor renal function in the setting of GAD use. CTA is yet another method that can be used to evaluate both the extracranial and intracranial carotid circulation. CTA disadvantages include radiation exposure and the need for intravenous injection of a contrast material, with a creatinine greater than 1.7 being a common limiting factor. Additionally, atherosclerotic calcifications with similar density to the contrast material may confound accurate measurements of the stenosis. On physical examination, a carotid bruit can reflect an underlying carotid stenosis; however, sensitivity is limited as evidenced by the NOMAS trial, in which auscultation had a sensitivity of 56% and a specificity of 98% [41].

4.1. Asymptomatic extracranial carotid stenosis

All patients with carotid stenosis have atherosclerosis that warrants intensive medical therapy that should be implemented as soon as possible. As mentioned, several methods exist to identify those patients with carotid stenosis who are at the greater risk for future events. Transcranial Doppler (TCD) embolus detection is a well-validated methodology exemplified by Spence et al. [42], where 10% of the 319 patients with asymptomatic carotid stenosis who have two or more microemboli in 1 h had a 1-year stroke risk of 15.6%. This was much higher than the complication rates of stenting and endarterectomy. Another telling result from that study was that a 1% one-year stroke risk was seen in 90% of patients without microemboli on TCD. This finding was replicated in a 2010 report of 468 patients [14], and further verified in the Asymptomatic Carotid Emboli Study (ACES) [43], among 467 patients. As mentioned previously, other methods exist to identify high-risk patients. As a general guideline, population screening for asymptomatic carotid artery stenosis is not recommended by the US Preventive Services Task Force, which found "no direct evidence that screening adults with duplex ultrasonography for asymptomatic stenosis reduces stroke [44]." In general, since ~2005, the risk of ipsilateral stroke with intensive medical therapy is much lower than the risk of CEA or CAS, this even in the carefully controlled clinical trials to be discussed. As such, in real-world practice the risk of an intervention would be even higher than in a clinical trial, meaning that CEA or CAS is *not indicated* for asymptomatic carotid stenosis, less the few patients at high risk of ipsilateral stroke that are potentially identifiable using TCD.

Endarterectomy for asymptomatic carotid stenosis: The Asymptomatic Carotid Atherosclerosis Study (ACAS) (see **Table 2**) was the first large-scale trial to compare CEA with best medical therapy vs. best medical therapy alone [45]. The study included 1662 patients from 34 centers and examined the composite of any stroke or death occurring in the perioperative period and ipsilateral cerebral infarction thereafter as its primary outcome. The trial was stopped early because of a clear benefit in favor of CEA. A contrast angiography showed diameter-reducing lesions of ≥60% based on the North American method for those patients randomized to surgery. The aggregate 5-year risk for ipsilateral stroke, any perioperative stroke, and death was 5.1% for the surgical patients compared to 11% for the medical patients (RR reduction, 53%; 95% CI, 22–72). The 30-day stroke morbidity and all-cause mortality for CEA, including a 1.2% rate of stroke with catheter angiography, were 2.3%. The rationale for including complications of angiography as part of the risk of surgery was that an angiogram otherwise would not have been performed if surgery was not considered.

The Asymptomatic Carotid Surgery Trial (ACST) (see **Table 2**) included 3120 patients with asymptomatic carotid stenoses of ≥60% as measured by duplex ultrasonography and compared patients undergoing immediate CEA vs. those with an indefinite deferral of the operation [46]. The trial used perioperative stroke, MI, or death, and non-perioperative stroke as the primary end points, which differed from those used in the aforementioned ACAS. Stroke risks were 4.1 vs. 10.0% at 5 years for immediate vs. deferred CEA, respectively, when excluding perioperative events and non-stroke mortality; this resulted in a gain of 5.9% (95% CI: 4.0–7.8). The 10-year stroke risks were 10.8 vs. 16.9% for immediate vs. deferred CEA, respectively; this resulted in a gain of 6.1% (95% CI: 2.7–9.4). Subgroup analysis demonstrated that the benefits of CEA were confined to patients <75 years of age.

Some caveats regarding these trials should be considered. First, it should be noted that both ACAS and ACST were conducted at times when best medical management was far less than the intensive medical therapy as outlined earlier in this chapter. Second, the surgeons were subject to intense screening, as such their skills may not be generalizable to the community at large. For instance, the complication rate of 30-day stroke and death for CEA in ACAS drops to 1.54% when angiography complications are removed from the analysis [47]. More recently, complication rates from the CREST trial were reported with CEA in asymptomatic patients carrying a combined risk of stroke and death of 1.4% [48]. These complication rates appear lower than what is seen in standard practice. In general, current surgical best practice restricts surgery for asymptomatic carotid stenosis to patients with ≥70% carotid stenosis if the surgery can be performed with ≤3% risk of perioperative complications. Further research regarding this topic is ongoing via the National Institute of Neurological Disorders and Stroke-sponsored Carotid Revascularization of Primary Prevention of Stroke (CREST-2) trial (see **Table 2**) which compares centrally managed patients receiving intensive medical therapy with or without CEA [49, 50].

Endovascular treatment for asymptomatic carotid stenosis: Carotid angioplasty and stenting (CAS) was initially evaluated in patients thought to be at high risk for CEA. The Stenting and Angioplasty with Protection in Patients at High Risk for Endarterectomy (SAPPHIRE) trial (see **Table 2**) evaluated CAS vs. CEA. The outcome measures included a composite of stroke, MI, or death within 30 days or death resulting from neurological cause or ipsilateral stroke between 31 and 365 days. The results showed that CAS was not inferior to CEA (within 3%; $p = 0.004$) [51]. Approximately, 70% of the subjects had an asymptomatic stenosis. The rates of stroke, MI, or death were 5.4% with CAS and 10.2% with CEA at 30 days ($p = 0.20$). The same composite outcome measures as above occurred in 9.9% of the CAS patients and 21.5% of the CEA patients after 1 year ($p = 0.02$). CAS had a significantly higher death rate (20.0%) than stroke rate (10.1%) after 3 years [52], raising questions about the long-term value of the procedure in this high-risk cohort. One glaring limitation to this study was the lack of a medically treated control group because the high complication rates in both Carotid Artery Stenosis (CAS) and CEA raise questions about the benefit of either intervention over medical therapy alone.

The CREST study (see **Table 2**) enrolled patients technically eligible for CEA or CAS with both symptomatic and asymptomatic carotid stenosis [53]. The inclusion criteria for asymptomatic patients were stenosis of ≥60% on angiography, ≥70% on ultrasonography, or ≥80% on CTA or MRA if the stenosis on ultrasonography was 50–69%. Composite of stroke, MI, or death resulting from any cause during the periprocedural period or any ipsilateral stroke within 4 years after randomization was the primary end point. The estimated 4-year occurrence of the composite primary end point between CAS (7.2%) and CEA (6.8%) demonstrated no difference (HR, 1.11; 95% CI, 0.81–1.51; $p = 0.51$). Symptom status showed no significant heterogeneity. The CREST study did, however, show an interaction of age on the primary end point. Patients aged >70 years showed a significant benefit for CEA over CAS. Patients >64 years old who

Topic/Trial Name/Years performed and published	Arms/Population/Primary outcome measure(s)	Results	Summary and implications on clinical practice
1. Cervical carotid atherosclerosis			
1a. Asymptomatic carotid stenosis			
ACAS: Endarterectomy for Asymptomatic Carotid Artery Stenosis [45] Enrollment Period: 12/1987–12/1993 Publication Year: 1995	**Arms**: Carotid endarterectomy (CEA) vs. aspirin and risk-factor modification (medical management). **Population**: Patients with at least 60% carotid stenosis and no stroke/TIA. **Outcome**: Primary end points were perioperative stroke and/or death or stroke in the study artery territory after the perioperative period.	-Primary end point was measured in the CEA arm 5.1 vs. 11.0% for medical therapy alone. -Patients who were good surgical candidates with at least 60% carotid stenosis showed decreased 5-year risk of stroke in the study carotid artery. They had 3% perioperative morbidity and mortality.	- Predominantly white males with ≥60% asymptomatic extracranial carotid stenosis benefited from CEA vs. medical management alone. - It is reasonable to perform CEA in asymptomatic patients who have more than 60% stenosis of the internal carotid artery and it was shown to be superior to medical management alone.
ACST: 10-year stroke prevention after successful carotid endarterectomy for asymptomatic stenosis: a multicenter randomized trial [46] Enrollment Period: 1993–2003 Publication Year: 2010	**Arms**: Immediate carotid endarterectomy (CEA) vs. deferral of any carotid procedure. **Population**: Patients with at least 60% carotid stenosis and no stroke/TIA within 6 months were eligible. **Outcome**: Primary end points were perioperative mortality/morbidity and non-perioperative stroke.	-Perioperative stroke risk or death within 30 days of CEA was 3.0%. -Non-perioperative stroke risk was 4.1 vs. 10.0% at 5 years and 10.8 vs. 16.9% at 10 years for immediate CEA vs. deferral of any carotid procedure, respectively. -The net risk was 6.9 vs. 10.9% at 5 years and 13.4 vs. 17.9% at 10 years for immediate CEA vs. deferral of any carotid procedure, respectively. -Patients with effective antihypertensive, antithrombotic, and lipid-lowering therapy and with little likelihood of death from other causes within 10 years had an absolute 10-year stroke reduction of 5%, with a number needed to treat of 20.	-The risk of CEA is greatest in the perioperative period, but in the long term it leads to decreased risk of non-perioperative stroke and shows an overall favorable net risk vs. deferral of CEA. - It is reasonable to perform CEA in asymptomatic patients who have more than 70% stenosis of the internal carotid artery.
SAPPHIRE: Protected Carotid-Artery Stenting vs. Endarterectomy in High-Risk Patients [51] Enrollment Period: 8/2000–7/2002 Publication Year: 2004	**Arms**: Carotid artery stenting (CAS) with embolic protection device vs. carotid endarterectomy (CEA). **Population**: Patients who presented with asymptomatic carotid stenosis with at least 80% carotid stenosis. **Outcome**: Non-inferiority study. Primary end point was cumulative major cardiovascular events at 1 year. This was composed of death, stroke, or MI within 30 days of intervention or stroke in the territory of the study vessel between days 31 and 1 year.	- For all comers (symptomatic and asymptomatic carotid stenosis), the primary end point was 12.2 (CAS) vs. 20.1% (CEA). Not statistically different for superiority but significant for non-inferiority. - For all comers, the 1-year revascularization rate was 0.6 (CAS) vs. 4.3% (CEA). - Asymptomatic carotid stenosis showed cumulative incidence of the primary end point at 1 year was 9.9 (CAS) vs. 21.5% (CEA), statistically significant. - Periprocedural stroke, MI, or death was 5.4 (CAS) vs. 10.2% (CEA), not statistically different, for asymptomatic carotid stenosis.	-CAS with embolic protection device was non-inferior to CEA in patients ≤80 years old with at least 80% asymptomatic extracranial carotid stenosis; however, subgroup analysis showed CAS to be superior to CEA at 1 year. - As an alternative to CEA, CAS with embolic protection device is indicated for patients at low or average surgical risk who have an anticipated rate of periprocedural stroke or mortality is less than 6% who have non-disabling stroke or TIA in the presence of ipsilateral ICA stenosis (≥70% by US/MRA/CTA or ≥50% by catheter angiogram); should undergo CEA within 6 months.

http://dx.doi.org/10.5772/65047

Topic/Trial Name/Years performed and published	Arms/Population/Primary outcome measure(s)	Results	Summary and implications on clinical practice
CREST-2: The Carotid Revascularization Endarterectomy vs. Stenting Trial 2 [49] Enrollment Period: Ongoing Publication Year: Pending	**Arms**: Intensive medical management alone vs. Carotid endarterectomy (CEA) + medical management vs. Carotid stenting (CAS) + medical management. **Population**: Enrollment goal is 2480 patients. Men and women 35 years and older who have at least 70% carotid narrowing in at least one carotid artery. **Outcome**: Composite of stroke plus death within 44 days after randomization and ipsilateral stroke thereafter up to 4 years.	Ongoing.	Ongoing.
1b. Symptomatic carotid stenosis			
NASCET: North American Symptomatic Carotid Endarterectomy Trial [25] Enrollment Period: 1/1988–2/1991 (stopped early) Publication Year: 1991	**Arms**: Medical therapy vs. CEA. **Population**: Patients with symptomatic carotid stenosis greater than or equal to 30% were randomized to medical therapy vs. CEA. **Outcome**: Cumulative risk of any ipsilateral stroke at 2 years.	- After a mean follow-up of 2 years, patients with *severe* stenosis showed a dramatic risk reduction of any ipsilateral stroke from 26% in the medical arm to 9% in the CEA arm. The absolute risk reduction was 17% ($p <$ 0.001), which translated to a number needed to treat six. - Among patients with *moderate* stenosis, CEA showed a lower, but significant, risk reduction from 22.2% in the medical arm to 15.7% in the CEA arm. The absolute risk reduction was 6.5% ($p = 0.045$), resulting in a number needed to treat 15.5 - Patients with *mild* stenosis of 30–49% did not achieve a significant risk reduction of any ipsilateral stroke following CEA.	- CEA + medical management showed lower risk of death and stroke compared to medical management alone in patients with symptomatic ICA stenosis 70–99%. - Based on NASCET and ECSS, the American Heart Association recommends that it is reasonable to perform CEA, when indicated, for patients with stroke or TIA within 2 weeks, rather than delaying surgery. - Surgery within 2 weeks may be contraindicated for patients who have very large infarctions at high risk of hemorrhagic conversion, or already have hemorrhagic conversion of their infarctions.
ECST: European Carotid Surgery Trial [54] Enrollment Period: 1981–1994 Publication Year: 1998	**Arms**: Carotid endarterectomy (CEA) vs. control (i.e., delay surgery if at all possible) with crossover from the control group. **Population**: Patients with some degree of ICA stenosis who had one or more carotid territory ischemic episodes within the previous 6 months. **Outcomes**: Primary end point was major stroke or death.	- Major stroke or death in 37.0 vs. 36.5% for CEA vs. control group, respectively. - For 2–3 years after randomization, severity of stenosis above 70–80% increased the risk of major ischemic stroke ipsilateral to the unoperated symptomatic carotid artery. - Kaplan-Meier estimates of the frequency of a major stroke or death at 3 years was 26.5 vs. 14.9 for control vs. CEA, respectively; thus, the absolute benefit of CEA was 11.6%.	- For patients at low or average surgical risk who have non-disabling stroke or TIA in the presence of ipsilateral ICA stenosis (≥70% by US/MRA/CTA or ≥50% by catheter angiogram) should undergo CEA within 6 months.

Topic/Trial Name/Years performed and published	Arms/Population/Primary outcome measure(s)	Results	Summary and implications on clinical practice
VACS: Carotid Endarterectomy and Prevention of Cerebral Ischemia in Symptomatic Carotid Stenosis [55] Enrollment period: 7/1988–2/1991 Publication Year: 1991	**Arms**: Carotid endarterectomy (CEA) and best medical therapy vs. best medical therapy alone. **Population**: Men who presented within 120 days of TIA or small ischemic stroke who had angiography confirmed carotid stenosis great than 50% ipsilateral to the presenting symptoms. **Outcome**: Crescendo TIA in the study vessel distribution or infarction or death within 30 days of randomization.	- Primary end point shown in 7.7 vs. 19.4% for CEA vs. medical therapy alone. - Further analysis revealed that there was an absolute risk reduction of 17.7% for those undergoing CEA in ICA stenosis of at least 70%. This benefit was apparent within 2 months of surgery.	- For patients at low or average surgical risk who have non-disabling stroke or TIA in the presence of ipsilateral ICA stenosis (≥70% by US/MRA/CTA or ≥50% by catheter angiogram) should undergo CEA within 6 months.
CREST: The Carotid Revascularization Endarterectomy vs. Stenting Trial [48] Enrollment Period: 12/2000–7/2008 Publication Year: 2010	**Arms**: Carotid endarterectomy (CEA) vs. Carotid artery stenting (CAS). **Population**: The study evaluated both symptomatic and asymptomatic carotid stenosis. Symptomatic carotid stenosis was defined as TIA, amaurosis fugax or minor non-disabling stroke in the distribution of the study artery within 180 days of randomization. For symptomatic patient the carotid artery stenosis had to be >50% by angiography, ≥70% by Ultrasound or ≥70% by CTA or MRA if US was 50–69%. Asymptomatic patients had to have stenosis of >60% by angiography, >70% by US or ≥80CTA or MRA if US 50–69%. Patients with previous disabling stroke or chronic atrial fibrillation were not included. **Outcome**: Primary end point was the occurrence of any stroke, MI, or death during the periprocedural period or ipsilateral stroke thereafter up to 4 years.	- There was no significant difference in primary end point between CAS and CEA (7.2 vs. 6.8%). - Periprocedural stroke occurred 4.1 vs. 2.3% for CAS vs. CEA. Periprocedural MI occurred 1.1 vs. 2.3% for CAS vs. CEA. Both were significant differences. There was no significant difference between CAS and CEA for ipsilateral stroke. - Risk for stroke and death was significantly higher for CAS in symptomatic patients but NOT asymptomatic.	- Older patients (>70) had better outcomes after CEA and younger patients (<70) had better outcomes after CAS. Patients had more strokes after CAS and more MIs after CEA. - For patients at low or average surgical risk who have non-disabling stroke or TIA in the presence of ipsilateral ICA stenosis (≥70% by US/MRA/CTA or ≥50% by catheter angiogram) should undergo CEA within 6 months. - For patients at low or average surgical risk who have non-disabling stroke or TIA in the presence of ipsilateral ICA stenosis (≥70% by US/MRA/CTA or ≥50% by catheter angiogram) should undergo CEA within 6 months. - As an alternative to CEA, CAS is indicated for patients at low or average surgical risk who have an anticipated rate of periprocedural stroke or mortality is less than 6% who have non-disabling stroke or TIA in the presence of ipsilateral ICA stenosis (≥70% by US/MRA/CTA or ≥50% by catheter angiogram) should undergo CEA within 6 months.

http://dx.doi.org/10.5772/65047

Topic/Trial Name/Years performed and published	Arms/Population/Primary outcome measure(s)	Results	Summary and implications on clinical practice
SAPPHIRE: Protected Carotid-Artery Stenting vs. Endarterectomy in High-Risk Patients [51] Enrollment Period: 8/2000–7/2002 Publication Year: 2004	**Arms**: Carotid artery stenting (CAS) with embolic protection device vs. carotid endarterectomy (CEA). **Population**: Patients who presented with symptomatic carotid stenosis with at least 50% carotid stenosis. **Outcome**: Non-inferiority study. Primary end point was cumulative major cardiovascular events at 1 year. This was composed of death, stroke, or MI within 30 days of intervention or stroke in the territory of the study vessel between days 31 and 1 year.	- For all comers (symptomatic and asymptomatic carotid stenosis) the primary end point was 12.2 (CAS) vs. 20.1% (CEA). Not statistically different for superiority but significant for non-inferiority. - For all comers, the 1-year revascularization rate was 0.6 (CAS) vs. 4.3% (CEA). - The cumulative incidence of primary end point in symptomatic carotid stenosis was 16.8 (CAS) vs. 16.5% (CEA), not statistically different. - Post-procedural incidence of primary end point in symptomatic carotid stenosis within 30 days was 2.1 (CAS) vs. 9.3% (CEA), not statistically different.	-CAS with embolic protection device was non-inferior to CEA in patients ≤80 years old with symptomatic carotid stenosis. - As an alternative to CEA, CAS with embolic protection device is indicated for patients at low or average surgical risk who have an anticipated rate of periprocedural stroke or mortality is less than 6% who have non-disabling stroke or TIA in the presence of ipsilateral ICA stenosis (≥70% by US/MRA/CTA or ≥50% by catheter angiogram) should undergo CEA within 6 months.
CAVATAS: Carotid and Vertebral Artery Transluminal Angioplasty Study: a randomized trial Endovascular vs. surgical treatment in patients with carotid stenosis in *CAVATAS: a randomized trial* [63] Enrollment Period: 3/1992–7/1997 Publication Year: 2001	**Arms**: Endovascular therapy (balloon angioplasty or stenting) vs. carotid endarterectomy (CEA). **Populations**: Patients with symptomatic carotid stenosis. **Outcome**: Primary outcome is any stroke or death within 30 days of treatment.	- Disabling stroke or death within 30 days occurred in 6.4 vs. 5.9% for endovascular procedure vs. CEA, respectively, not statistically significant. - Any stroke lasting more than 7 days or death occurred in 10.0 vs. 9.9% for endovascular therapy vs. CEA, respectively, not statistically significant. - Of the endovascular procedures, 26% underwent stenting and 74% underwent balloon angioplasty. - Cranial neuropath occurred in 8.7% of CEA patient but 0% in endovascular procedures, statistically significant. - The survival analysis up to 3 years after randomization showed no significant difference in rate or ipsilateral stroke.	- There was no significant difference in the major risks or effectiveness on ipsilateral stroke prevention in endovascular procedures compared to CEA.
2. Intracranial atherosclerosis			
WASID: Comparison of Warfarin and Aspirin for Symptomatic Intracranial Arterial Stenosis [69] Enrollment Period: 2/1999–7/2003 Publication Year: 2005	**Arms**: Warfarin (INR 2.0–3.0) vs. Aspirin 1300 mg daily. **Population**: Patients with TIA or ischemic stroke caused by angiography verified 50–99% stenosis in a major intracranial artery. **Outcome**: Ischemic stroke, brain hemorrhage, or death from vascular causes other than stroke.	- Death 9.7 vs. 4.3% in warfarin vs. aspirin arms. - Major hemorrhage 8.3 vs. 3.2% in warfarin vs. aspirin arms. - MI or sudden death 7.3 vs. 2.9% in warfarin vs. aspirin arms. -Primary end point occurred in 22.1 vs. 21.8% (not statistically significant) for aspirin vs. warfarin.	- Warfarin demonstrated no benefit over aspirin in the primary outcome of this trial and was associated with significantly higher major adverse events. - Aspirin should be used for treatment of intracranial arterial stenosis.

Topic/Trial Name/Years performed and published	Arms/Population/Primary outcome measure(s)	Results	Summary and implications on clinical practice
SAMMPRIS: Stenting vs. Aggressive Medical Therapy for Intracranial Arterial Stenosis [15] Enrollment Period: 11/2008–4/2011 Publication Year: 2011	**Arms**: Aggressive medical management alone vs. aggressive medical management plus percutaneous transluminal angioplasty and stenting. **Population**: Patients with recent TIA or stroke due to major intracranial artery stenosis (70–99%). **Outcome**: Stroke or death within 30 days of enrollment or after revascularization or stroke in the territory of the qualifying artery.	- Primary end point occurred in 20.0 vs. 12.2% for stenting vs. medical management, respectively. - Thirty-day stroke rate or death was 14.7 vs. 5.8% in stenting vs. medical management group.	- Aggressive medical management is superior to percutaneous transluminal angioplasty and stenting in patients with symptomatic carotid stenosis. - The risk of early stroke after stenting was high. - The risk of stroke with aggressive medical therapy alone was low.
3. Extracranial vertebral artery disease			
CAVATAS: Carotid and Vertebral Artery Transluminal Angioplasty Study: a randomized trial *Treatment of Vertebral Artery Stenosis in CAVATAS* [79] Enrollment Period: 12/1987–12/1993 Publication Year: 1995	**Arms**: Endovascular therapy (balloon angioplasty or stenting) vs. best medical treatment alone. **Populations**: 2. Patients with symptomatic vertebral artery stenosis. **Outcome**: Recurrent vertebrobasilar stroke after intervention.	- Only eight patients were randomized to each arm. - Two patients had TIA during endovascular treatment, but there were no perioperative deaths or strokes within 30 days of the procedure. - No patient in either group experienced a vertebrobasilar territory stroke. Three patients in each arm died as a result of either MI or carotid territory stroke.	- The trial did not show benefit of endovascular therapy for vertebral artery stenosis, but the sample size of 16 was small. - Patients were more likely to have carotid territory stroke or MI during the trial's follow-up period than vertebrobasilar stroke. - Patients with vertebrobasilar disease require reduction of vascular risk factors.
OXVASC: Oxford Vascular Study. Incidence and prognosis of ≥50% symptomatic vertebral or basilar artery stenosis: prospective population-based study [80] Enrollment Period: 3/1992–7/1997 Publication Year: 2007	**Arms**: Posterior circulation vs. carotid territory events. **Populations**: Population based study of 91,000 individuals in and around Oxford, UK. **Outcome**: 90-day recurrent stroke or TIA.	-The frequency of ≥50% vertebrobasilar stenosis is greater than the prevalence of ≥50% carotid stenosis in carotid territory events. - In patients with posterior circulation events, vertebrobasilar stenosis ≥50% was associated with multiple TIAs at presentation and significantly higher 90-day event rates.	- The presence of ≥50 vertebrobasilar stenosis is associated with an increased risk of early recurrent TIA or strokes.

http://dx.doi.org/10.5772/65047

Topic/Trial Name/Years performed and published	Arms/Population/Primary outcome measure(s)	Results	Summary and implications on clinical practice
VAST: Vertebral Artery Stenting Trial – A phase 2 trial randomly allocating patients in a 1:1 ratio to stenting plus best medical treatment or best medical treatment [81] Enrollment Period: 1/2008–4/2013 Publication Year: 2015	**Arms**: Vertebral artery stenting vs. medical treatment alone. **Populations**: Patients with symptomatic extracranial or intracranial vertebral artery stenosis ≥50% and vertebrobasilar transient ischemic attack or ischemic stroke in previous 6 months (n = 115, target n = 180†). **Outcome**: Vascular death, myocardial infarction, or any stroke within 30 days.	- Of the 57 patients randomly assigned to vertebral artery stenting, 50 underwent stent placement of which eight were placed in the intracranial vertebral artery. - Three (5%) of 57 patients had the primary outcome in the stenting group. - One (2%) of 58 patients had the primary outcome in the medical treatment group. - Median follow-up of 3 years revealed seven patients (12%) in the stenting group and four patients (7%) in the medical management group had strokes in the symptomatic vertebral artery distribution.	- Symptomatic vertebral artery stenosis was associated with periprocedural complications in about 5% of patients while medical therapy showed low risk in terms of major vascular complications as well as recurrent stroke. - Medical therapy is the preferred treatment of symptomatic vertebral artery stenosis.
VIST: Vertebral Artery Ischaemia Stenting Trial [82] Enrollment Period: 10/2008–2/2015 Publication Year: PENDING	**Arms**: Vertebral artery stenting/angioplasty vs. best medical therapy alone. **Populations**: Patients age 20 or older who have >50% vertebral artery stenosis and non-disabling stroke or TIA within 3 months of randomization. Total recruitment was 182 patients. **Outcome**: Perioperative risk and long term efficacy (not otherwise specified).	Completed; results pending.	

Table 2. Large artery atherosclerosis studies.

underwent CAS had a higher periprocedural stroke/death rate. Therefore, age is an important factor to consider when deciding between the two procedures. The results were further evaluated by comparing periprocedural rates stroke and MI for CAS vs. CEA. There was a significant difference ($p = 0.01$) for periprocedural stroke, which was higher in patients undergoing CAS (4.1%) vs. CEA (2.3%). The periprocedural rate of MI, however, was significantly lower ($p = 0.03$) for CAS (1.1%) compared with CEA (2.3%). However, CAS had significantly higher ($p = 0.03$) overall estimated 4-year rate of any periprocedural stroke or death or post-procedural ipsilateral stroke when compared to CEA with a HR, 1.50 (95% CI, 1.05–2.15). Both procedures had relatively low point estimates (2.5% in CAS vs. 1.4% for CEA, $p = 0.15$) for rates of any stroke or death in the periprocedural period among asymptomatic patients. There was a trend favoring CEA over CAS in symptomatic (HR, 1.37; 95% CI: 0.90–2.09; $p = 0.14$) and asymptomatic (HR, 1.86; 95% CI: 0.95–3.66; $p = 0.07$) patients, but the study was not powered for this evaluation. The advantage of revascularization over medical therapy by itself was not addressed by CREST, which did not randomize a group of asymptomatic subjects to medical therapy without revascularization. Unfortunately, as consistent with several of these trials, the lack of medically treated control groups complicates their interpretation. The ongoing National Institute of Neurological Disorders and Stroke-sponsored CREST-2 trial (**Table 2**) will be comparing centrally managed, intensive medical therapy with or without carotid stenting with embolic protection [49, 50].

In summary, the vast majority (~90%) of patients with asymptomatic carotid stenosis would be better served by intensive medical therapy than by endarterectomy or stenting. The ~10% who could possibly benefit from intervention can be identified by microemboli detection on transcranial Doppler or other techniques. Routine intervention for asymptomatic stenosis without such risk stratification is unwarranted. Most of the high-risk patients (~10%) would be better served by CEA than by CAS. The patients who are most appropriate for CAS within the high-risk group would be those at high risk of stroke and who have anatomical features that make CEA difficult. High-risk patients are those with severe cardiac, lung, and renal morbidities and changing anatomy. The specific details are listed in the AHA/ASA guidelines [11]. While anatomic high risk has generally been accepted, improving anesthetic and critical care management may alter medical high-risk criteria.

4.1.1. Asymptomatic carotid stenosis: recommendations (adapted from [10, 11])

1. Patients with asymptomatic carotid stenosis should be prescribed daily aspirin and a statin. Patients should also be screened for other treatable risk factors for stroke, and appropriate medical therapies and lifestyle changes should be instituted.

2. In patients who are to undergo CEA, aspirin is recommended peri- and postoperatively unless contraindicated.

3. CEA is a reasonable consideration in asymptomatic patients with >70% stenosis of the internal carotid artery (ICA) if the risk of perioperative stroke, MI, and death is <3%. The data that support this recommendation did not include the current standard for best medical management.

http://dx.doi.org/10.5772/65047

4. It is reasonable to repeat duplex ultrasonography annually by a qualified technologist in a certified laboratory to assess the progression or regression of disease and response to therapeutic interventions in patients with atherosclerotic stenosis of >50%.

5. The effectiveness of prophylactic CAS compared to medical therapy alone in asymptomatic carotid stenosis is not well established, but it can be considered in highly selected patients.

6. In asymptomatic patients at high risk of complications for carotid revascularization by either CEA or CAS, the effectiveness of revascularization vs. medical therapy alone is not well established.

7. Screening low-risk populations for asymptomatic carotid artery stenosis is not recommended.

4.2. Symptomatic carotid stenosis

Over the last half century, numerous clinical trials have compared CEA plus medical therapy to medical therapy alone in the setting of symptomatic carotid stenosis. Again, most of these studies predate the intensive medical therapy now recommended. Surgical techniques have also evolved. Furthermore, carotid angioplasty and stenting (CAS) has emerged as an alternative treatment for stroke prevention in patients in this setting.

Endarterectomy for symptomatic carotid stenosis: Three major randomized trials (see **Table 2**) have demonstrated the superiority of CEA plus medical therapy over medical therapy alone for symptomatic patients with a high-grade (>70% angiographic stenosis) atherosclerotic carotid stenosis, and include (1) the European Carotid Surgery trial (ECST) [54], (2) the North American Symptomatic Carotid Endarterectomy Trial (NASCET) [25], and (3) the Veterans Affairs Cooperative Study Program (VACS) [55]. Symptomatic patients included those who had >70% ipsilateral carotid stenosis with a non-disabling stroke, TIA, or transient monocular blindness. A pooled analysis of ECST, NASCET, and VACS found a 30-day stroke and death rate of 7.1% in surgically treated patients [56]. In patients with a *70–99% (severe)* stenosis, NASCET found that for every six patients treated, one major stroke would be prevented at 2 years (i.e., a number needed to treat (NNT) of six). Additionally, these three seminal trials showed that patients with stenoses *<50% (mild)* did not have benefit in terms of stroke risk reduction with surgical intervention. The role of CEA was less clear among patients with symptomatic stenosis in the *50–69% (moderate)* range. NASCET evaluated 858 symptomatic patients with a stenosis of 50–69%, and in the surgically treated patients the 5-year rate of any ipsilateral stroke was 15.7% compared with 22.2% in those treated medically ($p = 0.045$) [25]. Thus, the number needed to treat was 15 (i.e., 15 patients would have to undergo CEA to prevent one ipsilateral stroke during the 5-year follow-up period). Therefore, CEA is justified only in appropriate cases when the risk-benefit ratio is favorable for the patient when evaluating surgical and anesthesia risks. In NASCET, the rate of perioperative stroke or death was 6.7%, with more recent population-based studies reporting a rate of 6% [57]. Given that medical management has improved since NASCET, current guidelines advise proceeding with CEA in the setting of symptomatic stenosis only if the surgeon's rate for perioperative stroke or death is <6% [10, 11].

Patient-selection criteria influencing surgical risk often include gender and age. There is some concern, as based on the NASCET subgroup analyses, that CEA may not be beneficial in women with symptomatic carotid stenosis. Although women were not well represented and the effect of gender was not overwhelming [25], these data did demonstrate a significant difference (p = 0.008) suggesting that woman are more likely to have poorer outcomes as compared to men when undergoing CEA [58]. The surgical mortality, neurological morbidity, and recurrent carotid stenosis were 14% in women and 3.9% in men (p = 0.008) [58]. Notably, CREST was designed with pre-planned subgroup analysis intended to evaluate the effects of gender and age on the primary outcome end point. CREST included both symptomatic and asymptomatic patients, and found no significant interaction in the primary end point by gender. However, CREST did show superior results for CEA as compared with CAS in patients aged >70 years old [53, 59]. Of note, there are limited age-related data on the safety and efficacy of carotid revascularization because patients 80 years old or older were often excluded from trials, including NASCET. However, safe CEA in patients ≥80 years of age has been documented in case series [60]. Some studies comparing CAS and CEA have focused specifically on patients considered at high risk for surgical intervention and will be discussed in greater detail in the upcoming section on CAS. In summary, outcome differences in age and gender, along with medical comorbidities, should be considered when deciding whether or not to proceed with carotid revascularization. *The optimal timing of carotid revascularization via CEA* after a completed non-disabling stroke has been defined to be within 2 weeks if there are no contraindications. This time period is driven by data from the three major randomized controlled trials (RCTs) mentioned above, among others [25, 53, 59]. In these trials, patients were randomized to surgery within 2–14 days (median) and a third of the perioperative strokes occurred during this same time period. The first 2 weeks represented the greatest stroke risk in medically treated patients. After 2–3 years, the annual rate of stroke among the medically treated patients approached the rate observed for asymptomatic patients. Further analysis of patients with ≥70% carotid stenosis in ECST and NASCET showed a reduction in attributable risk from 30 to 18% when surgery occurred within 2 weeks vs. at 2–4 weeks, then to 11% for surgery at 4–12 weeks for any ipsilateral stroke or any stroke or death within 30 days of trial surgery [61]. These three trials included only patients with non-disabling stroke or TIA and reported low rates of ICH associated with surgery (0.2%). The risk for perioperative ICH may be increased with early surgery in patients with major cerebral infarction via a hyper- or reperfusion syndrome, this because of the sudden increase in perfusion of the vasculature distal to stenosis. Optimal control of blood pressure during and post-procedure is emphasized.

Endovascular treatment for symptomatic carotid stenosis: CAS has emerged as a therapeutic alternative to CEA for the treatment of extracranial carotid artery occlusive disease. The theoretical advantages of being a less invasive procedure resulting in decreased patient discomfort and a shorter recovery period were indeed born out in CREST, with an improved health-related quality of life in the perioperative period, although this difference was not sustained at 1 year [62]. As mentioned above in the asymptomatic carotid section, the historical use of CAS was typically reserved for patients considered at high risk for CEAs. Many of the reported trials have been industry sponsored and evaluated the efficacy of a single-stent/neuroprotection system in an effort to garner Food and Drug Administration (FDA) approval. The first large randomized trial was the Carotid and Vertebral Artery Transluminal Angioplasty Study (CAVATAS—see **Table 2**) [63]. CAVATAS randomized patients suitable for either stenting or surgery, and if patients were unsuitable for surgery, they were randomized to either stenting or medical management. The results showed that CAS and CEA had comparable results with 30-day rate of stroke or death of 6% in both groups. Preliminary analyses demonstrated no stroke rate differences 3 years after randomization. The major limitations were that a minority (55 of the 251 patients) in the endovascular group was treated with a stent and embolic protection devices were not used. Of note, embolic protection devices are now required in endovascular procedures reimbursed by the Centers for Medicare & Medicaid Services. Such devices aim to reduce periprocedural stroke rates. The Stenting and Angioplasty with Protection in Patients at High Risk for Endarterectomy (SAPPHIRE – see **Table 2**) had the primary objective of comparing the safety and efficacy of CAS with an embolic protection device to CEA; 334 symptomatic and asymptomatic high-risk patients were randomized [51]. The outcomes by which they studied safety included the cumulative incidence of stroke, myocardial infarction, or death. In the periprocedural period, the rate was 4.8% in patients assigned to receive a stent vs. 9.8% assigned to undergo endarterectomy in an intention-to-treat analysis ($p = 0.09$). Those patients who actually underwent stenting and CEA had primary outcomes incidence of 4.4 and 9.9%, respectively ($p = 0.06$). The 1-year rates of the aforementioned primary end point in addition to ipsilateral stroke or death of neurological causes within 31 days to 1 year were 20.1% for CEA and 12.2% for CAS ($p = 0.05$). The conclusion from the trial was that CAS was non-inferior to CEA in this specific high-risk patient cohort in spite of the fact that these differences primarily represented differences in periprocedural MI rates. Overall, the post-procedure morbidity and mortality for asymptomatic patients in both CAS and CEA were high enough to question the benefit of either procedure compared with medical management.

There have been several other RCTs comparing CEA and CAS for symptomatic patients. These trials include EVA-3S (Endarterectomy vs. Angioplasty in Patients with Symptomatic Severe Carotid Stenosis), SPACE (Stent-Supported Percutaneous Angioplasty of the Carotid Artery vs. Endarterectomy), and ICSS (International Carotid Stenting Study) trials [64]. In a meta-analysis of these studies, the rate of stroke and death at 120 days after randomization was significantly higher for CAS (8.9%) compared to CEA (5.8%) with HR 1.53 ($p = 0.0006$). Notably subgroup analyses revealed a higher rate of stroke or death at 120 days for CAS (12.0%) vs. CEA (5.9%) among patients aged ≥70 (HR, 2.04; $p = 0.0053$). No significant difference was observed in patients younger than 70 years of age [65].

CREST is an important recent RCT that compared the efficacy of CAS with that of CEA [48, 53]. In CREST, 2502 symptomatic and asymptomatic patients with carotid stenosis were recruited from the US and Canadian centers. Carotid stenosis was defined as >70% by ultrasonography or >50% by angiography. The primary outcome was a composite measure of 30-day rate of stroke, death, and MI and 4-year ipsilateral stroke. The primary outcome was observed at a rate of 7.2% in CAS and 6.8% in CEA ($p = 0.51$). The 4-year rate of the primary end point in asymptomatic patients was 5.6% with CAS vs. 4.9% with CEA (HR 1.17; 95% CI: 0.69–1.98; $p = 0.56$). By comparison, the rates were 8.6% with CAS vs. 8.4% with CEA in symptomatic patients (HR 1.08; 95% CI: 0.74–1.59; $p = 0.69$). Analysis of symptomatic and asymptomatic patients together showed an interaction between age and treatment efficacy ($p = 0.02$). The HR for the primary outcome increased (CAS compared to CEA) when stratifying by age; HR was 0.6 (95% CI, 0.31–1.18) for patients <65 years of age, 1.08 (95% CI, 0.65–1.78) for patients 65–74 years old, and 1.63 (95% CI, 0.99–2.69) for patients aged ≥75 years. The risk of MI did not increase with age for either CEA or CAS. The effect of age was primarily driven by stroke risk, with greater stroke risk by age, with this effect stronger in the CAS group as compared to the CEA group. The HR became 1.0 at ≈70 years old for the primary outcomes and 64 years old for stroke. Gender was examined for periprocedural events, there was a trend for fewer events in women undergoing CEA compared to CAS; no periprocedural differences were seen in men. Periprocedural complication rates were lower in CREST as compared to prior trials. In the first 30 days, the rate of any stroke, MI, or death was 5.2% with CAS vs. 4.5% with CEA (HR 1.18; 95% CI: 0.82–1.68). Analyses regarding the type of periprocedural complications identified important differences. First, patients who had CAS had lower rates of MI than patients who had CEA (1.1% vs. 2.3%; HR: 0.50; 95% CI: 0.26–0.94) but higher rates of stroke (4.1% vs. 2.3%; HR: 1.79; 95% CI: 1.14–2.82). Second, complication rates also differed according to the surgical indication; asymptomatic patients had a rate of 3.5% for CAS vs. 3.6% with CEA, and symptomatic patients had a rate of 6.7% with CAS and 5.4% with CEA [48, 53].

Other considerations: strong evidence regarding follow-up imaging and re-stenosis after CEA or CAS is lacking. The Asymptomatic Carotid Atherosclerosis Study (ACAS) trial demonstrated that risk for re-stenosis after CEA was highest in the first 18 months after surgery (7.6%). The incidence decreased to 1.9% in the next 42 months. These data are comparable to the CEA arm of the CREST trial 18-month estimates which showed 6.3% risk of re-stenosis (>70% stenosis) after 24 months of observation. Other smaller studies have variable re-stenosis rates after CEA, but there are many limitations to these studies including the imaging technique utilized, length of follow-up, stenosis criterion, patient loss rates, and case mix. According to a recent narrative review, the rate of hemodynamically significant re-stenosis after CEA is probably 5–7% during variable periods of follow-up [53]. In older trials, the rates of re-stenosis were reportedly higher after CAS than after CEA. In the SPACE trial [64], the rate of re-stenosis (≥70% luminal occlusion) was 10.7% for CAS compared with 4.6% for CEA after 2 years. In CAVATAS, the rates after 5 years were 30.7% for CAS as compared with 10.5% for CEA. In a relatively recent review of 2191 CREST patients with follow-up at 2 years, highly standardized ultrasonography data were used to examine the incidence of re-stenosis and found no differences [66], although independent predictors of re-stenosis including DM, hypertension, and female sex were identified. Smoking was also an independent predictor for re-stenosis, but only with CEA, not CAS. In summary, the most current data suggest that rates of re-stenosis are similar between CEA and CAS. Moreover, there is no clear association between re-stenosis and increased risk for stroke. Therefore, routine surveillance for re-stenosis in asymptomatic patients is not well established.

http://dx.doi.org/10.5772/65047

Extracranial-intracranial bypass. The International Cooperative Study of Extracranial/Intracranial Arterial Bypass (EC/IC Bypass Study) was the first major trial of EC/IC bypass surgery. The trial randomized 1377 patients within 3 months of a TIA or minor ischemic stroke to either surgery or best medical care [67]. Patients who were eligible for inclusion in the study had narrowing or occlusion of the ipsilateral middle cerebral artery (MCA), stenosis of the (surgically inaccessible) ipsilateral distal internal carotid artery (ICA) or the occlusion of the ipsilateral mid-cervical ICA. The primary outcome was fatal or nonfatal stroke. After nearly 5 years, the primary outcome was more common in patients who underwent surgery. A later trial [68] selected a high-risk group to examine with the goal to evaluate the effectiveness of EC/IC bypass for the prevention of ipsilateral stroke. The trial enrolled 195 patients who had evidence on positron emission tomography (PET) scanning of hemodynamic cerebral ischemia distal to a symptomatic ipsilateral carotid occlusion [68]. TIA or ischemic stroke within 4 months of randomization, such as the previous study, was required for eligibility. The trial was terminated early for futility given a 30-day rate of ipsilateral stroke of 14.4% in the surgical group and 2.0% in the non-surgical group. The same outcome at 2 years was similar in both groups, 21.0% in the surgical group and 22.7% in the nonsurgical group ($p = 0.78$).

4.2.1. Symptomatic extracranial carotid disease: recommendations (adapted from [10, 11])

1. CEA is recommended for patients with a TIA or ischemic stroke within the past 6 months who have severe ipsilateral (70–99%) carotid artery stenosis when the perioperative morbidity and mortality risk is estimated to be <6%.

2. CEA is recommended for patients with patient-specific factors (i.e., age, sex, medical comorbidities) when they have had a recent TIA or ischemic stroke as well as moderate ipsilateral (50–69%) carotid stenosis and the perioperative morbidity and mortality risk is estimated to be <6%.

3. When the *degree of stenosis is <50%*, CEA and CAS are not recommended.

4. When revascularization is indicated for patients with TIA or minor, non-disabling stroke, it is reasonable to perform the procedure within 2 weeks of the index event rather than delay surgery if there are no contraindications to early revascularization.

5. CAS can be considered as an alternative to CEA for symptomatic patients at average or low risk of complications associated with endovascular intervention when the anticipated rate of periprocedural stroke or death is <6%.

6. Age should be considered when deciding which procedure is appropriate in symptomatic carotid stenosis. CEA was associated with improved outcomes in patients older than 70 years especially when anatomy is unfavorable for CAS. The periprocedural risk due to stroke, MI, or death and long-term risk for ipsilateral stroke are equivalent for CAS and CEA in younger patients.

7. In patients at high of complications of surgery due to anatomical or medical factors, CAS is a reasonable alternative compared to CEA for patients with symptomatic severe stenosis (>70%).

8. The accepted periprocedural stroke and mortality rates for symptomatic carotid stenosis are <6% for operators performing CAS and/or CEA.

9. Routine, long-term follow-up imaging of the extracranial carotid circulation with carotid duplex ultrasonography is not recommended.

10. For patients with a recent (within 6 months) TIA or ischemic stroke ipsilateral to a stenosis or occlusion of the middle cerebral or carotid artery, EC/IC bypass surgery is not recommended.

11. EC/IC bypass is considered investigational in patients on optimal medical therapy with recurrent/progressive ischemic symptoms ipsilateral to a stenosis/occlusion of surgically inaccessible portions of the carotid artery.

12. Optimal medical therapy including antiplatelet therapy, statin therapy, and risk-factor modification is recommended for all patients with carotid artery stenosis and a TIA or stroke.

5. Intracranial atherosclerosis

Intracranial atherosclerosis is a common cause of stroke carrying a high risk for recurrence. To date, there have only been a few large, multicenter randomized trials evaluating stroke-preventive therapies for this disease, the two primary trials include WASID [69] and SAMPPRIS [15] (see **Table 2**).

The WASID study was a double-blind trial that included 569 patients. Patients included in the study were required to have stroke or TIA attributable to 50–99% intracranial stenosis of the MCA, intracranial ICA, intracranial vertebral artery, or basilar artery. The patients were randomized to receive either aspirin 1300 mg or warfarin with a target international normalized ratio (INR) between 2 and 3. WASID was stopped early because of higher rates of death and major hemorrhage in the warfarin arm. The primary end point, the composite rate of ischemic stroke, brain hemorrhage, and non-stroke vascular death occurred in 22% of patients in both treatment arms over a mean follow-up of 1.8 years. The 1- and 2-year rates of stroke in the territory of the stenotic artery occurred in the aspirin arm 12 and 15% at 1- and 2-years, respectively. The 1- and 2-year rates of stroke in the warfarin arm were 11 and 13%, respectively. Both arms demonstrated higher rates of stroke in the territory of the stenotic artery with higher degrees of intracranial stenosis. For patients with ≥70% stenosis, the stroke rate at 1 year was 18% and the rate was 7–8% in patients with 50–69% stenosis [70]. This was supported by a multivariate analysis, which demonstrated that the risk of stroke in the territory of the stenotic artery was highest for severe stenosis (≥70%) and for patients enrolled early (≤17 days, which was the median time to enrollment in the trial) after their qualifying event. Analyses also showed that women appeared to be at increased risk. No subgroup in the post hoc analyses benefited from warfarin. Controlling BP and LDL-C may reduce the risk of subsequent stroke based on WASID results. Contrary to the argument that BP lowering may impair cerebral blood flow and thus increase stroke risk in patients with large artery stenosis, post hoc analysis showed that patients with mean SBP of ≥140 mmHg had a significantly increased risk of recurrent stroke compared with patients with mean SBP of <140 mmHg (HR 1.63; $p = 0.01$) [71]. Additionally, the patients with high LDL-C levels (mean ≥100 mg/dL) were 1.72 times more likely ($p = 0.03$) to have stroke compared to lower LDL-C levels (mean <100 mg/dL). A low rate of vascular events was observed in the small subset of patients with LDL-C of <70 mg/dL [72].

The SAMMPRIS trial compared endovascular therapy with medical therapy for the prevention of recurrent stroke in patients with symptomatic intracranial arterial stenosis [15]. In SAMMPRIS, patients with TIA or stroke within the past 30 days related to 70–99% stenosis of a major intracranial artery were randomized to aggressive medical management alone or aggressive medical management plus percutaneous transluminal angioplasty and stenting (PTAS, self-expanding Wingspan stent). Intensive medical therapy was aspirin of 325 mg/d, clopidogrel of 75 mg/d for 90 days after enrollment, intensive risk-factor management that primarily targeted SBP of <140 mmHg (<130 mmHg in patients with DM) and LDL-C of <70 mg/dL, and a lifestyle modification program. Enrollment was stopped early after 451 patients because the primary end point of stroke and death was significantly higher in the PTAS arm at 30 days ($p = 0.002$), 14.7% in PTAS arm and 5.8% in medical arm. The rate of the primary end point at 1 year was also significantly higher in the PTAS arm (20.0%) vs. 12.2% for the medical arm ($p = 0.009$). These 1-year event rate differences were driven by the increased 30-day events in the PTAS arm. Periprocedural ischemic strokes were associated with older age, diabetes mellitus, basilar stenosis, and non-smoking. Of the strokes that occurred within 30 days, 10 of 33 (30.3%) in the PTAS arm and none of 12 (0%) in the medical arm were symptomatic brain hemorrhages ($p = 0.04$). Estimated 1-year rates of major hemorrhage (any brain hemorrhage or major non-stroke-related hemorrhage) were 9.0% in the stenting arm and 1.8% in the medical arm ($p < 0.001$). Of note in SAMMPRIS, the event rates in the PTAS arm (14.7%) were significantly higher than anticipated from the Wingspan stent registry (4.5%) [73]. The results of the medical arm demonstrated better than expected event rates as compared with WASID at 1 month (5.8% observed rate in SAMMPRIS vs. 10.7% expected based on WASID) and at 1 year (12.2% observed vs. 25% expected). These improved outcomes were deemed related to the intensive medical therapy utilized in the trial. Importantly, 284 of the 451 patients (63%) enrolled in SAMMPRIS had their qualifying event while undergoing antithrombotic therapy. In this subgroup of the SAMMPRIS cohort, the rates of the primary end point were 16.0% in the stenting arm and 4.3% in the medical arm at 30 days. At 1 year, the rates were 20.9 and 12.9% for the stenting and medical arms, respectively ($p = 0.028$) [74]. These results indicate that stenting (with the Wingspan system) is *not* a safe or effective rescue treatment for patients who experience a TIA or stroke while already being treated with antithrombotic therapy. Results from extended follow-up of the SAMMPRIS cohort were published in 2014 and demonstrated persistence of the early benefit of medical management over stenting with the Wingspan device [75]. In comparison, patients in the WASID trial were treated with aspirin of 1300 mg/d. In the SAMMPRIS trial, the medical arm used aspirin of 325 mg/d (in combination with clopidogrel of 75 mg/d) and achieved favorable rates of stroke outcome compared with the intervention arm. Lower doses of aspirin were effective in other large trials of secondary prevention, most of which enrolled patients with more heterogeneous subtypes of stroke. In aggregate, these data suggest that doses lower than 1300 mg/d are probably effective in patients with intracranial stenosis and that dual antiplatelet therapy while optimizing vascular risk-factor control is reasonable. Of note, the SAMMPRIS results are a major contributor to the current recommendations regarding the intensive medical therapy now recommended in many societal and professional stroke-prevention guidelines [76].

A subsequent detailed analysis of the 30-day events in the SAMMPRIS PTAS arm revealed that a large number of the ischemic strokes occurred from occlusion of perforators (basilar perforators to the pons or lenticulostriate perforators from the middle cerebral artery) with the PTAS occluding the perforator 'takeoffs' (i.e., ostium). Other periprocedural risks demonstrated by SAMMPRIS included those associated with wire-vessel perforation causing subarachnoid hemorrhage (SAH) and ICH as associated with dual antiplatelet therapy in the setting of increased perfusion of an ischemic vascular bed. Balloon angioplasty alone without stenting has been proposed as a method to reduce perforator strokes; however, no randomized trials have compared angioplasty against intensive medical management. Re-stenosis rates after angioplasty alone or PTAS in this setting are uncertain.

One other notable study in the setting of intracranial stenosis is the previously described International Cooperative Study of Extracranial/Intracranial Arterial Bypass (EC/IC Bypass Study) [67]. This study included patients with MCA stenosis and ICA stenosis above the second cervical vertebra in addition to the symptomatic patients with extracranial carotid occlusion. The patient population included 109 patients with ≥70% MCA stenosis and 149 patients with ≥70% ICA stenosis. These groups were randomized to bypass surgery or medical treatment with aspirin of 1300 mg/d. The mean follow-up was 55.8 months. The rates of stroke during follow-up in patients with ≥70% MCA stenosis were significantly lower in the medical arm (23.7%) compared to the bypass arm (44%). There was no statistically significant difference in patients with ≥70% ICA stenosis above C2 between the medical arm (36.1%) and bypass arm (37.7%). The results of this study have led to EC/IC bypass being largely abandoned as a treatment for intracranial stenosis.

5.1. Intracranial atherosclerosis: recommendations (adapted from [10, 11])

1. For patients with a stroke or TIA caused by 50–99% stenosis of a major intracranial artery, aspirin of 325 mg/d is recommended in preference to warfarin.

2. For patients with recent stroke or TIA (within 30 days) attributable to severe stenosis (70–99%) of a major intracranial artery, the addition of clopidogrel of 75 mg/d to aspirin for 90 days might be reasonable.

3. There are insufficient data for the usefulness of clopidogrel alone, aspirin + dipyridamole or cilostazol alone in patients with stroke or TIA attributable to 50–99% stenosis of a major intracranial artery.

4. For patients with a stroke or TIA attributable to 50–99% stenosis of a major intracranial artery, the maintenance of SBP below 140 mmHg and high-intensity statin therapy are recommended.

http://dx.doi.org/10.5772/65047

5. Angioplasty or stenting is not recommended in patients with stroke or TIA attributable to moderate stenosis (50–69%). Medical management is the recommended treatment.

6. Irrespective of whether a patient is on antithrombotic therapy at the time of the stroke or TIA, the Wingspan stent system is not recommended as the initial treatment for patients with severe stenosis (70–99%).

7. For patients with stroke or TIA attributable to severe stenosis (70–99%) of a major intracranial artery, the usefulness of angioplasty alone or placement of stents other than the Wingspan stent is unknown and is considered investigational.

8. In patients with recurrent TIA or stroke after maximization of medical management (aspirin or clopidogrel therapy, SBP of <140 mmHg and high-intensity statin therapy) in patients with severe stenosis (70–99%) of a major intracranial artery, the usefulness of angioplasty alone or the placement of a Wingspan stent or other stent is unknown and is considered investigational.

9. In patients with actively progressive symptoms despite starting aspirin and clopidogrel, the usefulness of angioplasty alone or the placement of a Wingspan stent or other stents is not known and considered investigational in patients with severe stenosis (70–99%) of a major intracranial artery.

10. For patients with stroke or TIA attributable to 50–99% stenosis of a major intracranial artery, EC/IC bypass surgery is not recommended.

6. Extracranial vertebral artery disease

Extracranial vertebral artery stenosis (ECVAS) is a well-recognized cause of posterior circulation stroke. Proximal vertebral (V1 segment) lesions may account for ~9% of all posterior circulation strokes [77], while vertebral artery ostial lesions may account for another third [78]. As consistent with the anterior circulation, there are two primary stroke mechanisms including (1) plaque rupture with subsequent artery to artery thromboembolism and (2) hemodynamic insufficiency. Treatment options for symptomatic ECVAS include intensive medical therapy, endovascular stenting, and in rare cases open surgical revascularization. Unfortunately, scant RCTs results exist specific to this setting. There was a small subset of 16 CAVATAS trial (see **Table 2**) participants with symptoms in the vascular territory supplied by a stenosed vertebral artery that were randomized to receive either endovascular therapy (angioplasty or stenting) or medical management alone [79]. Participants had a mean follow-up of 4.7 years. No patient in either group experienced a vertebrobasilar stroke. Among the eight patients in the endovascular group, six patients underwent percutaneous transluminal angioplasty alone while the other two had stenting, two periprocedural TIAs in the endovascular group. The investigators concluded that medical treatment should focus on global vascular risk reduction after three patients in each arm of the study died of MI or carotid territory stroke during follow-up. The Oxford Vascular Study (OXVASC) (see **Table 2**) is a population-based study of incidence and prognosis of ≥50% symptomatic vertebral or basilar artery stenosis [80]. Medical therapy was determined by the patient's general practitioners. Of the 141 patients with posterior circulation events (26.2%) had ≥50% vertebral and basilar stenosis, compared with 41 (11.5%) patients with ≥50% ipsilateral carotid stenosis. The presence of ≥50% vertebral and basilar stenosis was unrelated to age, sex, or vascular risk factors. Carotid stenosis of ≥50% was associated with the evidence of coronary/peripheral atherosclerosis but not vertebral and basilar stenosis of ≥50%. In patients with posterior circulation events, ≥50% vertebral and basilar stenosis was associated with multiple transient ischemic attacks at presentation and with a significantly higher 90-day risk of recurrent events (OR 3.2; $p = 0.006$), reaching 22% for stroke and 46% for transient ischemic attack and stroke combined. These rates were higher than the recurrence rates of events in patients with carotid stenosis, although to re-emphasize, the medical therapy was not standardized in this study. A more recent phase 2 study performed in the Netherlands, the Vertebral Artery Stenting Trial (VAST) (see **Table 2**) identified patients with a recent transient ischemic attack or minor stroke associated with an extracranial (or intracranial) vertebral artery stenosis of at least 50% and randomized patients to stenting plus best medical treatment or best medical treatment alone [81]. All patients received 'best medical treatment' at the discretion of the treating neurologist, including antithrombotic agents, a statin, and 'rigorous control' of other vascular risk factors. The primary outcome was the composite of vascular death, myocardial infarction, or any stroke within 30 days after the start of treatment. The trial was stopped after inclusion of 115 patients because of new regulatory requirements. Fifty-seven patients were assigned to stenting and 58 were assigned to medical treatment alone. The primary outcome was observed in three patients in the stenting group within 30 days after the start of treatment (5%, 95% CI: 0–11) vs. one patient in the medical treatment group (2%, 95% CI: 0-5). During the complete period of follow-up (4 years), there were 60 serious adverse events (eight strokes) in the stenting group and 56 (seven strokes) in the medical treatment alone group. The investigators concluded that stenting of symptomatic vertebral artery stenosis was associated with a major periprocedural vascular complication in about one in 20 patients and the risk of recurrent vertebrobasilar stroke under best medical treatment alone was low, with these results leading the authors to question the need for a phase 3 study. Another study that recently completed enrollment in February 2015 is the Vertebral Artery Ischaemia Stenting Trial (VIST) [82]. This is a UK-based multiple-center RCT that will compare vertebral artery stenting/angioplasty vs. the best medical therapy alone in patients with symptomatic vertebral artery stenosis of >50%. Recruitment was stopped early due to a cessation of funding as related to a low recruitment rate. A total of 182 patients were recruited. The stated primary end points were perioperative risk and long-term efficacy, not further specified; results are forthcoming. Lastly, one can also infer from the SAMMPRIS trial [15], which evaluated the similar condition of recently symptomatic large-vessel intracranial stenosis, that aggressive medical therapy strategy including dual antiplatelet therapy for 3 months, along with statin therapy, blood pressure, and glycemic control, and risk-factor modification is highly effective for secondary prevention of stroke. It remains unclear if aggressive medical therapy would be as effective for patients with symptoms caused by hemodynamic compromise from ECVAS.

Specific to stenting in the setting of ECVAS, there has been numerous retrospective, non-randomized case series published. One review including 980 patients from 27 studies demonstrated a technical success rate of 99%, with a periprocedural risk of 1.2% for stroke and 0.9% for TIA [83]. In this study, participants were followed up for an average of 21 months perioperatively, with vertebrobasilar territory stroke or TIA only occurring in 1.3 and 6.5%, respectively. A prospective database of 114 patients undergoing stenting for symptomatic vertebral ostial stenosis demonstrated a recurrence of symptoms at 1 year after stenting of just 2% [78]. In another review of 300 endovascular interventions in symptomatic vertebral artery origin stenosis, periprocedural neurologic complications occurred in 5.5% and the re-stenosis rate was 26% [84]. Nevertheless, at long-term follow-up (mean 14.2 months), the risk of death was 0.3%, and the risk for posterior stroke was 0.7%. In general, the risks of adverse events are higher with distal vertebral or basilar interventions and when interventions are performed in the setting of urgent revascularization.

Symptomatic re-stenosis rates in this setting are ECVAS stenting, which remain uncertain and a topic of study. A recent pooled analyses [85] of five studies comparing drug-eluting (DES) vs. bare-metal stents (BMS) found no significant difference in the technical success (OR 1.53; $p = 0.62$), clinical success (OR 1.92; $p = 0.27$), and periprocedural complications (OR 0.74; $p = 0.61$) between the two stent types. An OR of 0.388 for no re-stenosis in the BMS to DES arms ($p = 0.001$) indicated a significantly higher re-stenosis rate in the BMS group relative to the DES group (33.57 vs. 15.49%). When compared with the DES group, the BMS group had a significantly higher rate of recurrent symptoms (2.76 vs. 11.26%; OR 3.32; $p = 0.01$). In summary, a significantly lower rate of re-stenosis and recurrent symptoms was noted in the DES group compared with the BMS group.

Open surgical procedures for revascularization of ECVAS include vertebral artery endarterectomy and vertebral artery transposition. While such procedures are performed rarely, they can be considered in patients with persistent symptoms despite intensive medical therapy. In one older series of 27 patients, there was no perioperative stroke or death [86]. In that same series, there were two permanent neurological complications: one case of Horner syndrome and one case of vocal hoarseness. Additionally, two patients developed neurological symptoms localizable to the posterior circulation after the perioperative period [86]. In closing, larger randomized trials will be necessary to better define evidence-based recommendations for ECVAS patients and to assess whether vertebral artery stenting is of relevance as a primary treatment strategy in patients with symptomatic ECVAS.

6.1. Extracranial vertebrobasilar disease: recommendations (adapted from [10, 11])

1. Routine preventive therapy with emphasis on antithrombotic therapy, lipid lowering, BP control, and lifestyle optimization is recommended for all patients with recently symptomatic extracranial vertebral artery stenosis.

2. Endovascular stenting of patients with extracranial vertebral stenosis may be considered when patients are having symptoms despite optimal medical treatment.

3. Open surgical procedures, including vertebral endarterectomy and vertebral artery transposition, may be considered when patients are having symptoms despite optimal medical treatment.

7. Conclusion

Extracranial and intracranial large artery atherosclerosis is a common cause of ischemic stroke and TIA. Lifelong vascular risk-factor optimizations via sustained behavioral modifications and intensive medical therapy are the key elements to reduce future stroke risk in these settings. Intensive medical therapy achieves low rates of stroke and death in asymptomatic carotid stenosis. Evidence indicates that patients with moderate to severe symptomatic carotid stenosis should undergo carotid revascularization sooner rather than later and that the risk of stroke or death is lower using carotid endarterectomy than carotid stenting. Specific to stenting, the risk of stroke or death is greatest among older patients and women. When considering a revascularization procedure for carotid stenosis, patient demographics, comorbidities, as well as the periprocedural risks of stroke and death should be carefully considered.

8. Acknowledgements

Dr. Cole is supported by research grants from the US Department of Veterans Affairs and the American Heart Association—Cardiovascular Genome-Phenome Study (#15GPSPG23770000).

Author details

John W. Cole[1,2*] and Christopher A. Stack[1,2]

*Address all correspondence to: jcole@som.umaryland.edu

1 UMD SOM, Baltimore, MD, USA

2 Baltimore VAMC, Baltimore, MD, USA

References

[1] Gounis MJ, van der Marel K, Marosfoi M, Mazzanti ML, Clarençon F, Chueh JY, Puri AS, Bogdanov AA Jr. Imaging Inflammation in Cerebrovascular Disease. Stroke. 2015;46(10):2991–2997. doi: 10.1161/STROKEAHA.115.008229.

[2] CDC. Detailed Tables for the National Vital Statistics Report (NVSR) "Deaths: Final Data for 2013". 2013, http://www.cdc.gov/nchs/data/nvsr/nvsr64/nvsr64_02.pdf

[3] Goff DC, Lloyd-Jones DM, Bennet G, O'Donnell CJ, Coady S, Robinson J, et al. 2013 ACC/AHA guideline on the assessment of cardiovascular risk: a report of the American

College of Cardiology/American Heart Association Task Force on Practice Guidelines. Circulation. 2014;129(25 Suppl 2):S49–S73. doi: 10.1161/01.cir.0000437741.48606.98.

[4] Eckel RH, Jakicic JM, Ard JD, Miller NH, Hubbard VS, Nonas CA, et al. 2013 AHA/ACC guideline on lifestyle management to reduce cardiovascular risk. Circulation. 2014;129(25 Suppl 2):S76–S99. doi: 10.1161/01.cir.0000437740.48606.d1.

[5] Stone NJ, Robinson J, Lichtenstein AH, Merz NB, Lloyd-Jones DM, Blum CB, et al. 2013 ACC/AHA guideline on the treatment of cholesterol to reduce atherosclerotic cardiovascular risk in adults: a report of the American College of Cardiology/American Heart Association Task Force on Practice Guidelines. Circulation. 2014;129(25 Suppl 2):S1–S45. doi: 10.1161/01.cir.0000437738.63853.7a.

[6] Jensen MD, Ryan DH, Apovian CM, Loria CM, Ard JD, Millen BE, et al. 2013 AHA/ACC/TOS guideline for the management of overweight and obesity in adults. Circulation. 2014;129(25 Suppl 2):S10–S38. doi: 10.1161/01.cir.0000437739.71477.ee.

[7] Go AS, Bauman MA, Coleman King SM, Fonarow GC, Lawrence W, Williams KA, et al. An effective approach to high blood pressure control. A science advisory from the American Heart Association, the American College of Cardiology, and the Centers for Disease Control and Prevention. Hypertension. 2014;63(4):878–885. doi: 10.1161/HYP.0000000000000003.

[8] James PA, Oparil S, Carter BL, Cushman WC, Dennison-Himmelfarb C, Handler J, et al. 2014 evidence-based guideline for the management of high blood pressure in adults. Report from the panel members appointed to the Eight Joint National Committee (JNC 8). JAMA. 2014;311(5):507–520. doi: 10.1001/jama.2013.284427.

[9] Weber MA, Schiffrin EL, White WB, Mann S, Lindholm LH, Kenerson JG, et al. Clinical practice guidelines for the management of hypertension in the community. A statement by the American Society of Hypertension and the International Society of Hypertension. J Clin Hypertens (Greenwich). 2014;16(1):14–26. doi: 10.1111/jch.12237.

[10] Meschia JF, Bushnell C, Boden-Albala B, Braun LT, Bravata DM, Chaturvedi S, et al. Guidelines for the primary prevention of stroke: a statement for healthcare professionals from the American Heart Association/American Stroke Association. Stroke. 2014;45:3754–3832.

[11] Kernan WN, Ovbiagele B, Black HR, Bravata DM, Chimowitz MI, et al. Guidelines for the prevention of stroke in patients with stroke and transient ischemic attack: a guideline for healthcare professionals from the American Heart Association/American Stroke Association. Stroke. 2014;45(7):2160–2236. doi: 10.1161/STR.0000000000000024.

[12] Spence JD. Management of patients with an asymptomatic carotid stenosis-medical management, endovascular treatment, or carotid endarterectomy? Curr Neurol Neurosci Rep. 2016;16(1):3. doi: 10.1007/s11910-015-0605-6.

[13] Spence JD. Lessons from Africa: the importance of measuring plasma renin and aldosterone in resistant hypertension. Can J Cardiol. 2012;28(3):254–257. doi:10.1016/j.cjca.2011.11.010.

[14] Spence JD, Coates V, Li H, Tamayo A, Munoz C, Hackam DG, et al. Effects of Intensive medical therapy on microemboli and cardiovascular risk in asymptomatic carotid stenosis. Arch Neurol. 2010;67(2):180–186.

[15] Chimowitz MI, Lynn MJ, Derdeyn CP, et al. Stenting versus aggressive medical therapy for intracranial arterial stenosis. N Engl J Med 2011;365(11):993Y1003.

[16] Grosser T, Fries S, Lawson JA, Kapoor SC, Grant GR, FitzGerald GA. Drug resistance and pseudoresistance: an unintended consequence of enteric coating aspirin. Circulation. 2013;127(3):377–378.

[17] CAPRIE Steering Committee. A randomised, blinded, trial of clopidogrel versus aspirin in patients at risk of ischaemic events (CAPRIE). Lancet. 1996;348(9038):1329–1339.

[18] Sacco RL, Diener HC, Yusuf S, et al; PRoFESS Study Group. Aspirin and extended-release dipyridamole versus clopidogrel for recurrent stroke. N Engl J Med. 2008;359(12):1238–1251.

[19] Wang Y, Wang Y, Zhao X, et al; CHANCE Investigators. Clopidogrel with aspirin in acute minor stroke or transient ischemic attack. N Engl J Med. 2013;369(1):11–19.

[20] Wang Y, Pan Y, Zhao X, et al; CHANCE Investigators. Clopidogrel with aspirin in acute minor stroke or transient ischemic attack (CHANCE) trial: one-year outcomes. Circulation. 2015;132(1):40–46.

[21] Wang X, Lin WH, Zhao YD, et al. The effectiveness of dual antiplatelet treatment in acute ischemic stroke patients with intracranial arterial stenosis: a subgroup analysis of CLAIR study. Int J Stroke. 2013;8(8):663–668.

[22] POINT Investigators 2016. General Information about ongoing trial, Platelet-Oriented Inhibition and minor ischemic stroke (POINT) Trial. http://www.pointtrial.org/.

[23] Markus HS, Droste DW, Kaps M, et al. Dual antiplatelet therapy with clopidogrel and aspirin in symptomatic carotid stenosis evaluated using Doppler embolic signal detection: the Clopidogrel and Aspirin for Reduction of Emboli in Symptomatic Carotid Stenosis (CARESS) trial. Circulation. 2005;111(17):2233–2240.

[24] Diener HC, Bogousslavsky J, Brass LM, et al; MATCH Investigators. Aspirin and clopidogrel compared with clopidogrel alone after recent ischaemic stroke or transient ischaemic attack in high risk patients (MATCH): randomised, double-blind, placebo controlled trial. Lancet. 2004;364(9431):331–337.

[25] Barnett HJM, Taylor DW, Eliasziw M, et al. Benefit of carotid endarterectomy in patients with symptomatic moderate or severe carotid stenosis. (NASCET) N Engl J Med. 1998;339(20):1415–1425.

[26] De Caterina R, Scarano M, Marfisi R, Lucisano G, Palma F, Tatasciore A, Marchioli R. Cholesterol-lowering interventions and stroke: insights from a meta-analysis of randomized controlled trials. J Am Coll Cardiol. 2010;55:198–211.

[27] Grundy SM, Mok HY, Zech L, Berman M. Influence of nicotinic acid on metabolism of cholesterol and triglycerides in man. J Lipid Res 1981;22:24.

[28] Illingworth DR, Stein EA, Mitchel YB, et al. Comparative effects of lovastatin and niacin in primary hypercholesterolemia. A prospective trial. Arch Intern Med 1994;154:1586.

[29] AIM-HIGH Investigators, Boden WE, Probstfield JL, et al. Niacin in patients with low HDL cholesterol levels receiving intensive statin therapy. N Engl J Med 2011;365:2255.

[30] HPS2-THRIVE Collaborative Group, Landray MJ, Haynes R, et al. Effects of extended-release niacin with laropiprant in high-risk patients. N Engl J Med 2014;371:203.

[31] James PA, Oparil S, Carter BL, Cushman WC, Dennison-Himmelfarb C, Handler J, Lackland DT, LeFevre ML, MacKenzie TD, Ogedegbe O, Smith SC Jr, Svetkey LP, Taler SJ, Townsend RR, Wright JT Jr, Narva AS, Ortiz E. 2014 Evidence-based guideline for the management of high blood pressure in adults: report from the panel members appointed to the Eighth Joint National Committee (JNC 8). JAMA. 2014;311:507–520.

[32] Chambless LE, Folsom AR, Davis V, et al. Risk factors for progression of common carotid atherosclerosis: the Atherosclerosis Risk in Communities Study, 1987-1998. Am J Epidemiol. 2002;155(1):38–47.

[33] Banerjee C, Moon YP, Paik MC, Rundek T, Mora-McLaughlin C, Vieira JR, Sacco RL, Elkind MS. Duration of diabetes and risk of ischemic stroke: the Northern Manhattan Study. Stroke. 2012;43:1212–1217.

[34] Paraskevas KI, Mikhailidis DP, Veith FJ, Spence JD. Definition of best medical treatment23 in asymptomatic and symptomatic carotid artery stenosis. Angiology. 2016 67(5):411–9.

[35] Koo BB, Bravata DM, Tobias LA, Mackey JS, Miech EJ, Matthias MS, Stahl SM, Sico JJ, Vaz Fragoso CA, Williams LS, Lampert R, Qin L, Yaggi HK. Observational study of obstructive sleep apnea in wake-up stroke: the SLEEP TIGHT study. Cerebrovasc Dis. 2016;41(5-6):233–241.

[36] Seminog OO, Goldacre MJ. Gout as a risk factor for myocardial infarction and stroke in England: evidence from record linkage studies. Rheumatology (Oxford). 2013;52(12): 2251–2259. doi: 10.1093/rheumatology/ket293. Epub 2013 September 17.

[37] Larsen KS, Pottegård A, Lindegaard HM, Hallas J. Effect of allopurinol on cardiovascular outcomes in hyperuricemic patients: a cohort study. Am J Med. 2016. 129(3):299–306.

[38] Stewart R, West M. Increasing evidence for an association between periodontitis and cardiovascular disease. Circulation. 2016.133(6):549–51.

[39] NINDS Stroke Genetics Network (SiGN); International Stroke Genetics Consortium1 (ISGC). Loci associated with ischaemic stroke and its subtypes (SiGN): a genome-wide2 association study. Lancet Neurol. 2016. 15(2):174–184.

[40] Kaufmann TJ, Huston J 3rd, Mandrekar JN, Schleck CD, Thielen KR, Kallmes DF. Complications of diagnostic cerebral angiography: evaluation of 19,826 consecutive patients. Radiology. 2007;243:812–819.

[41] Ratchford EV, Jin Z, Di Tullio MR, Salameh MJ, Homma S, Gan R, Boden-Albala B, Sacco RL, Rundek T. Carotid bruit for detection of hemodynamically significant carotid stenosis: the Northern Manhattan Study. Neurol Res. 2009;31:748–752.

[42] Spence JD, Tamayo A, Lownie SP, Ng WP, Ferguson GG. Absence of microemboli on transcranial Doppler identifies low-risk patients with asymptomatic carotid stenosis. Stroke. 2005;36(11):2373–2378.

[43] Markus HS, King A, Shipley M, Topakian R, Cullinane M, Reihill S, et al. Asymptomatic embolisation for prediction of stroke in the Asymptomatic Carotid Emboli Study (ACES): a prospective observational study. Lancet Neurol. 2010;9(7):663–671.

[44] US Preventive Services Task Force. Screening for carotid artery stenosis: U.S. Preventive Services Task Force recommendation statement. Ann Intern Med. 2007;147:854–859.

[45] Endarterectomy for asymptomatic carotid artery stenosis: Executive Committee for the Asymptomatic Carotid Atherosclerosis Study. JAMA. 1995;273:1421–1428. http://www.ncbi.nlm.nih.gov/pubmed/7723155

[46] Halliday A, Mansfield A, Marro J, Peto C, Peto R, Potter J, Thomas D; MRC Asymptomatic Carotid Surgery Trial (ACST) Collaborative Group. Prevention of disabling and fatal strokes by successful carotid endarterectomy in patients without recent neurological symptoms: randomized controlled trial. Lancet. 2004;363:1491–1502.

[47] Moore WS, Young B, Baker WH, Robertson JT, Toole JF, Vescera CL, Howard VJ. Surgical results: a justification of the surgeon selection process for the ACAS trial: the ACAS Investigators. J Vasc Surg. 1996;23:323–328.

[48] Voeks JH, Howard G, Roubin GS, Malas MB, Cohen DJ, Sternbergh WC 3rd, Aronow HD, Eskandari MK, Sheffet AJ, Lal BK, Meschia JF, Brott TG; CREST Investigators. Age and outcomes after carotid stenting and endarterectomy: the Carotid Revascularization Endarterectomy Versus Stenting Trial. Stroke. 2011;42:3484–3490.

[49] Lal BK, Meschia JF, Brott TG. CREST-2: Guiding treatments for asymptomatic carotid disease. Endovascular Today. 2013:73–76. http://evtoday.com/2013/09/crest-2-guiding-treatments-for-asymptomatic-carotid-disease/

[50] Rubin MN, Barrett KM, Brott TG, Meschia JF. Asymptomatic carotid stenosis: What we can learn from the next generation of randomized clinical trials. JRSM Cardiovasc Dis. 2014;3:2048004014529419. doi: 10.1177/2048004014529419.

[51] Yadav JS, Wholey MH, Kuntz RE, Fayad P, Katzen BT, Mishkel GJ, Bajwa TK, Whitlow P, Strickman NE, Jaff MR, Popma JJ, Snead DB, Cutlip DE, Firth BG, Ouriel K; Stenting and Angioplasty With Protection in Patients at High Risk for Endarterectomy Investigators. Protected carotid-artery stenting versus endarterectomy in high-risk patients. N Engl J Med. 2004;351:1493–1501.

[52] Gurm HS, Yadav JS, Fayad P, Katzen BT, Mishkel GJ, Bajwa TK, Ansel G, Strickman NE, Wang H, Cohen SA, Massaro JM, Cutlip DE, SAPPHIRE Investigators. Long-term results of carotid stenting versus endarterectomy in high-risk patients. 2008;358:1572–1579.

[53] Brott TG, Hobson RW 2nd, Howard G, Roubin GS, Clark WM, Brooks W, Mackey A, Hill MD, Leimgruber PP, Sheffet AJ, Howard VJ, Moore WS, Voeks JH, Hopkins LN, Cutlip DE, Cohen DJ, Popma JJ, Ferguson RD, Cohen SN, Blackshear JL, Silver FL, Mohr JP, Lal BK, Meschia JF; CREST Investigators. Stenting versus endarterectomy for treatment of carotid-artery stenosis. N Engl J Med. 2010;363:11–23.

[54] European Carotid Surgery Trialists Collaborative Group. MRC European Carotid Surgery Trial: interim results for symptomatic patients with severe (70–99%) or with mild (0–29%) carotid stenosis. Lancet. 1991;337:1235–1243.

[55] Mayberg MR, Wilson SE, Yatsu F, Weiss DG, Messina L, Hershey LA, Colling C, Eskridge J, Deykin D, Winn HR; Veterans Affairs Cooperative Studies Program 309 Trialist Group. Carotid endarterectomy and prevention of cerebral ischemia in symptomatic carotid stenosis. JAMA. 1991;266:3289–3294.

[56] Rothwell PM, Eliasziw M, Gutnikov SA, Fox AJ, Taylor DW, Mayberg MR, Warlow CP, Barnett HJ; Carotid Endarterectomy Trialists' Collaboration. Analysis of pooled data from the randomised controlled trials of endarterectomy for symptomatic carotid stenosis. Lancet. 2003;361:107–116.

[57] Tu JV, Wang H, Bowyer B, Green L, Fang J, Kucey D; for the Participants in the Ontario Carotid Endarterectomy Registry. Risk factors for death or stroke after carotid endarterectomy: observations from the Ontario Carotid Endarterectomy Registry. Stroke. 2003;34:2568–2573.

[58] Hugl B, Oldenburg WA, Neuhauser B, Hakaim AG. Effect of age and gender on restenosis after carotid endarterectomy. Ann Vasc Surg. 2006;20:602–608.

[59] Howard VJ, Lutsep HL, Mackey A, Demaerschalk BM, Sam AD, 2nd, Gonzales NR, Sheffet AJ, Voeks JH, Meschia JF, Brott TG; for the CREST Investigators. Influence of sex on outcomes of stenting versus endarterectomy: a subgroup analysis of the Carotid Revascularization Endarterectomy versus Stenting Trial (CREST). Lancet Neurol. 2011;10:530–537.

[60] Hingorani A, Ascher E, Schutzer R, Tsemkhim B, Kallakuri S, Yorkovich W, Jacob T. Carotid endarterectomy in octogenarians and nonagenarians: is it worth the effort? Acta Chir Belg. 2004;104:384–387.

[61] Rothwell PM, Eliasziw M, Gutnikov SA, Warlow CP, Barnett HJ; Carotid Endarterectomy Trialists Collaboration. Endarterectomy for symptomatic carotid stenosis in relation to clinical subgroups and timing of surgery. Lancet. 2004;363:915–924.

[62] Cohen DJ, Stolker JM, Wang K, Magnuson EA, Clark WM, Demaerschalk BM, Sam AD Jr, Elmore JR, Weaver FA, Aronow HD, Goldstein LB, Roubin GS, Howard G, Brott TG; on behalf of the CREST Investigators. Health-related quality of life after carotid stenting versus carotid endarterectomy: results from CREST (Carotid Revascularization Endarterectomy Versus Stenting Trial). J Am Coll Cardiol. 2011;58:1557–1565.

[63] CAVATAS Investigators. Endovascular versus surgical treatment in patients with carotid stenosis in the Carotid and Vertebral Artery Transluminal Angioplasty Study (CAVATAS): a randomised trial. Lancet. 2001;357:1729–1737.

[64] International Carotid Stenting Study Investigators; Ederle J, Dobson J, Featherstone RL, Bonati LH, van der Worp HB, de Borst GJ, Lo TH, Gaines P, Dorman PJ, Macdonald S, Lyrer PA, Hendriks JM, McCollum C, Nederkoorn PJ, Brown MM. Carotid artery stenting compared with endarterectomy in patients with symptomatic carotid stenosis (International Carotid Stenting Study): an interim analysis of a randomised controlled trial [published correction appears in Lancet. 2010;376:90]. Lancet. 2010;375:985–997.

[65] Carotid Stenting Trialists' Collaboration; Bonati LH, Dobson J, Algra A, Branchereau A, Chatellier G, Fraedrich G, Mali WP, Zeumer H, Brown MM, Mas JL, Ringleb PA. Short-term outcome after stenting versus endarterectomy for symptomatic carotid stenosis: a preplanned meta-analysis of individual patient data. Lancet. 2010;376:1062–1073.

[66] Lal BK, Beach KW, Roubin GS, Lutsep HL, Moore WS, Malas MB, Chiu D, Gonzales NR, Burke JL, Rinaldi M, Elmore JR, Weaver FA, Narins CR, Foster M, Hodgson KJ, Shepard AD, Meschia JF, Bergelin RO, Voeks JH, Howard G, Brott TG; CREST Investigators. Restenosis after carotid artery stenting and endarterectomy: a secondary analysis of CREST, a randomised controlled trial. Lancet Neurol. 2012;11:755–763.

[67] The EC/IC Bypass Study Group. Failure of extracranial-intracranial arterial bypass to reduce the risk of ischemic stroke: results of an international randomized trial. N Engl J Med. 1985;313:1191–1200.

[68] Powers WJ, Clarke WR, Grubb RL Jr, Videen TO, Adams HP Jr, Derdeyn CP; COSS Investigators. Extracranial-intracranial bypass surgery for stroke prevention in hemodynamic cerebral ischemia: the Carotid Occlusion Surgery Study randomized trial [published correction appears in JAMA. 2011;306:2672]. JAMA. 2011;306:1983–1992.

[69] Chimowitz MI, Lynn MJ, Howlett-Smith H, Stern BJ, Hertzberg VS, Frankel MR, Levine SR, Chaturvedi S, Kasner SE, Benesch CG, Sila CA, Jovin TG, Romano JG; for the Warfarin-Aspirin Symptomatic Intracranial Disease Trial Investigators. Comparison of

warfarin and aspirin for symptomatic intracranial arterial stenosis. N Engl J Med. 2005;352:1305–1316.

[70] Kasner SE, Chimowitz MI, Lynn MJ, Howlett-Smith H, Stern BJ, Hertzberg VS, Frankel MR, Levine SR, Chaturvedi S, Benesch CG, Sila CA, Jovin TG, Romano JG, Cloft HJ; for the Warfarin Aspirin Symptomatic Intracranial Disease (WASID) Trial Investigators. Predictors of ischemic stroke in the territory of a symptomatic intracranial arterial stenosis. Circulation. 2006;113:555–563.

[71] Turan TN, Cotsonis G, Lynn MJ, Chaturvedi S, Chimowitz M; for the Warfarin-Aspirin Symptomatic Intracranial Disease (WASID) Trial Investigators. Relationship between blood pressure and stroke recurrence in patients with intracranial arterial stenosis. Circulation. 2007;115:2969–2975.

[72] Chaturvedi S, Turan TN, Lynn MJ, Kasner SE, Romano J, Cotsonis G, Frankel M, Chimowitz MI; WASID Study Group. Risk factor status and vascular events in patients with symptomatic intracranial stenosis. Neurology. 2007;69:2063–2068.

[73] Bose A, Hartmann M, Henkes H, Liu HM, Teng MM, Szikora I, Berlis A, Reul J, Yu SC, Forsting M, Lui M, Lim W, Sit SP. A novel, self-expanding, nitinol stent in medically refractory intracranial atherosclerotic stenoses: The wingspan study. Stroke. 2007;38:1531–1537.

[74] Fiorella D, Derdeyn CP, Lynn MJ, Barnwell SL, Hoh BL, Levy EI, Harrigan MR, Klucznik RP, McDougall CG, Pride GL Jr, Zaidat OO, Lutsep HL, Waters MF, Hourihane JM, Alexandrov AV, Chiu D, Clark JM, Johnson MD, Torbey MT, Rumboldt Z, Cloft HJ, Turan TN, Lane BF, Janis LS, Chimowitz MI; for the SAMMPRIS Trial Investigators. Detailed analysis of periprocedural strokes in patients undergoing intracranial stenting in Stenting and Aggressive Medical Management for Preventing Recurrent Stroke in Intracranial Stenosis (SAMMPRIS). Stroke. 2012;43:2682–2688.

[75] Derdeyn CP, Chimowitz MI, Lynn MJ, Fiorella D, Turan TN, Janis LS, Montgomery J, Nizam A, Lane BF, Lutsep HL, Barnwell SL, Waters MF, Hoh BL, Hourihane JM, Levy EI, Alexandrov AV, Harrigan MR, Chiu D, Klucznik RP, Clark JM, McDougall CG, Johnson MD, Pride GL, Lynch JR, Zaidat OO, Rumboldt Z, Cloft HJ; for the Stenting and Aggressive Medical Management for Preventing Recurrent Stroke in Intracranial Stenosis Trial Investigators. Aggressive medical treatment with or without stenting in high-risk patients with intracranial artery stenosis (SAMMPRIS): the final results of a randomised trial. Lancet. 2014;383:333–341.

[76] Klucznik RP, Clark JM, McDougall CG, Johnson MD, Pride GL, Lynch JR, Zaidat OO, Rumboldt Z, Cloft HJ; for the Stenting and Aggressive Medical Management for Preventing Recurrent Stroke in Intracranial Stenosis Trial Investigators. Aggressive medical treatment with or without stenting in high-risk patients with intracranial artery stenosis (SAMMPRIS): the final results of a randomised trial. Lancet. 2014;383:333–341.

[77] Wityk RJ, Chang HM, Rosengart A, Han WC, DeWitt LD, Pessin MS, Caplan LR. Proximal extracranial vertebral artery disease in the New England Medical Center Posterior Circulation Registry. Arch Neurol. 1998;55:470–478.

[78] Al-Ali F, Barrow T, Duan L, Jefferson A, Louis S, Luke K, Major K, Smoker S, Walker S, Yacobozzi M. Vertebral artery ostium atherosclerotic plaque as a potential source of posterior circulation ischemic stroke: result from Borgess Medical Center Vertebral Artery Ostium Stenting Registry. Stroke. 2011;42:2544–2549.

[79] Coward LJ, McCabe DJ, Ederle J, Featherstone RL, Clifton A, Brown MM; CAVATAS Investigators. Long-term outcome after angioplasty and stenting for symptomatic vertebral artery stenosis compared with medical treatment in the Carotid And Vertebral Artery Transluminal Angioplasty Study (CAVATAS): a randomized trial. Stroke. 2007;38:1526–1530.

[80] Marquardt L, Kuker W, Chandratheva A, et al. Incidence and prognosis of 9 or = 50% symptomatic vertebral or basilar artery stenosis: prospective population-based study. Brain 2009;132(pt 4):982Y988.

[81] Compter A, van der Worp HB, Schonewille WJ, Vos JA, Boiten J, Nederkoorn PJ, Uyttenboogaart M, Lo RT, Algra A, Kappelle LJ; VAST investigators. Stenting versus medical treatment in patients with symptomatic vertebral artery stenosis: a randomised open-label phase 2 trial. Lancet Neurol. 2015;14(6):606–614. doi: 10.1016/S1474-4422(15)00017-4.

[82] VIST 2016. Overview of The Vertebral Artery Ischaemia Stenting Trial (VIST). http://www.vist.org.uk/84. Stayman AN, Nogueira RG, Gupta R. A systematic review of stenting and angioplasty of symptomatic extracranial vertebral artery stenosis. Stroke. 2011;42:2212–2216.

[83] Stayman AN, Nogueira RG, Gupta R. A systematic review of stenting and angioplasty of symptomatic extracranial vertebral artery stenosis. Stroke. 2011;42(8):2212–2216.

[84] Eberhardt O, Naegele T, Raygrotzki S, et al. Stenting of vertebrobasilar arteries in symptomatic atherosclerotic disease and acute occlusion: case series and review of the literature. J Vasc Surg 2006;43(6):1145Y1154.

[85] Tank VH, Ghosh R, Gupta V, Sheth N, Gordon S, He W, Modica SF, Prestigiacomo CJ, Gandhi CD. Drug eluting stents versus bare metal stents for the treatment of extracranial vertebral artery disease: a meta-analysis. J Neurointerv Surg. 2016. 8(8):770–4.

[86] Berguer R, Bauer RB. Vertebral artery reconstruction: a successful technique in selected patients. Ann Surg. 1981;193:441–447.

Chapter 11

Complementary Therapy with Traditional Chinese Medicine for Ischemic Stroke

Po-Yu Huang, Yu-Chiang Hung and Wen-Long Hu

Additional information is available at the end of the chapter

http://dx.doi.org/10.5772/64585

Abstract

Stroke has remained the leading cause of morbidity or mortality worldwide over the past decade. Stroke survivors suffer various degrees of disability and also contribute to the large socioeconomic disease burden. Traditional Chinese medicine (TCM) serves as an important alternative or complementary therapy in many countries. This chapter aims to explore the utility of TCM for ischemic stroke, including a review of recent literature on the mechanisms of herbal medicine and acupuncture therapy on ischemic stroke, a summary of clinical trial results for the safety and efficacy of acupuncture, and finally a discussion of acupuncture as a preventive therapy for ischemic stroke in clinical practice. On the basis of these reports, more and more scientific evidences suggest that TCM use was safe for ischemic stroke at acute and subacute stages. Moreover, TCM has benefit for stroke recovery as well as it reduces the likelihood of hospital readmission for cardiovascular or subsequent stroke events.

Keywords: ischemic stroke, traditional Chinese medicine, acupuncture

1. Introduction

Stroke has remained the leading cause of death worldwide over the past decade despite a gradual decline in stroke mortality in many industrialized countries. Stroke survivors suffer various degrees of disability, including urinary incontinence, dysarthria, limb deficits, swallowing deficits, dysphasia, and consciousness disorders. Stroke also contributes to the largest socioeconomic disease burden together with ischemic heart disease [1, 2]. Additional treatment strategies are needed to improve poststroke recovery. Traditional Chinese medicine (TCM) serves as an important alternative or complementary healthcare option in many countries. The purpose of this review was to investigate and discuss the utility of TCM as a complementary therapy for ischemic stroke. English and Chinese articles on TCM and acupuncture for ischemic stroke published between 2006 and 2015 were sourced from the Cochrane Library, PubMed, and China National Knowledge Infrastructure databases. On the basis of these reports, this chapter presents a brief description of the pathophysiology of ischemic stroke, a review of recent literature on the mechanisms of herbal medicine and acupuncture therapy in ischemic stroke, a summary of clinical trial results for the safety and efficacy of acupuncture, and finally a discussion of acupuncture as a preventive therapy for ischemic stroke in clinical practice.

2. Ischemic stroke

2.1. Pathophysiology of ischemic stroke

Ischemic stroke accounts for approximately 80% of stroke events and is an acute neurological injury that occurs as a result of reduced cerebral blood flow [3]. Reductions in cerebral blood flow in ischemic stroke can be due to decreased systemic perfusion, severe stenosis, or blood vessel occlusion. Decreased systemic perfusion can be the result of low blood pressure, heart failure, or blood loss. An infarcted brain is initially pale due to a lack of perfusion. Within hours to days, the gray matter of an infarcted brain becomes congested with engorged, dilated blood vessels, and minute petechial hemorrhages. When an embolus blocking a major vessel migrates, lyses, or disperses, recirculation into the infarcted area can cause an additional hemorrhagic infarction and may aggravate edema formation due to disruption of the blood-brain barrier (BBB) [3]. Given the diversity of stroke characteristics, an accurate determination of the type of stroke can influence the treatment indicated.

2.2. Stroke subtypes

Acute ischemic stroke subtypes have been classified in clinical studies using a system developed by the Trial of Org 10172 in Acute Stroke Treatment (TOAST) trial [4]. The TOAST classification denotes five subtypes of ischemic stroke according to underlying cause: (1) large-artery atherosclerosis, (2) cardioembolism, (3) small-vessel occlusion, (4) stroke of other determined etiology, and (5) stroke of undetermined etiology.

2.3. Cerebral autoregulation during stroke

Cerebral autoregulation is the maintenance of cerebral blood flow at a relatively constant level despite moderate variations in perfusion pressure. Importantly, cerebral autoregulation is impaired during ischemic stroke. Normally, as cerebral perfusion pressure falls, cerebral blood vessels dilate to increase cerebral blood flow. However, a decrease in perfusion pressure beyond the compensatory ability of blood vessels results in an overall reduction in cerebral blood flow. In response to the impairment of cerebral autoregulation, the oxygen extraction fraction is initially increased in order to maintain necessary levels of oxygen delivery to the brain. With time, these mechanisms fail and a state of ischemia occurs [5–7].

2.4. Mechanisms of ischemic cell injury and death

The human brain is exquisitely sensitive and susceptible to even short durations of ischemia. Because the brain contains little or no energy stores of its own, it relies on blood flow for the delivery of important resources. Thus, even brief blood flow deprivation can lead to cellular death in affected brain tissue.

During ischemic stroke, reduced blood flow results in simultaneous glucose and oxygen deprivation [3]. Ischemic cell injury initiates a cascade of events that finally lead to cell death including adenosine triphosphate (ATP) depletion, changes in intracellular ionic concentrations of sodium, potassium, and calcium, increased lactate formation, acidosis, accumulated oxygen free radicals, intracellular accumulation of water, and the activating proteolytic processes [8, 9].

2.5. Loss of brain structural integrity

Cerebral ischemia and infarction lead to decreases in the structural integrity of the affected brain tissue and blood vessels [9]. This process of tissue damage and neurovascular disruption is mediated in part by the release of various proteases including matrix metalloproteases (MMPs) that degrade components of the basal lamina [8]. Loss of vascular integrity leads to breakdown of the blood-brain barrier and the development of cerebral edema.

2.6. Cerebral edema

Cerebral edema occurring as a complication of stroke can cause secondary damage via several mechanisms, including increased intracranial pressure. Intracranial pressure can lead to decreases in cerebral blood flow and the life-threatening displacement of brain tissue from one compartment to another (i.e., herniation).

Two types of cerebral edema can follow ischemic stroke [9]. Cytotoxic edema is caused by the failure of ATP-dependent sodium and calcium ion transport across the cell membrane. The result is cellular water accumulation and swelling of neurons, glia, and endothelial cells. Alternatively, vasogenic edema is caused by breakdown of the vascular endothelial cells and tight junctions that constitute the BBB [10]. Increases in the permeability of the BBB during vasogenic edema allow proteins and other macromolecules to enter the extracellular space, resulting in increased extracellular fluid volume.

3. Mechanisms of herbal medicines in ischemic stroke

3.1. Limiting postischemic inflammation as a mechanism of neuroprotection

Astrocytes, endothelial cells, and pericytes constitute a neurovascular network that attends the metabolic requirements of neurons. These cells contribute to postischemic inflammation during different stages of ischemia [11]. Upon ischemia onset, resident microglia and astrocytes as well as infiltrating immune cells become activated and release inflammatory factors including cytokines, chemokines, enzymes, free radicals, and other small molecules. These inflammatory factors not only mediate further brain damage but also affect brain repair.

Recent research indicates that postischemic inflammation is an important therapeutic target for stroke [12–14]. In this context, TCM and related natural compounds are recognized as important resources for drug discovery. In the past decade, significant progress has been made in the identification of active compounds from herbal medicines useful for limiting postischemic inflammation [11]. In the subsequent sections, we discuss the different roles of inflammatory pathways in ischemic stroke, from initial arterial occlusion to brain repair, and review active ingredients observed to have antiinflammatory and neuroprotective properties relevant to ischemic stroke.

4. Chinese herbal formulas used in patients with ischemic stroke

4.1. Di Huang Yin Zi (DHYZ)

A double-blind randomized controlled trial (RCT) was conducted to investigate the safety and therapeutic efficacy of the Di Huang Yin Zi (DHYZ) herbal formula in patients affected by ischemic stroke [15]. In this study, 100 patients with an ischemic stroke event occurring in the previous 30 days were randomly assigned to receive either DHYZ treatment or placebo for 12 weeks. Both groups also received rehabilitation therapy during the study period. The results indicated that there were increases in both Fugl-Meyer Assessment (FMA) scores and Barthel index (BI) scores in both groups at 4, 8, and 12 weeks relative to baseline. However, FMA scores in the DHYZ group were statistically better than those in the placebo group at 8 and 12 weeks ($P < 0.05$), and BI scores were significantly higher in the DHYZ group at 12 weeks ($P < 0.05$). By the end of the study, DHYZ produced significantly greater improvements in FMA score than placebo (44.4% vs. 23.8%, respectively, $\chi^2 = 4.09$, $P < 0.05$). It was concluded that DHYZ showed good efficacy, safety, and tolerability in patients affected by ischemic stroke [15].

4.2. Bu-yang-huan-wu-tang (BYHWT) and Dan Shen

A study was conducted to investigate the prescription patterns and combinations of traditional Chinese herbal products (CHPs) for ischemic stroke in Taiwan. Every CHP prescription with a leading diagnosis of ischemic stroke between the years 2000 and 2010 (15,896 patients) was obtained from the National Health Insurance Research Database (NHIRD) of Taiwan and included for analysis. Bu-yang-huan-wu-tang (BYHWT) was by far the most frequently prescribed CHP formula for ischemic stroke (40.32%), while BYHWT with Shu-jin-huo-xue-tang (SJHXT) was the most commonly prescribed CHP formula combination (4.40%). Dan Shen was the most commonly prescribed single CHP for ischemic stroke (16.50%), and Shi Chang Pua with Yuan Zhi was the most commonly prescribed single-CHP combination (4.79%). These results provide information about individualized stroke therapy and propose specific CHP components and formulas for further pharmacological investigation and clinical evaluation [16].

http://dx.doi.org/10.5772/64585

4.3. Rhubarb root and rhizome (RRR)-based Chinese herbal prescriptions

Rhubarb root and rhizome (RRR)-based Chinese herbal prescription is one of the principal treatments for stroke. A systematic literature search of six databases was performed to identify RCTs comparing RRR-based prescriptions with Western conventional medicine (WCM) for the treatment of acute ischemic stroke [17]. A total of 968 participants were included from 12 eligible studies. The methodological quality of RCTs was assessed independently based on the 12 criteria recommended by the Cochrane Back Review Group. While all trials were deemed to have high a risk of bias, RRR-based prescriptions had a significantly better effect clinical efficacy rate (n = 10) and improved Barthel index scores (n = 5), National Institutes of Health Stroke Scale scores (n = 2), Glasgow Coma Scale scores (n = 1), and neurological deficit scores (n = 5) relative to WCM ($P < 0.05$ or $P < 0.01$) in the included studies. Six trials reported no adverse events for RRR-based prescriptions, while the remaining studies did not report adverse effect monitoring. Despite these positive findings, it is premature to recommend the routine use of RRR-based prescriptions for acute ischemic stroke due to methodological flaws in the aforementioned studies. However, RRR-based treatments merit further development and research. Larger sample sizes and more rigorously designed RCT paradigms are required in the future **(Table 1)**.

Study	*N*	Design	Chinese herbal formulas	Outcomes
Yu et al. (2015) [15]	45:42	Double-blind RCT	DHYZ	DHYZ significantly improved FMA scores after 12 weeks of treatment relative to placebo control. DHYZ showed good efficacy, safety, and tolerability.
Hung et al. (2015) [16]	15,896	Observational study from NHIRD	BYHWT and Dan Shen	BYHWT and Dan Shen were the most frequently prescribed formula and single CHP, respectively, for ischemic stroke.
Lu et al. (2014) [17]	968	Systematic review of RCT	RRR-based prescriptions	RRR-based prescriptions had a significantly better effect clinical efficacy rate (n = 10) and improved BI scores (n = 5), NIHSS scores (n = 2), GCS scores (n = 1), and neurological deficit scores (n = 5) relative to WCM ($P < 0.05$ or $P < 0.01$).

NHIRD: National Health Insurance Research Database

Table 1. Chinese herbal formulas used in patients with ischemic stroke.

5. The mechanism of acupuncture therapy in ischemic stroke

5.1. Acupuncture promotes neurogenesis in experimental ischemic stroke

Previous studies have reported that acupuncture enhances stroke recovery by promoting neurogenesis. A systematic review and metaanalysis of preclinical studies assessing acupuncture in ischemic stroke identified a total of 1617 animals in 34 eligible studies [18]. Neurogenesis markers including BrdU, Nestin, PSA-NCAM, NeuN, and GFAP were selected as major outcomes. The pooled results of 15 studies evaluating BrdU incorporation showed a significant positive effect of acupuncture on proliferation relative to control ($P < 0.01$); 13 studies evaluating Nestin labeling corroborated this finding ($P < 0.01$). Four studies examining PSA-NCAM identified a significant positive effect of acupuncture on cell migration ($P < 0.01$) while four studies examining NeuN labeling demonstrated a significant effect of acupuncture on neuronal differentiation ($P < 0.01$). These findings suggest that acupuncture is a prospective therapy for targeting neurogenesis in ischemic stroke.

5.2. Neuroprotective effects of electroacupuncture (EA) in experimental stroke

It is well established that EA has neuroprotective effects in animals [19]. A series of studies have proposed EA as a promising method for reducing brain damage after stroke and inducing brain ischemic tolerance prior to a stroke event. The mechanism of action for EA has been reported to involve the promotion of angiogenesis, alleviation of the inflammatory response, regulation of the BBB, and inhibition of apoptosis.

5.3. Acupuncture regulates cerebral glucose metabolism in functional regions

A previous study using (18)FDG PET-CT analyzed the relevance between acupuncture and cerebral glucose metabolism in functional regions of the brain in poststroke patients [20]. Forty-three patients with ischemic stroke were randomly assigned to five groups: a Waiguan (TE5) needling group, a TE5 sham needling group, a sham point needling group, a sham point and sham needling group, and a nonneedling group. Needling at TE5 resulted in the activation of Brodmann area (BA) 30. Sham needling at a sham point led to the deactivation of BA6, whereas needling or sham needling at TE5 or needling at the sham point did not deactivate any cerebral areas. Compared with sham needling at TE5, needling at TE5 activated BA13, BA19, and BA47, but did not deactivate any areas. Compared with needling at the sham point, needling at TE5 did not activate any areas but did deactivate BA9. This study concluded that needling at TE5 has a regulatory effect on cerebral glucose metabolism that potentially relates to its impact on poststroke recovery in patients [20].

5.4. Effects of acupuncture on motor function and white matter microstructure

Evidence shows that ischemic stroke can induce structural reorganization of the brain. One study used diffusion tensor imaging (DTI) to evaluate 14 ischemic stroke patients one month after either conventional treatment or acupuncture treatment [21]. While significant functional improvements as measured by FMA score were observed in the acupuncture group relative to the conventional treatment group, no significant differences in DTI indices were identified between the two groups. However, postpair *t*-tests in each group revealed that diffusion indices were significantly altered in the body of the corpus callosum, bilateral corticospinal tracts, inferior longitudinal fasciculus, inferior frontooccipital fasciculus, superior longitudinal fasciculus, forceps minor, cingulum gyrus, and thalamic radiation one month after treatment intervention. These data indicate that while successful treatment produced alterations in white matter regions of the brain, the changes did not correlate with differences in functional improvement.

Study	N	Design	Possible mechanisms
Lu et al. (2016) [18]	1617	1. Systematic review and metaanalysis 2. Neurogenesis markers 3. Animals model	Neurogenesis markers including BrdU, Nestin, PSA-NCAM, NeuN, and GFAP are increased after acupuncture.
Feng et al. (2014) [19]		1. Review study 2. Animal model	EA reduces brain damage and induces brain ischemic tolerance by promoting angiogenesis, alleviating the inflammatory response, regulating the BBB, and inhibiting apoptosis.
Huang et al. (2012) [20]	43	1. Functional neuroimaging (F-18 FDG PET/CT) 2. Acupoint: Waiguan (TE5) 3. Five groups: TE5 needling group, the TE5 sham needling group, the sham point needling group, the sham point sham needling group and the nonneedling group.	Needling at TE5 regulates cerebral glucose metabolism functional areas of the brain.
Li et al. (2015) [21]	*7:7*	1. *Diffusion tensor imaging* studies 2. Acupoints: Baihui (GV20), Fengchi (GB20, bilateral), Xuanzhong (GB39, bilateral), Quchi (LI11 bilateral), Hegu (LI4, bilateral), Zusanli (ST36, bilateral), and Sanyinjiao (SP6, bilateral). 3. Conventional treatment group (CG) and acupuncture treatment group (AG).	Acupuncture had better functional benefits than conventional stroke therapy, but white matter microstructure changes were not significantly different from those elicited by conventional therapy.
Li et al. (2015) [22]	5:5	1. Functional magnetic resonance imaging study 2. Acupoint: Waiguan (SJ5) 3. Deqi group, non-Deqi group	Deqi can be observed as a change in brain activity during acupuncture. Cerebellar activation may be a central mechanism of the beneficial effect of acupuncture in stroke.

Table 2. The possible mechanisms of acupuncture therapy in ischemic stroke.

5.5. Brain activation in response to acupuncture and Deqi

The Deqi response in acupuncture (obtaining Qi, causing the acupuncture needle to elicit the patient's feeling of soreness, numbness, distension, heaviness, or even electric shock sensation around the acupuncture point together with the practitioner's feeling of tenseness around the needle) during acupuncture is a key factor that influences treatment outcome. Recent studies have mainly focused on the functional effects of Deqi in a physiological brain state. A functional magnetic resonance imaging (fMRI) study was conducted on 12 ischemic stroke patients receiving acupuncture at Waiguan (SJ5) and patients were group according to Deqi sensation [22]. In the Deqi group, the activated and deactivated areas were the left superior temporal gyrus (BA39) and the right anterior lobe of the cerebellum as well as left thalamus, respectively.

In the non-Deqi group, activated areas included the medial frontal gyrus of the right frontal lobe (BA11), right limbic lobe (BA30, 35), and left frontal lobe (BA47), while the right parietal lobe (BA40) was deactivated. Compared with the non-Deqi group, the Deqi group exhibited marked activation of the right anterior lobe of the cerebellum and right limbic lobe (BA30). These findings confirm that Deqi is a clinically measurable effect of acupuncture. Given the importance of Deqi for treatment outcome, cerebellar activation may be a central mechanism of the beneficial effect of acupuncture on ischemic stroke **(Table 2)**.

6. Clinical studies of acupuncture therapy in ischemic stroke

6.1. A case match-controlled study of acupuncture in acute and subacute ischemic stroke

In order to reduce the healthcare burden of stroke, the Taiwan Department of Health initiated the Pilot Scheme of the Health Policy in Stroke Adjuvant Acupuncture Therapy (HPSAAT) in 2006. This study was conducted with cross-sectional, hospital-based, case match-controlled method retrospectively analyzed the clinical characteristics of acute and subacute ischemic stroke patients who electively joined the HPSAAT between 2006 and 2008 [23]. The study also evaluated the safety and clinical benefits of adjuvant acupuncture in acute and subacute ischemic stroke. Adjuvant acupuncture was concluded to be safe in the acute and subacute stages of ischemic stroke; however, due to uneven baseline severity between the 26 HPSAAT participants and 52 age- and sex-matched controls, the ability of acupuncture to reduce neurological deficits and improve functional recovery was not determined by this study [23].

6.2. Prospective RCTs of acupuncture in acute ischemic stroke

In a study of 290 first onset acute ischemic stroke patients aged 40–75 years old, patients initially (after 24 hours but within 14 days of the stroke event) received standard treatment and were then randomly allocated into an intervention group (treated with resuscitating acupuncture) or a control group (treated with sham acupuncture) [24]. Primary outcome measures included the Barthel index (BI), relapse, and mortality within a six-month period. There was one case of mortality in the intervention group and two cases in the control group ($P = 0.558$). Six patients experienced relapse in the intervention group whereas 34 patients experienced relapse in the control group ($P < 0.001$). The mean values for BI at six months were 70.25 ± 20.37 and 57.43 ± 19.61 for the intervention and control groups, respectively ($P < 0.01$). The mean values for NIHSS score were also significantly different between groups at four weeks (4.15 ± 2.032 vs. 6.35 ± 3.131, respectively, $P < 0.01$) but not at two weeks. Acupuncture also produced greater improvements via the Chinese Stroke Scale (CSS) at four weeks (9.40 ± 4.51 vs. 13.09 ± 5.80, respectively, $P < 0.001$) and via the Stroke-Specific Quality-of-Life Scale (SS-QOL) at six months (166.63 ± 45.70 vs. 143.60 ± 50.24, respectively, $P < 0.01$). The results of this clinical trial therefore identified not only a clinically relevant decrease in relapse in patients treated with six months of resuscitating acupuncture, but also demonstrated improvements in self-care ability and quality of life as evaluated by the BI, NIHSS, CSS, Oxford Handicap Scale (OHS), and SS-QOL at various time points during and after treatment [24].

Another prospective RCT of acupuncture in 120 ischemic stroke inpatients and outpatients was conducted at Huashan Hospital and Fudan University in China [25]. Acupuncture, physiotherapy, and combined acupuncture with physiotherapy were utilized. Motor function of the limbs was measured using the FMA and the modified Barthel index (MBI) was used to rate activities of daily living. On the first day of therapy, FMA and MBI scores did not differ significantly among the treatment groups. By day 28 of therapy, the mean FMA scores for the physiotherapy, acupuncture, and combined treatment groups had increased relative to baseline by 65.6, 57.7, and 67.2%, respectively, and the mean MBI scores had increased by 85.2, 60.4, and 63.4%, respectively. FMA scores did not differ significantly among groups. By day 56, FMA scores had increased by 88.1, 64.5, and 88.6%, respectively ($P < 0.05$) and MBI scores had increased by 108.0, 71.2, and 86.2% at day 56, respectively ($P < 0.05$). FMA and MBI scores in the physiotherapy group were statistically higher than those in the acupuncture group ($P < 0.05$). No significant differences were identified between the combined treatment group and the other groups; in addition, FMA subscores for the upper extremities did not reflect any significant improvement in any group on day 56 of treatment [25]. The results of this study indicated that acupuncture is less effective than physiotherapy for rehabilitation. Moreover, the therapeutic effect of combined acupuncture and physiotherapy was not superior to that of physiotherapy alone. A larger-scale clinical trial is necessary to confirm these findings.

6.3. A pilot RCT of triple stimulation EA in ischemic stroke

A pilot study was conducted to objectively assess the effect of triple stimulation technique (TST) EA on motor functional recovery in patients with acute ischemic stroke [26]. Patients received either EA plus WCM ($n = 32$) or WCM alone ($n = 31$) for 14 days. EA plus WCM had a statistically higher total clinical effective rate than WCM alone ($P < 0.01$) and furthermore produced better improvements in FMA score, NIHSS score, and TST ratio ($P < 0.01$). Both before and after treatment, there was a positive correlation between the TST ratio and the NIHSS score ($P < 0.01$) and a negative correlation between the TST ratio and the FMA score ($P < 0.01$). Furthermore, there were no statistical differences in adverse events, electrocardiogram data, liver function, or kidney function between treatment groups. EA was concluded to be generally safe and beneficial for the motor functional recovery of patients with acute ischemic stroke. Moreover, TST was validated as a quantitative indicator of motor functional recovery that can objectively analyze the injury and recovery of corticospinal tract impairments.

6.4. A metaanalysis of EA RCTs in acute ischemic stroke

A systematic review was conducted to assess the effectiveness and safety of EA for acute ischemic stroke [27]. Eight databases were searched for relevant RCTs published prior to June 2013. Ultimately, 67 studies were identified and 1411 individuals from 18 studies were included in the analysis. According to the GRADE approach, the quality of evidence was mostly high or moderate. A significant difference in the total clinical efficacy rate was identified between EA and WCM, and significant effects of EA were observed on the BI score, FMA score, NIHSS score, and Revised Scandinavian Stroke Scale score relative to WCM. EA was well tolerated in the six studies that monitored adverse events. Thus, this metaanalysis produced evidence supporting the use of EA acute ischemic stroke.

6.5. A multicentered RCT of EA in China

As aforementioned, acupuncture is frequently used as a complementary treatment for ischemic stroke in China; however, evidence available from previous RCTs was considered to be inconclusive. Thus, a more robustly designed, larger-scale trial was conducted. A multi-centered, single-blinded RCT of 862 hospitalized patients with limb paralysis between 3 and 10 days after ischemic stroke onset was treated with either acupuncture plus routine care or routine care alone [28]. Acupuncture therapy was conducted five times per week for 3–4 weeks. The primary outcomes were defined as follows: (1) death/disability according to BI score and (2) death/institutional care at 6 months. Fewer patients were classified as having death/disability in the acupuncture group (20.7%) than in the control group (25.8%) at 6 months (odds ratio [OR], 0.75; 95% confidence interval [CI], 0.54–1.05). In a subgroup receiving ≥10 sessions of acupuncture (OR, 0.68; 95% CI, 0.47–0.98) was found therapeutic benefit. There was no significant difference in death/institutional care between two groups (OR, 1.06; 95% CI, 0.63–1.79). Severe adverse events occurred in 7.6 and 8.3% of patients in the acupuncture and control groups, respectively. The study concluded that acupuncture appeared to be safe in the subacute phase of ischemic stroke. However, confirmation of the observed therapeutic benefit is necessary in order to facilitate the widespread use of acupuncture in subacute ischemic stroke **(Table 3)**.

Trial	*N*	Design	Test group	Control group	Acupoints	Outcomes/conclusion
Wei et al. (2011) [23]	26:52	Case controlled study	Acupuncture plus WCM	WCM	NA	Acupuncture was concluded to be safe for use in the acute and subacute stages of ischemic stroke. The clinical benefits in reducing neurological deficits and functional recovery were not concluded.
Shen et al. (2012) [24]	145:145	RCT	Acupuncture	Sham-acupoints	PC6, DU26, SP6, HT1, BL40, LU5. auxiliary acupoints: GB20, TE17, GB12, LI4, CV23, EX-HN 12, EX-HN 13; cross-foot, puncture–GB40 toward KI 6.	(1) BI at six months ($P < 0.01$). (2) NIHSS at four weeks ($P < 0.01$). (3) CSS at four weeks ($P < 0.001$). (4) SS-QOL at six months ($P < 0.01$).
Bai et al. (2013) [25]	39:40:41	RCT	(1) Acupuncture group (2) Combined therapy group	Physiotherapy only	GV20, LI15, SI9, LI11, TE5, LI4, GB34, BL60, GB39, GB30, GB31, PC6, SP5,	FMA and MBI scores did not significantly differ between the physiotherapy and the combined therapy groups. The therapeutic effect of combined acupuncture

Trial	N	Design	Test group	Control group	Acupoints	Outcomes/conclusion
					LR3, SP9, SP6, KI10, PC7, LI4, SI3, HT1, LU5, PC3.	and physiotherapy was not superior to that of physiotherapy alone.
Tan et al. (2013) [26]	32:31	Pilot RCT	EA plus WCM	WCM	LI15 and TE14, LI11 and LI4, LU5 and PC6 ST36 and GB34, ST40 and GB39, SP6 and LR3 (at hemiparetic limb).	(1) FMA score ($P < 0.01$). (2) NIHSS ($P < 0.01$). (3) TST_{ratio} ($P < 0.01$). EA was concluded to be safe and beneficial for motor functional recovery.
Liu et al. (2015) [27]	1411	Systematic review and metaanalysis of RCT	EA	WCM	NA	(1)BI ($P < 0.00001$). (2)FMA score ($P < 0.00001$). (3)NIHSS ($P < 0.00001$). (4) RSSS ($P < 0.00001$). This metaanalysis produced evidence supporting the use of EA for acute ischemic stroke.
Zhang et al. (2015) [28]	427: 435	Multicentered, RCT	Acupuncture plus WCM	WCM	DU26, PC6, SP6, DU20, ST36, ST40, LK3, LL5, GB20, RN6	Acupuncture appeared to be safe in the subacute phase of ischemic stroke. Subgroup analysis showed that only when patients who received ≥ 10 sessions of acupuncture had a significant difference in death or dependency at 6 months (OR, 0.68; 95% CI, 0.47–0.98; NNT 15).

CSS, Chinese Stroke Scale; EA, electroacupuncture; FMA, Fugl-Meyer assessment; MBI, modified Barthel index; NNT, number needed to treat; RSSS, Revised Scandinavian Stroke Scale; SS-QOL, Stroke-Specific Quality-of Life-Scale; WCM, Western *conventional* medicine.

Table 3. Clinical trials of acupuncture therapy in ischemic stroke.

7. Scalp acupuncture (SA)

Scalp acupuncture (SA) is one of the several specialized acupuncture techniques. Although SA has been practiced for thousands of years, SA was only developed for clinical use in recent decades. In 1984 and 1989, a standard nomenclature for acupuncture points was developed and redesigned to combine the teachings of different schools of SA, and resulted in the proposal of 14 therapeutic lines or zones [29]. Subsequently, "*A Proposed Standard International Acupuncture Nomenclature:* 3.6 Scalp acupuncture lines" was formally published by the World Health Organization in 1991 [30]. SA therapy for both ischemic stroke and hemorrhagic stroke has been empirically established and is now widely used in clinics around the world [31, 32].

7.1. A metaanalysis of SA RCTs in acute ischemic stroke

A metaanalysis of RCTs of SA in acute ischemic stroke was conducted [33]; a total of 538 acute ischemic stroke patients from eight eligible studies were included [34–41]. The main findings were that SA therapy improved neurological deficits and had a better clinical effective rate relative to WCM. However, this evidence was insufficient to warrant a clinical recommendation due to the generally low methodological quality of included studies.

7.2. Baihui (GV20)-based SA in experimental ischemic stroke

A systematic review and metaanalysis was conducted to assess current evidence for a beneficial effect of Baihui (GV20)-based SA in animal models of focal cerebral ischemia [42]. Six databases were searched for relevant studies published prior to June 2013. Primary outcomes were infarct size and neurobehavioral outcome. Ultimately, a total of 1816 animals from 54 eligible studies were included in the analysis. Twelve studies reported significant effects of Baihui (GV20)-based SA on infarct volume in middle cerebral artery occlusion ($P < 0.01$), and 32 studies reported significant beneficial effects of Baihui (GV20)-based SA on neurological function relative to control ($P < 0.01$). Therefore, in conclusion, Baihui (GV20)-based SA may specifically improve infarct volume and neurological function in experimental ischemic stroke **(Table 4)**.

Study	N	Study design	Test group	Control group	Outcomes/conclusion
Wang et al. (2012) [33]	538	Metaanalysis of SA RCTs	SA	WCM	6 RCTs improving neurological deficit scores ($P < 0.01$); 4 RCTs favoring the clinical effective rate ($P < 0.01$).
Wang et al. (2014) [42]	1816	1. Systematic review and metaanalysis 2. Animal model	GV20-based SA	MCAo group	12 studies improving infarct volume ($P < 0.01$) 32 studies improving the neurological function score ($P < 0.01$). Baihui (GV20)-based SA improves infarct volume and neurological function in experimental ischemic stroke.

MCAo, middle cerebral artery occlusion.

Table 4. Scalp acupuncture in ischemic stroke.

8. Specific acupuncture points studied in the context of ischemic stroke

8.1. Waiguan (SJ5)

Sixteen patients with ischemic stroke were randomly assigned to receive either true point acupuncture at right SJ5 or sham point acupuncture during fMRI. SJ5 acupuncture produced

http://dx.doi.org/10.5772/64585

activation in the right parietal lobe (BA7 and BA19), right temporal lobe (BA39), right limbic lobe (BA23), and bilateral occipital lobes (BA18) as well as deactivation of the bilateral frontal lobes (BA4, BA6, and BA45), right parietal lobe (BA1 and BA5), and left temporal lobe (BA21). Sham point acupuncture produced activation in the precuneus of the right parietal lobe (BA7) and deactivation of the left superior frontal gyrus (BA10). Compared with sham point acupuncture, SJ5 acupuncture inhibited the contralateral BA5 in stroke patients. These results suggested that altered specificity of the sensation-associated cortex (BA5) is a possible mechanism of the beneficial effect of SJ5 acupuncture in stroke patients [43].

8.2. Hegu (LI4)

A 14-day treatment study was conducted to determine the clinical efficacy of acupuncture at LI4 in central facial nerve paralysis after ischemic stroke and to explore the dose-response effect of different stimulation intensities [44]. Patients received either different stimulation intensities of acupuncture at LI4 combined with facial paralysis acupoints including Yingxiang (LI20), Dicang (ST4), Jiache (ST6), and Quanliao (SI18), acupuncture at facial paralysis acupoints alone, acupuncture at stroke acupoints including Neiguan (PC6), Shuigou (GV26), and Sanyinjiao (SP6), or medication treatment. The House-Brackmann Facial Nerve Grading System (H-B), Toronto Facial Grading System (TFGS), Degrees of Facial Nerve Paralysis (DFNP), Facial Disability Index (FDI), and clinical efficacy were used as outcome measures. Various intensities of LI4 stimulation improved H-B score, TFGS score, DFNP score, and FDI physical function score ($P < 0.05$), but LI4 stimulation had no effect on FDI social function score. No changes were observed in the control group. The study concluded that LI 4 acupuncture had clinical efficacy in central facial nerve paralysis after ischemic stroke and that oblique needle insertion along the opposite direction of the meridian with five seconds of twirling manipulation had the best clinical effect **(Table 5)**.

Study	N	Study design	Test group	Control group	Acupoint	Outcomes/conclusion
Qi et al. (2014) [43]	7:7	fMRI	SJ5 acupuncture	Sham acupoint	Waiguan (SJ5)	SJ5 acupuncture altered specificity of the sensation-associated cortex (BA5) is a possible mechanism of the beneficial effect in stroke patients.
Li et al. (2014) [44]	50	Case controlled study	Hegu 1 Hegu 2 Hegu 3 Hegu 4	WCM	Hegu (LI4) combined with facial paralysis acupoints	H-B in the Hegu 1 to 4 groups ($P < 0.05$). TFGS in the Hegu 2 group ($P < 0.05$). DFNP in the Hegu 1 and Hegu 2 groups ($P < 0.05$). LI4 acupuncture had clinical efficacy in central facial nerve paralysis after ischemic stroke.

H-B, The House-Brackmann facial never grading systems; TFGS, Toronto facial grading system; DFNP, degrees of facial never paralysis; FDI, facial disability index.

Table 5. Specific acupuncture point study.

9. The role of acupuncture therapy in preventive medicine

On average, the annual risk of ischemic stroke after an initial ischemic stroke event or transient ischemic attack is 3–4% [45, 46]. Antiplatelet therapy is a preventive medical option that has utility for the prevention of hypertension, atrial fibrillation, arterial obstruction, and hyperlipidemia [1]. However, preventive options for ischemic stroke are limited. Therefore, the role of acupuncture therapy in preventive medicine was explored in a preliminary study.

9.1. The effect of acupuncture on stroke recurrence

A retrospective study evaluated 30,058 cases of first onset ischemic stroke between the years 2000 and 2004 based on claims history from the Taiwan National Health Insurance Research Database [47]. Uses of acupuncture treatment and stroke recurrences were identified in a follow-up period between 2000 and 2009. Use of acupuncture treatment was associated with a decrease in the rate of stroke recurrence from 71.4 to 69.9 cases per 1000 person-years ($P < 0.001$). Acupuncture treatment was also associated with a reduced risk of stroke recurrence (hazard ratio [HR], 0.88; 95% CI, 0.84–0.91). The effect of acupuncture on stroke recurrence was noted in patients independent of medical treatment for stroke prevention: the HRs of stroke recurrence for those had medical treatment, acupuncture, and both were 0.42 (95% CI, 0.38–0.46), 0.50 (95% CI, 0.43–0.57), and 0.39 (95% CI, 0.35–0.43), respectively. However, the effect of acupuncture on stroke recurrence decreased with patient age. This study raises the possibility that acupuncture may have utility for preventing stroke recurrence after an initial event, even in patients already taking medications for stroke prevention. Confirmation in the form of a prospective RCT is required to establish the efficacy of acupuncture as a preventive practice in ischemic stroke [47].

9.2. The effect of acupuncture on acute myocardial infarction (AMI) risk after stroke

A retrospective study evaluated 23,475 stroke patients aged 40–79 years who received acupuncture treatment and 46,950 propensity score-matched control stroke patients who did not receive acupuncture treatment between the years 2000 and 2004 based on claims history from the Taiwan National Health Insurance Research Database [48]. Both stroke cohorts were followed until the end of 2009. Stroke patients who received acupuncture therapy (9.2 per 1000 person-years) had a lower incidence of AMI compared with those who did not receive acupuncture therapy (10.8 per 1000 person-years), with an HR of 0.86 (95% CI, 0.80–0.93) after adjustment for age, sex, low income, coexisting medical conditions, and medications. These results reveal that acupuncture therapy may be useful for the prevention of AMI in stroke patients aged 50–69. However, the study was limited by lack of information relating to stroke severity and acupuncture points. Further prospective randomized trials are required to establish the efficacy of acupuncture for preventing AMI after stroke.

9.3. The effect of acupuncture on stroke risk after traumatic brain injury (TBI)

Patients with TBI are subject to an increased risk of stroke. A retrospective study evaluated 7409 TBI patients who received acupuncture treatment and 29,636 propensity score-matched control TBI patients who did not receive acupuncture treatment between the years 2000–2008 based on claims history from the Taiwan National Health Insurance Research Database. Both TBI cohorts were followed until the end of 2010. TBI patients who received acupuncture treatment (4.9 per 1000 person-years) had a lower incidence of stroke compared with those who did not receive acupuncture treatment (7.5 per 1000 person-years), with an HR of 0.59 (95% CI, 0.50–0.69) after adjusting for sociodemographic information, coexisting medical conditions, and medication use. Moreover, TBI patients who received acupuncture treatment during the follow-up period had a lower probability of stroke than those who did not receive acupuncture treatment ($P < 0.0001$). However, this study was limited by lack of information regarding lifestyle, biochemistry results, TBI severity, and acupuncture points [45].

10. Conclusions

The use of complementary therapies in stroke is increasing due to a rising demand for better poststroke rehabilitation and management. TCM is a popular complementary therapy in East Asia and throughout the world. Increasing scientific evidence suggests that TCM can significantly improve stroke recovery as well as reduce the likelihood of hospital readmission for cardiovascular or subsequent stroke events. Therefore, patients can benefit from comprehensive treatment plans that combine standard and complementary therapies to address immediate medical concerns, minimize the occurrence of future complications, and ultimately decrease medical costs. Further studies on the therapeutic targets mediating the beneficial actions of TCM may additionally lead to the development of novel therapeutic strategies.

Abbreviations

ATP	adenosine triphosphate
BA	Brodmann Area
BBB	blood brain barrier
BI	Barthel index
BYHWT	Bu-yang-huan-wu-tang
CHPs	Chinese herbal products
DHYZ	Di Huang Yin Zi
DTI	Diffusion Tensor Imaging
EA	electro-acupuncture
FMA	Fugl-Meyer Assessment
FDG PET-CT	Fluoro-2-Deoxy-D-Glucose Positron Emission Tomography and Computed

ATP	adenosine triphosphate
	Tomography
fMRI	Functional magnetic resonance imaging
MMP	matrix metalloproteases
OGD	oxygen-glucose deprivation
SA	Scalp acupuncture
SJHXT	Shu-jin-huo-xue-tang
TCM	Traditional Chinese medicine
TOAST	the Trial of Org 10172 in Acute Stroke Treatment
TST	triple-stimulation technique

Author details

Po-Yu Huang[1], Yu-Chiang Hung[1,2] and Wen-Long Hu[1,3,4*]

*Address all correspondence to: oolonghu@gmail.com

1 Department of Chinese Medicine, Kaohsiung Chang Gung Memorial Hospital and School of Traditional Chinese Medicine, Chang Gung University College of Medicine, Kaohsiung, Taiwan

2 School of Chinese Medicine for Post Baccalaureate, I-Shou University, Kaohsiung, Taiwan

3 Kaohsiung Medical University College of Medicine, School of Medicine, Kaohsiung, Taiwan

4 Fooyin University College of Nursing, School of Nursing, Kaohsiung, Taiwan

References

[1] Kernan, W.N., et al., Guidelines for the prevention of stroke in patients with stroke and transient ischemic attack: a guideline for healthcare professionals from the American Heart Association/American Stroke Association. Stroke, 2014. 45(7): 2160–2236.

[2] Mozaffarian, D., et al., Heart disease and stroke statistics-2016 update: a report from the American Heart Association. Circulation, 2016. 133(4): e38–e360.

[3] LR., C., Basic pathology, anatomy, and pathophysiology of stroke. In: Caplan's Stroke: A Clinical Approach, 4th ed., Saunders Elsevier, Philadelphia, 2009: p. 22.

[4] Adams, H.P., Jr., et al., Classification of subtype of acute ischemic stroke. Definitions for use in a multicenter clinical trial. TOAST Trial of Org 10172 in Acute Stroke Treatment. Stroke, 1993. 24(1): 35–41.

[5] Eames, P.J., et al., Dynamic cerebral autoregulation and beat to beat blood pressure control are impaired in acute ischaemic stroke. J Neurol Neurosurg Psychiatry, 2002. 72(4): 467–472.

[6] Atkins, E.R., et al., Dynamic cerebral autoregulation is compromised acutely following mild ischaemic stroke but not transient ischaemic attack. Cerebrovasc Dis, 2010. 29(3): 228–235.

[7] Aries, M.J., et al., Cerebral autoregulation in stroke: a review of transcranial Doppler studies. Stroke, 2010. 41(11): 2697–2704.

[8] Doyle, K.P., R.P. Simon, and M.P. Stenzel-Poore, Mechanisms of ischemic brain damage. Neuropharmacology, 2008. 55(3): 310–318.

[9] Deb, P., S. Sharma, and K.M. Hassan, Pathophysiologic mechanisms of acute ischemic stroke: an overview with emphasis on therapeutic significance beyond thrombolysis. Pathophysiology, 2010. 17(3): 197–218.

[10] Yang, Y. and G.A. Rosenberg, Blood-brain barrier breakdown in acute and chronic cerebrovascular disease. Stroke, 2011. 42(11): 3323–3328.

[11] Gu, Y., J. Chen, and J. Shen, Herbal medicines for ischemic stroke: combating inflammation as therapeutic targets. J Neuroimmune Pharmacol, 2014. 9(3): 313–339.

[12] Carden, D.L. and D.N. Granger, Pathophysiology of ischaemia-reperfusion injury. J Pathol, 2000. 190(3): 255–266.

[13] Barone, F.C., et al., Tumor necrosis factor-alpha. A mediator of focal ischemic brain injury. Stroke, 1997. 28(6): 1233–1244.

[14] Abulafia, D.P., et al., Inhibition of the inflammasome complex reduces the inflammatory response after thromboembolic stroke in mice. J Cereb Blood Flow Metab, 2009. 29(3): 534–544.

[15] Yu, M., et al., The beneficial effects of the herbal medicine Di-Huang-Yin-Zi (DHYZ) on patients with ischemic stroke: a randomized placebo controlled clinical study. Complement Ther Med, 2015. 23(4): 591–597.

[16] Hung, I.L., et al., Chinese herbal products for ischemic stroke. Am J Chin Med, 2015. 43(7): 1365–1379.

[17] Lu, L., et al., Rhubarb root and rhizome-based Chinese herbal prescriptions for acute ischemic stroke: a systematic review and meta-analysis. Complement Ther Med, 2014. 22(6): 1060–1070.

[18] Lu, L., et al., Acupuncture for neurogenesis in experimental ischemic stroke: a systematic review and meta-analysis. Sci Rep, 2016. 6: 19521.

[19] Feng, R. and F. Zhang, The neuroprotective effect of electro-acupuncture against ischemic stroke in animal model: a review. Afr J Tradit Complement Altern Med, 2014. 11(3): 25–29.

[20] Huang, Y., et al., Acupuncture regulates the glucose metabolism in cerebral functional regions in chronic stage ischemic stroke patients-—a PET-CT cerebral functional imaging study. BMC Neurosci, 2012. 13: 75.

[21] Li, Y., et al., The Effect of acupuncture on the motor function and white matter microstructure in ischemic stroke patients. Evid Based Complement Altern Med, 2015. 2015: 164792.

[22] Li, M.K., et al., Acupuncture for ischemic stroke: cerebellar activation may be a central mechanism following Deqi. Neural Regen Res, 2015. 10(12): 1997–2003.

[23] Wei, Y.C., et al., Pilot scheme of health policy in stroke adjuvant acupuncture therapy for acute and subacute ischemic stroke in taiwan. Evid Based Complement Altern Med, 2011. 2011: 689813.

[24] Shen, P.F., et al., Acupuncture intervention in ischemic stroke: a randomized controlled prospective study. Am J Chin Med, 2012. 40(4): 685–693.

[25] Bai, Y.L., et al., Prospective randomized controlled trial of physiotherapy and acupuncture on motor function and daily activities in patients with ischemic stroke. J Altern Complement Med, 2013. 19(8): 684–689.

[26] Tan, F., et al., A randomized controlled pilot study of the triple stimulation technique in the assessment of electroacupuncture for motor function recovery in patients with acute ischemic stroke. Evid Based Complement Altern Med, 2013. 2013: 431986.

[27] Liu, A.J., et al., Electroacupuncture for acute ischemic stroke: a meta-analysis of randomized controlled trials. Am J Chin Med, 2015. 43(8): 1541–1566.

[28] Zhang, S., et al., Acupuncture efficacy on ischemic stroke recovery: multicenter randomized controlled trial in China. Stroke, 2015. 46(5): 1301–1306.

[29] Liu, Z., et al., History and mechanism for treatment of intracerebral hemorrhage with scalp acupuncture. Evid Based Complement Altern Med, 2012. 2012: 895032.

[30] WHO Scientific Group on International Acupuncture Nomenclature. A Proposed Standard International Acupuncture Nomenclature. Report of a WHO Scientific Group, World Health Organization, Geneva, Switzerland, 1991.

[31] Zheng, G.Q., et al., Meta-analysis of scalp acupuncture for acute hypertensive intracerebral hemorrhage. J Altern Complement Med, 2011. 17(4): 293–299.

[32] Hsing, W.T., et al., Clinical effects of scalp electrical acupuncture in stroke: a sham-controlled randomized clinical trial. J Altern Complement Med, 2012. 18(4): 341–346.

[33] Wang, Y., et al., Scalp acupuncture for acute ischemic stroke: a meta-analysis of randomized controlled trials. Evid Based Complement Altern Med, 2012. 2012: 480950.

[34] Tang QS, S.S., Clinical and experimental research on acute cerebral infartion treated by needing Shu Xue on head. J Beij Coll Trad Chin Med, 1996. 19(4): 37–39.

[35] Yu CD, W.B., Hong AH, Bei JY, Yu Z., Changes of serum MDA content and neurological rehabil itation in cerebral infarction patients treated with scalp acupuncture plus medication. Acupuncture Res, 2004. 29(3): 222–226.

[36] Wei TH, X.T., Tang Q., The evaluation of scalp acupuncture combined with recovery techniques on the movement dysfunction after cerebral infarction. Chin J Rehabilit Theor Pract, 2005. 11(7): 522–523.

[37] Xu HB, Z.G., Li NP, et al., Treatment of acute cerebral infarction with scalp acupuncture combined with Yinxingdamo injection. J Clin Exp Med, 2007. 6(8): 140–141.

[38] Chen J, J.L., Clinical application of cluster needling of scalp point therapy combined with swallowing functional training in treatment of dysphagia after acute cerebral infarction. Chin J Trau Dis Med, 2008. 16(5): 70–71.

[39] Yu CD, W.G., Wu BH, Li ZW, Song HM, Yu Ze., Effects of cranial sutures acupuncture plus drugson recovery of neural function and serum SOD and MDA in acute cerebral infarction patients with phlegm syndrome. J Fuj Univ TCM, 2010. 20(2): 7–9.

[40] Zhang LR, S.B., Luo HL, Dong GR, Bao CL, Guo YQ., Effect of bilateral scalp-acupoint penetrating acupuncture on serum levels of VEGF. Chin J Rehabilita, 2011. 26(3): 214–215.

[41] Zhu GQ, H.S., Effect of Xingnaoyinyang penetration needling method on the level of Ca2+ in serum of patients with acute cerebral infarction. J Emerg Trad Chin Med, 2011. 20(1): 9–11.

[42] Wang, W.W., et al., A systematic review and meta-analysis of Baihui (GV20)-based scalp acupuncture in experimental ischemic stroke. Sci Rep, 2014. 4: 3981.

[43] Qi, J., et al., Acupuncture at Waiguan (SJ5) and sham points influences activation of functional brain areas of ischemic stroke patients: a functional magnetic resonance imaging study. Neural Regen Res, 2014. 9(3): 293–300.

[44] Li, L.X., et al., Different stimulation intensities of acupuncture at Hegu (LI 4) for central facial nerve paralysis after ischemic stroke: a randomized controlled trial. Zhongguo Zhen Jiu, 2014. 34(7): 669–674.

[45] Dhamoon, M.S., et al., Recurrent stroke and cardiac risks after first ischemic stroke: the northern manhattan study. Neurology, 2006. 66(5): 641–646.

[46] Hong, K.S., et al., Declining stroke and vascular event recurrence rates in secondary prevention trials over the past 50 years and consequences for current trial design. Circulation, 2011. 123(19): 2111–2119.

[47] 47. Shih, C.C., et al., A retrospective cohort study comparing stroke recurrence rate in ischemic stroke patients with and without acupuncture treatment. Med (Baltimore), 2015. 94(39): e1572.

[48] Chuang, S.F., et al., Decreased risk of acute myocardial infarction in stroke patients receiving acupuncture treatment: a nationwide matched retrospective cohort study. BMC Complement Altern Med, 2015. 15: 318.